Contemporary Diagnosis and Management in *Preventive Cardiology*®

Patrick McBride, MD, MPH
Professor, Department of Medicine
and Family Medicine
Co-Director, Preventive Cardiology Program
Associate Dean for Students
University of Wisconsin Medical School,
Madison

James H. Stein, MD
Associate Professor of Medicine
Co-Director, Preventive Cardiology Program
University of Wisconsin Medical School

First Edition
Published by
Handbooks in Health Care Co., Newtown, Pennsylvania, USA.

This book has been prepared and is presented as a service to the medical community. The information provided reflects the knowledge, experience, and personal opinions of the authors, Patrick McBride, MD, MPH, Professor, Department of Medicine and Family Medicine, and Co-Director, Preventive Cardiology Program, University of Wisconsin Medical School, Madison, and James H. Stein, MD, Associate Professor of Medicine, Co-Director, Preventive Cardiology Program, University of Wisconsin Medical School.

This book is not intended to replace or to be used as a substitute for the complete prescribing information prepared by each manufacturer for each drug. Because of possible variations in drug indications, in dosage information, in newly described toxicities, in drug/drug interactions, and in other items of importance, reference to such complete prescribing information is definitely recommended before any of the drugs discussed are used or prescribed.

Dedications

I dedicate this book to my children, Sean and Gabrielle, and especially to my wife, Kim, whose support and patience are invaluable for my work. (PEM)

I dedicate this book to Andrea, Hannah, and Jacob, whose love and support make my career possible; to my parents, Ken and Diana; and to my grandfather Leo, who taught me that hard work, compassion, and loving kindness are pillars upon which our world is built. (JHS)

Acknowledgment

We wish to thank Donna Miceli, a medical writer, for her assistance in the research and writing of this book.

International Standard Book Number: 1-931981-23-X

Library of Congress Catalog Card Number: 2005935352

Table of Contents

Cardiovascular Disease Prevention

The purpose of this handbook is to help physicians reduce premature cardiovascular disease (CVD) and recurrent cardiovascular events in patients with known atherosclerosis. The need for heart disease prevention and the potential for reducing CVD events are significant. More than 80% of patients with CVD have at least one of the conventional risk factors (cigarette smoking, hyperlipidemia, hypertension, or diabetes).[1,2] More than half of the impressive decline in CVD death and disability is attributable to the decline in the common risk factors.[3]

The number of patients who need treatment for the prevention of coronary heart disease (CHD) and other forms of atherosclerosis is rising substantially in the United States and in the rest of the world. CHD is the leading cause of death and disability for men and women in the United States, and the annual cost of CHD is estimated to exceed $60 billion.[4] Over the next several decades, the prevalence of CHD and the number of patients eligible for aggressive preventive therapy are expected to increase drastically. More than 6% of the US population has diabetes, and the prevalence is increasing. In 1990, four states had diabetes rates of 6% or higher; by 2000, the number of states had grown to 43.[5,6] In addition, obesity is prevalent among US adults, and its incidence is increasing. Between 1991 and 2000, the prevalence of obesity rose 61%, with increases in nearly every population subgroup.[7]

The presence of atherosclerosis identifies a high-risk patient. With atherosclerosis, the risk of future cardiovascular events is high, and aggressive prevention treatment is recommended. Risk factor treatment is highly effective for patients with known CVD.[8]

There is significant potential for the prevention of CVD events in primary care patients through routine screening and managing for CVD.[9,10] Primary care practices are essential to the delivery of comprehensive preventive health services because most patients see their primary care provider at least once, and often several times, annually. Although nearly all physicians agree on the importance of primary and secondary CHD prevention, less than half of the patients in the United States with hypertension, hyperlipidemia, or diabetes mellitus are now being treated.[11,12]

Many reasons account for the underuse of therapy. It is not simply that physicians forget or that patients are not motivated or cannot afford the treatment. It is essential to systematically screen for and identify high-risk patients. This handbook outlines organizational strategies to identify high-risk patients who are most likely to benefit from CHD prevention treatment. Studies demonstrate that medical practices can make changes in their delivery of health care that result in significant increases in preventive services.[13,14]

The many advances in CVD care have had a significant impact on the reduction of CHD mortality. Most of that reduction has been achieved by applying current knowledge, including lifestyle changes and increased use of therapeutic treatments. Although it is important to discover new risk factors and treatments for CHD, it is imperative that all providers, practices, and patients apply current knowledge about CHD prevention and therapy by changing practice methods and systems. Using current knowledge and screening procedures to clearly identify high-risk patients could result in major reductions in CHD morbidity and mortality.[9]

This handbook addresses the best approaches to identifying high-risk patients, options for treating them, strategies for improving adherence, and practice strategies for increasing prevention services and obtaining reimbursement. We hope that health-care practitioners will apply all the best interventions to ensure that our patients lead full and healthy lives.

References

1. Greenland P, Knoll MD, Stamler J, et al: Major risk factors as antecedents of fatal and nonfatal coronary heart disease events. *JAMA* 2003;290:891-897.

2. Khot UN, Khot MB, Bajzer CT, et al: Prevalence of conventional risk factors in patients with coronary heart disease. *JAMA* 2003;290:898-904.

3. Goldman L, Phillips KA, Coxson P, et al: The effect of risk factor reductions between 1981 and 1990 on coronary heart disease incidence, prevalence, mortality and cost. *J Am Coll Cardiol* 2001;38:1012-1017.

4. American Heart Association 2001 Heart and Stroke Statistical Update 2001. Dallas, TX. American Heart Association.

5. American Diabetes Association: Screening for type 2 diabetes. *Diabetes Care* 2003;26(suppl 1):S21-S24.

6. American Diabetes Association Web site. Available at: http://www.diabetes.org. Accessed January 19, 2006.

7. Centers for Disease Control Web site. Available at: http://www.cdc.gov. Accessed January 19, 2006.

8. Gluckman TJ, Baranowski B, Ashen D, et al: A practical and evidence-based approach to cardiovascular disease risk reduction. *Arch Intern Med* 2004;164:1490-1500.

9. Levenson JW, Skerrett PJ, Gaziano JM: Reducing the global burden of cardiovascular disease: the role of risk factors. *Prev Cardiol* 2002;5:188-189.

10. Keevil JG, Stein JH, McBride PE: Cardiovascular disease prevention. *Prim Care Clin Office Pract* 2002;29:667-696.

11. Gibbons RJ, Smith S, Antman E: American College of Cardiology/American Heart Association clinical practice guidelines: Part I: where do they come from. *Circulation* 2003;107:2979-2986.

12. Fonarow GC, French WJ, Parsons LS, et al: Use of lipid-lowering medications at discharge in patients with acute myocardial infarction: data from the National Registry of Myocardial Infarction 3. *Circulation* 2001;103:38-44.

13. McBride PE, Underbakke G, Plane MB, et al: Improving prevention systems in primary care practices: The Health Education and Research Trial (HEART). *J Fam Prac* 2000;49:115-125.

14. Ockene IS, Hebert JR, Ockene JK, et al: Effect of training and a structured office practice on physician-delivered nutrition counseling: the Worcester-Area Trial for Counseling in Hyperlipidemia (WATCH). *Am J Prev Med* 1996;12:252-258.

CHAPTER 1

Cardiovascular Risk Factors and Risk Assessment: Who's at Risk?

Identifying and reducing risk factors substantially reduce age-adjusted death rates from coronary heart disease (CHD).[1] Although the optimal goal is primary prevention of CHD, preventing cardiac events in patients already diagnosed with heart disease (secondary prevention) is vital, and most risk reduction therapies are cost-effective and strongly recommended in this population.

A risk factor is 'a clearly defined characteristic that has been associated with the increased rate of subsequently occurring disease.'[2] Cardiovascular research has focused on risk factors for many years, and the lists of modifiable and nonmodifiable risk factors are well established (Table 1-1). As research continues, new risk factors are being added, but aggressive modification of the core risk factors can dramatically reduce future risk in those with known CHD. Risk factor modification is the essence of primary and secondary prevention. Every patient should be screened for each risk factor at recommended intervals, and modification goals should be identified and updated as needed. Patient education is a key element of adherence to prevention therapies.

Nonmodifiable Risk Factors

Age, gender, and family history play significant roles in the estimation of background risk and provide the con-

Table 1-1: Established Risk Factors for CHD

Unmodifiable	*Modifiable*
• Age	• Smoking
• Male gender	• Diabetes
• Family history of premature atherosclerosis*	• Hypertension
	• Dyslipidemia – Elevated LDL-C – Elevated VLDL-C (triglycerides) – Low HDL-C – Elevated non-HDL-C
	• Obesity/overweight
	• Sedentary lifestyle
	• Psychosocial stressors

* Parent, sibling, grandparent, or child with CHD diagnosis at age <60 years.

LDL-C= low-density lipoprotein cholesterol
VLDL-C= very low-density lipoprotein cholesterol
HDL-C= high-density lipoprotein cholesterol

text around which decisions about treatment of modifiable risk factors must be made. Age is a powerful predictor of CHD and, although it cannot be modified, it should be considered in assessing risk. For example, controlling for all other factors, a 75-year-old is three times more likely to have a CHD event than a 50-year-old.[3] Depending on issues such as health and quality of life, it may be advisable to treat risk factors in older adults.

Gender also has important implications for the development of CHD. Males, on average, develop CHD 10 years

Table 1-2: Emerging Risk Factors*

- Homocysteine
- Lipoprotein (a) [Lp(a)]
- High-sensitivity C-reactive protein (Hs-CRP)
- Fibrinogen
- Interleukin-6 (IL-6)
- Number of low-density lipoprotein particles and lipoprotein density

* See Chapter 11 for an explanation of these emerging risk factors.

before females. However, the risk for women who experience surgical menopause at a young age nearly equals that of males.[4] Risk-factor screening for women should include age at menopause (natural or surgical) and presence or absence of the uterus.

The risk associated with a family history of early CHD is not always specific. It may be a genetic dyslipidemia or a predisposition to hypertension, or a genetic link to one of the emerging risk factors (Table 1-2). Family history may also be a learned behavior such as tobacco use, sedentary lifestyle, overeating, or other behaviors.

Modifiable Risk Factors

Smoking is the most preventable cause of premature death and disability, including all forms of heart disease. Approximately one in five CHD deaths is attributed to smoking,[5] and nonsmokers exposed to secondhand smoke, or those smoking as few as one to four cigarettes per day, have a significantly increased risk of CHD.[6] Although public awareness has decreased smoking rates overall, the percentage of teenagers and minorities who smoke continues

Table 1-3: Classification of Blood Pressure for Adults Aged 18 or Older

BP Classification	SBP mm Hg	DBP mm Hg
Normal	<120 and	<80
Prehypertension	120-129 or	80-90
Stage 1 hypertension	140-159 or	90-99
Stage 2 hypertension	≥160	≥100

BP= blood pressure; SBP= systolic blood pressure; DBP= diastolic blood pressure

to rise.[7] Screening for smoking and secondhand smoke exposure should occur at every medical visit and should be recorded as a vital sign.

Diabetes mellitus (DM) is a major, independent risk factor for CHD.[8,9] According to the Third Report of the National Cholesterol Education Program (NCEP) Expert Panel on Detection, Evaluation, and Treatment of High Blood Cholesterol in Adults (Adult Treatment Panel III [ATP III]) guidelines, DM is a CHD risk equivalent, because people with DM carry a risk for CHD events similar to those with established CHD.[10] In terms of secondary prevention, patients with a known history of heart disease and diabetes have a significantly higher risk of death compared to those with heart disease alone.[11] More than 90% of patients with diabetes in the United States have type-2 DM, which is strongly linked to obesity, another important risk factor for CHD. Because the percentage of Americans meeting the criteria for obesity is steadily increasing, the incidence of type 2 diabetes is expected to double in the next decade.[8,9]

The link between hypertension and the risk of CHD is strong and continuously graded.[4] Although there has been

Table 1-4: ATP III Classification of Total, LDL, and HDL Cholesterol and Triglycerides

Total Cholesterol	
<200	Desirable
200-239	Borderline high
>240	High
LDL Cholesterol—Primary Target of Therapy	
<70	Optional for high risk
<100	Optimal
100-129	Near optimal/above optimal
130-159	Borderline high
160-189	High
>190	Very high
HDL Cholesterol	
<40	Low
>60	High
Triglycerides	
<150	Normal
150-199	Borderline high
200-500	High
>500	Very high

LDL = low-density lipoprotein
HDL= high-density lipoprotein

some improvement in awareness and treatment of hypertension, it is still undertreated in the United States. Obesity and a sedentary lifestyle, two independent risk factors for CHD, have an important impact on hypertension. The Seventh Report of the Joint National Committee of

Table 1-5: Guide to Primary Prevention of Cardiovascular Disease and Stroke: Risk Assessment[41]

Risk Assessment	Recommendations
Risk factor screening goal: Adults should know the levels and significance of risk factors as routinely assessed by their primary care provider.	• Risk factor assessment in adults should begin at age 20. • Family history of CHD should be regularly updated. • Smoking status, diet, alcohol intake, and physical activity should be assessed at every routine evaluation. • Blood pressure, body mass index, waist circumference, and pulse (to screen for atrial fibrillation) should be recorded at each visit (at least every 2 years). • Fasting serum lipoprotein profile (or total HDL cholesterol if fasting is unavailable) and fasting blood glucose should be measured according to patient's risk for hyperlipidemia and diabetes, respectively (at least every 5 years; if risk factors are present, every 2 years).

Risk Assessment	Recommendations
Global risk estimation All adults ≥40 years of age should know their absolute risk of developing CHD. Goal: as low risk as possible.	• Every 5 years (or more frequently if risk factors change); adults, especially those ≥40 years of age or those with ≥2 risk factors, should have their 10-year risk for CHD assessed with a multiple risk score. • Risk factors used in global risk assessment include age, sex, smoking status, systolic (and sometimes diastolic) blood pressure, total (and sometimes LDL) cholesterol, HDL cholesterol,[10,42] and in some risk scores, diabetes.[43,44] • Persons with diabetes or 10-year risk >20% can be considered at a level of risk similar to a patient with established cardiovascular disease (CHD risk equivalent) • Equations for calculation of 10-year stroke risk are also available.

CHD = coronary heart disease; HDL = high-density lipoprotein; LDL = low-density lipoprotein

Table 1-6: Compilation of Risk Factors Used in Both Hypertension and Cholesterol Guidelines

Risk Factor	NCEP ATP III
Smoking	X
Diabetes mellitus	X
HDL-C <40 mg/dL	X
Family history of CHD	X
Age and gender	X
Hypertension	X
Dyslipidemia	*
Target organ damage	
CHD risk equivalent	

This table is a compilation of the risk factors used in both the cholesterol and hypertension guidelines. Many risks are similar in both guidelines but some apply to one or the other. These risks are used when counting risks as part of the second step in absolute risk assessment.

* Guidelines assume this risk is present.

JNC 7	Comment
X	Most powerful 'preventable' risk factor.
X	NCEP ATP III: Diabetes mellitus is a 'CHD equivalent.'
X	Increased from 35 mg/dL in NCEP ATP II
X	Father, brother, son <55 years; mother, sister, daughter <65 years
X	NCEP ATP III: men ≥45 years; women ≥55 years; JNC 7: >60 years men, postmenopausal women
*	BP ≥140/90 mm Hg or on antihypertensive medication
X	
X	CVA, TIA, nephropathy, hypertensive retinopathy, PAD, prior CABG, angina, prior MI, LVH
X	Angina, MI, CABG, symptomatic carotid artery disease, PAD, abdominal aortic aneurysm

CHD = coronary heart disease; HDL-C = high-density lipoprotein cholesterol; BP = blood pressure; PAD = peripheral artery disease; MI = myocardial infarction; CABG = coronary artery bypass graft; CVA = cerebrovascular accident; TIA = transient ischemic attack; LVH = left ventricular hypertrophy

Table 1-7: Framingham Point Scores Estimate of 10-Year Risk for Men

Age, years	Points
20-34	-9
35-39	-4
40-44	0
45-49	3
50-54	6
55-59	8
60-64	10
65-69	11
70-74	12
75-79	13

Total cholesterol, mg/dL	Points *Age 20-39y*	*Age 40-49y*	*Age 50-59y*	*Age 60-69y*	*Age 70-79y*
<160	0	0	0	0	0
160-199	4	3	2	1	0
200-239	7	5	3	1	0
240-279	9	6	4	2	1
≥280	11	8	5	3	1

Prevention, Detection, Evaluation and Treatment of High Blood Pressure (JNC 7) classifies optimal blood pressure as shown in Table 1-3.

An overwhelming body of evidence shows the causal relationship between dyslipidemia and CHD.[10] Additionally, multiple studies have linked improved choles-

	Points				
	Age 20-39y	*Age 40-49y*	*Age 50-59y*	*Age 60-69y*	*Age 70-79y*
Nonsmoker	0	0	0	0	0
Smoker	8	5	3	1	1

HDL-C, mg/dL	Points
≥60	-1
50-59	0
40-49	1
<40	2

Systolic BP, mm Hg	If untreated	If treated
<120	0	0
120-129	0	1
130-139	1	2
140-159	1	2
≥160	2	3

(continued on next page)

terol levels—accomplished either by lifestyle changes or pharmacologic therapy—to reduction of CHD events and all-cause mortality.[12] NCEP ATP III guidelines identify low-density lipoprotein cholesterol (LDL-C) as the primary target for cholesterol-lowering therapy, but secondary prevention goals for lipids are also important for

Table 1-7: Framingham Point Scores Estimate of 10-Year Risk for Men *(continued)*

Point total	10-year risk (%)
<0	<1
0	1
1	1
2	1
3	1
4	1
5	2
6	2
7	3
8	4
9	5
10	6
11	8
12	10
13	12
14	16
15	20
16	25
≥17	≥30

non-HDL-C and triglycerides with patients who have CHD, diabetes, and atherosclerosis. Table 1-4 presents the ATP III classification of LDL, total and HDL cholesterol, and triglycerides.

Obesity is one of the most serious and common health problems in the United States. Epidemiologic studies have

Table 1-8: Framingham Point Scores Estimate of 10-Year Risk for Women

Age, years	Points
20-34	-7
35-39	-3
40-44	0
45-49	3
50-54	6
55-59	8
60-64	10
65-69	12
70-74	14
75-79	16

Total cholesterol, mg/dL	Points				
	Age 20-39y	*Age 40-49y*	*Age 50-59y*	*Age 60-69y*	*Age 70-79y*
<160	0	0	0	0	0
160-199	4	3	2	1	1
200-239	8	6	4	2	1
240-279	11	8	5	3	2
≥280	13	10	7	4	2

(continued on next page)

shown that increasing abdominal girth is strongly correlated with an increased incidence of CHD.[13-15] In addition, the metabolic consequences of obesity contribute to hypertension, insulin resistance, elevated triglycerides, and

Table 1-8: Framingham Point Scores Estimate of 10-Year Risk for Women *(continued)*

	Points				
	Age 20-39y	***Age 40-49y***	***Age 50-59y***	***Age 60-69y***	***Age 70-79y***
Nonsmoker	0	0	0	0	0
Smoker	9	7	4	2	1

HDL-C, mg/dL	Points
≥60	-1
50-59	0
40-49	1
<40	2

Systolic BP, mm Hg	If untreated	If treated
<120	0	0
120-129	1	3
130-139	2	4
140-159	3	5
≥160	4	6

decreased levels of HDL-C.[16,17] When this combination of metabolic changes is present, it is called the metabolic syndrome, which is an added risk factor for CHD. (See Chapter 8 for an explanation of the metabolic syndrome.)

Sedentary lifestyle, or lack of physical activity, is an independent risk factor for CHD, and there is a dose-response relationship between exercise and mortality.[18-22]

Point total	10-year risk (%)
<9	<1
9	1
10	1
11	1
12	1
13	2
14	2
15	3
16	4
17	5
18	6
19	8
20	11
21	14
22	17
23	22
24	27
≥25	≥30

Studies indicate that, following a myocardial infarction, patients who modify their behavior to include regular exercise demonstrate improved rates of survival.[23,24] Patients who remain sedentary have the highest risk for all-cause and CHD mortality.[25] Exercise does not need to be vigorous to be beneficial. Clinicians should tell patients that even moderate activity can reduce CHD and

Table 1-9: Classification, Measurement Frequency, and Therapy of Hypertension in Children and Adolescents[*,50]

	SBP or DBP Percentile**	Frequency of BP Measurement
Normal	<90th	Recheck at next scheduled physical examination
Prehypertension	90th to <95th or if BP exceeds 120/80 mm Hg even if <90th percentile up to <95th percentile[†]	Recheck in 6 mo
Stage 1 hypertension	95th-99th percentile plus 5 mm Hg	Recheck in 1-2 wk or sooner if the patient is symptomatic; if persistently elevated on 2 additional occasions, evaluate or refer to source of care within 1 month

Therapeutic Lifestyle Changes	Pharmacologic Therapy
Encourage healthy diet, sleep, and physical activity	—
Weight-management counseling if overweight; introduce physical activity and diet management[‡]	None unless compelling indications such as chronic kidney disease, diabetes mellitus, heart failure, or LVH exist
Weight-management counseling if overweight; introduce physical activity and diet management	Initiate therapy based on the following indications: symptomatic hypertension, secondary hypertension, hypertensive target-organ damage, diabetes (type 1 or 2), persistent hypertension despite nonpharmacologic measures *or* if compelling indications (as shown above) exist

(continued on next page)

Table 1-9: Classification, Measurement Frequency, and Therapy of Hypertension in Children and Adolescents[*,50] *(continued)*

	SBP or DBP Percentile**	Frequency of BP Measurement
Stage 2 hypertension	>99th percentile plus 5 mm Hg	Evaluate or refer to source of care within 1 wk or immediately if the patient is symptomatic

* Hypertension in children and adolescents is defined as systolic blood pressure (SBP) and/or diastolic blood pressure (DBP) that is >95th percentile on repeated measurement. To be consistent with the *Seventh Report of the Joint National Committee on the Prevention, Detection, Evaluation, and Treatment of High Blood Pressure,* BP between the 90th and 95th percentiles is now termed 'prehypertensive' and is an indication for lifestyle modifications.

** For gender, age, and height measured on at least 3 separate occasions; if systolic and diastolic categories are different, categorize by the higher value.

encourage sedentary people to begin some simple exercise, such as walking.

Extensive literature has established that psychosocial factors, including depression, anxiety, personality factors and character traits, social isolation, and chronic life stress, contribute significantly to the pathogenesis and manifes-

Therapeutic Lifestyle Changes	**Pharmacologic Therapy**
Weight-management counseling if overweight; introduce physical activity and diet management[‡]	Initiate therapy[§]

[†] This typically occurs at age 12 years for SBP and at age 16 years for DBP.

[‡] Parents and children trying to modify their eating plan to the Dietary Approaches to Stop Hypertension Study eating plan may benefit from consultation with a registered or licensed nutritionist.

[§] More than one drug may be required.

tation of CHD.[26] Psychosocial stresses tend to cluster, compounding their health-damaging effects. This can result in a substantially elevated risk that equates to that of previously established risk factors, such as hypertension and dyslipidemia.[26] Depression is associated with both hypercortisolemia [27-29] and impaired platelet function,[30,31]

Table 1-10: Cholesterol Classifications for Children and Adolescents Aged 2 to 19 Years*[51,52]

Category	Total Cholesterol (mg/dL)	LDL Cholesterol (mg/dL)
Acceptable	<170	<110
Borderline	170-199	110-129
High	≥200	≥130

* High-density lipoprotein levels should be ≥35 mg/dL, and triglycerides should be ≤150 mg/dL.

LDL = low-density lipoprotein

which, when combined, help establish the theoretic basis for explaining the proatherogenic effects of depression on CHD. Depression and anxiety disorders contribute to reduced heart rate variability[32,33] and impaired vagal control,[32,34,35] which may also contribute to enhanced arrhythmia potential and sudden death.[36] Hostility and social isolation are also correlated with CHD.[37] Patients with high levels of hostility have a greater rate of restenosis after angioplasty,[38] experience more rapid atherosclerosis progression during serial carotid ultrasonography,[39] and manifest more ischemia during exercise testing than other CHD patients.[40]

Clinical Risk Factor Assessment

It is vital to prevent the first episode of coronary disease or stroke, because many first heart attacks and strokes are fatal or disabling. According to a 2002 update of American Heart Association (AHA) Guidelines for Primary Prevention of Cardiovascular Disease and Stroke, physicians should routinely assess patients' general risk of cardiovascular disease beginning at age 20 (Table 1-5). The updated guidelines also recommend that physicians calculate the 10-year risk for people older than 40 years or for anyone who has multiple risk factors.[41]

Because heart disease is a result of many factors, it is important to simultaneously consider all risk factors when estimating a patient's CHD risk. Focusing on single-factor assessment results in too much emphasis being placed on elevations of a single risk factor rather than on the overall risk level based on a combination of risk factors. Groups of risk factors can multiply the risk so that an individual with a number of modest risk factors may have a considerably higher risk than a person with one high-risk factor.[45]

Obviously, patients with clinically manifest CHD are already at risk for further coronary or vascular events. The focus for these patients should be on modifying risk factors related to lifestyle, managing other risk factors, and using drug therapies appropriately. Calculating the risk of CHD for healthy individuals is a two-step procedure. First, the number of risk factors is counted (Tables 1-1 and 1-6). A more detailed description of the risk factors and how to use them for patients with high cholesterol or hypertension is presented in Table 1-6. Second, for individuals with two or more risk factors, a 10-year risk assessment is conducted using Framingham scoring (Tables 1-7 and 1-8) to identify those whose short-term risk warrants intensive treatment. Estimating the 10-year risk goes a step beyond risk-factor counting, but it is justified because it makes it easier to target people who will benefit from intensive treatment. Framingham scoring is not necessary for persons with 0 to 1 risk factor, because the 10-year risk seldom reaches levels requiring intensive intervention.[10]

Subsequent chapters of this book provide detailed information on clinical assessment for each of the established CHD risk factors.

Table 1-11: Selected Resources Available on the World Wide Web

Organization	Web Site
American Heart Association	www.americanheart.org
American College of Cardiology	www.acc.org
National Cholesterol Education Program (NCEP)	www.nhlbi.nih.gov www.nhlbi.nih.gov/guidelines/cholesterol/profmats.htm
American Diabetes Association	www.diabetes.org/home.jsp
JNC 7-Hypertension	www.nhlbi.nih.gov/guidelines/index.htm
Obesity guidelines	www.nhlbi.nih.gov and www.obesity.org
Smoking cessation	www.ahcpr.gov/clinic and www.guidelines.gov
Palm/handheld resources	www.handheldmed.com
General	www.guidelines.gov

Assessing Risk Factors in Children

Risk factors that we know are important in adults are common in children and adolescents.[46] Since 1990, the prevalence of tobacco use, obesity, and sedentary lifestyle has steadily increased among children and adolescents in the United States. The number of young people who smoke has increased each year since 1991 and, every day, more

Comments

Comprehensive Web site for professionals and patients

Shares guidelines with American Heart Association plus more

NCEP guidelines including adult and pediatric panels and calculators

Useful clinical guidelines

The best overview of hypertension treatment guidelines

Guidelines from NHLBI and American Obesity Association—practical and current

Commercial sites with abundant medical palm software

National Guideline Clearinghouse

than 3,000 adolescents start smoking. More than 20% of adolescents in the United States are now overweight, which is a more than 50% increase in prevalence since 1980. These declines in the health status of adolescents in the United States have important implications for future rates of cardiovascular disease. Cardiovascular disease will soon be the leading cause of premature death and disability worldwide.[46]

Family physicians are in a unique position to screen for children at risk. Although screening for hyperlipidemia in children and medically treating high blood cholesterol levels and blood pressure in this age group remain controversial,[47] pathologic studies suggest that atherosclerosis is diffuse and advanced as early as adolescence.[48,49] Based on the risk associated with prolonged extreme elevations of blood pressure or LDL-C levels, expert panels have concluded that adolescents who have blood pressure or LDL-C levels greater than the 90th percentile should receive medication if they are not responding to lifestyle changes.[47,49] Tables 1-9 and 1-10 show blood pressure and cholesterol classifications for children.

It is difficult to extrapolate health care recommendations for children from the results of adult clinical trials, and long-term trials of risk factor modification in children to prevent future cardiovascular events are not available. Because of problems related to sample sizes, expense, and the length of time required for meaningful results, it is unlikely that clinical trials assessing risk modification in children will ever be conducted. The fact still remains that primary prevention of atherosclerosis is important because more than 40% of cardiovascular events occur in people younger than 65 years of age, and nearly 50% of these events are fatal.[44] The question is: At what age do we start medical treatment? From the perspective of a primary care physician, it seems reasonable to make every effort to ensure that our children avoid tobacco, are physically active, and have a healthy diet. It also seems reasonable to treat extreme risk that is highly likely to result in premature cardiovascular disease.

Risk Factor Tools

Many tools are available from the AHA, NIH, and other organizations that you may find useful in assessing your patients' risk for CHD. We have included a few of them in this chapter (Table 1-11).

References

1. Levenson JW, Skerrett PJ, Gaziano JM: Reducing the global burden of cardiovascular disease: the role of risk factors. *Prev Cardiol* 2002;5:188-189.

2. *Dorland's Illustrated Medical Dictionary*. Friel JP, ed: WB Saunders, Philadelphia, 2000.

3. Assmann G, Cullen P, Schulte H: Simple scoring scheme for calculating the risk of acute coronary events based on the 10-year follow-up of the prospective cardiovascular Munster (PROCAM) study. *Circulation* 2002;105:310-315.

4. Keevil JG, Stein JH, McBride PE: Cardiovascular disease prevention. *Prim Care* 2002;29:667-696.

5. American Heart Association: *2001 Heart and Stroke Statistical Update 2001*. Dallas, TX, American Heart Association, 2001.

6. McBride PE: The health consequences of smoking. Cardiovascular diseases. *Med Clin North Am* 1992;76:333-353.

7. Fiore MC, Hatsukami DK, Baker TB: Effective tobacco dependence treatment. *JAMA* 2002;288:1768-1771.

8. American Diabetes Association: Clinical practice recommendations 2003. *Diabetes Care* 2003;26:S21-S24.

9. American Diabetes Association: Clinical Practice Recommendations 2003. Web site http://diabetes.org/home.jsp. Accessed April 19, 2005.

10. Expert Panel on Detection, Evaluation and Treatment of High Blood Cholesterol in Adults: Executive summary of the third report of the National Cholesterol Education Program (NCEP) Expert Panel on Detection, Evaluation and Treatment of High Blood Cholesterol in Adults (Adult Treatment Panel III). *JAMA* 2001;285:2486-2497.

11. Haffner SM, Lehto S, Ronnemaa T, et al: Mortality from coronary heart disease in subjects with type 2 diabetes and in nondiabetic subjects with and without prior myocardial infarction. *N Engl J Med* 1998;339:229-234.

12. Wilson PW, D'Agostino RB, Levy D, et al: Prediction of coronary heart disease using risk factor categories. *Circulation* 1998;97:1837-1847.

13. Grundy SM: The optimal ratio of fat-to-carbohydrate in the diet. *Annu Rev Nutr* 1999;19:325-341.

14. Harlan WR, Landis JR, Flegal KM, et al: Secular trends in body mass in the United States, 1960-1980. *Am J Epidemiol* 1988;128:1065-1074.

15. Williamson DF, Kahn HS, Remington PL, et al: The 10-year incidence of overweight and major weight gain in US adults. *Arch Intern Med* 1990;150:665-672.

16. Bouchard C, Bray GA, Hubbard VS: Basic and clinical aspects of regional fat distribution. *Am J Clin Nutr* 1990;52:946-950.

17. Bjorntorp P: The associations between obesity, adipose tissue distribution and disease. *Acta Med Scand Suppl* 1988;723: 121-134.

18. Blair SN, Kohl HW 3rd, Paffenbarger RS Jr, et al: Physical fitness and all-cause mortality. A prospective study of healthy men and women. *JAMA* 1989;262:2395-2401.

19. Blair SN, Kohl HW 3rd, Barlow CE, et al: Changes in physical fitness and all-cause mortality. A prospective study of healthy and unhealthy men. *JAMA* 1995;273:1093-1098.

20. Lee IM, Hsieh CC, Paffenbarger RS Jr: Exercise intensity and longevity in men. The Harvard Alumni Health Study. *JAMA* 1995;273:1179-1184.

21. Morris JN, Clayton DG, Everitt MG, et al: Exercise in leisure time: coronary attack and death rates. *Br Heart J* 1990;63:325-334.

22. Powell KE, Thompson PD, Caspersen CJ, et al: Physical activity and the incidence of coronary heart disease. *Annu Rev Public Health* 1987;8:253-287.

23. O'Connor GT, Buring JE, Yusuf S, et al: An overview of randomized trials of rehabilitation with exercise after myocardial infarction. *Circulation* 1989;80:234-244.

24. Oldridge NB, Guyatt GH, Fischer ME, et al: Cardiac rehabilitation after myocardial infarction. Combined experience of randomized clinical trials. *JAMA* 1988;260:945-950.

25. Fletcher GF, Balady G, Blair SN, et al: Statement on exercise: benefits and recommendations for physical activity for all Americans. A statement for health professionals by the Committee on Exercise and Cardiac Rehabilitation of the Council on Clinical Cardiology. American Heart Association. *Circulation* 1996;94:857-862.

26. Rozanski A, Blumenthal JA, Kaplan J: Impact of psychological factors on the pathogenesis of cardiovascular disease and implications for therapy. *Circulation* 1999;99:2192-2217.

27. Carroll BJ, Curtis GC, Davies BM, et al: Urinary free cortisol excretion in depression. *Psychol Med* 1976;6:43-50.

28. Gold PW, Loriaux DL, Roy A, et al: Responses to corticotropin-releasing hormone in the hypercortisolism of depression and Cushing's disease. Pathophysiologic and diagnostic implications. *N Engl J Med* 1986;314:1329-1335.

29. Veith RC, Lewis N, Linares OA, et al: Sympathetic nervous system activity in major depression. Basal and desipramine-induced alterations in plasma norepinephrine kinetics. *Arch Gen Psychiatry* 1994;51:411-422.

30. Musselman DL, Tomer A, Manatunga AK, et al: Exaggerated platelet reactivity in major depression. *Am J Psychiatry* 1996;153:1313-1317.

31. Laghrissi-Thode F, Wagner WR, Pollock BG, et al: Elevated platelet factor 4 and beta-thromboglobulin plasma levels in depressed patients with ischemic heart disease. *Biol Psychiatry* 1997;42:290-295.

32. Carney RM, Saunders RD, Freedland KE, et al: Association of depression with reduced heart rate variability in coronary artery disease. *Am J Cardiol* 1995;76:562-564.

33. Kawachi I, Sparrow D, Vokonas PS, et al: Decreased heart rate variability in men with phobic anxiety (data from the Normative Aging Study). *Am J Cardiol* 1995;75:882-885.

34. Martin GJ, Magid NM, Myers G, et al: Heart rate variability and sudden death secondary to coronary artery disease during ambulatory electrocardiographic monitoring. *Am J Cardiol* 1987;60:86-89.

35. Rich MW, Saini JS, Kleiger RE, et al: Correlation of heart rate variability with clinical and angiographic variables and late mortality after coronary angiography. *Am J Cardiol* 1988;62(10 Pt 1):714-717.

36. Lown B, Verrier R, Corbalan R: Psychologic stress and threshold for repetitive ventricular response. *Science* 1973;182:834-836.

37. Blumenthal JA, Barefoot J, Burg MM, et al: Psychological correlates of hostility among patients undergoing coronary angiography. *Br J Med Psychol* 1987;60(Pt 4):349-355.

38. Goodman M, Quigley J, Moran G, et al: Hostility predicts restenosis after percutaneous transluminal coronary angioplasty. *Mayo Clin Proc* 1996;71:729-734.

39. Matsumoto Y, Uyama O, Shimizu S, et al: Do anger and aggression affect carotid atherosclerosis? *Stroke* 1993;24:983-986.

40. Helmers KF, Krantz DS, Howell RH, et al: Hostility and myocardial ischemia in coronary artery disease patients: evaluation by gender and ischemic index. *Psychosom Med* 1993;55:29-36.

41. Pearson TA, Blair SN, Daniels SR, et al: AHA Guidelines for Primary Prevention of Cardiovascular Disease and Stroke: 2002 Update: Consensus panel guide to comprehensive risk reduction for adult patients without coronary or other atherosclerotic vascular disease. American Heart Association Science Advisory and Coordinating Committee. *Circulation* 2002;106:388-391.

42. Third Report of the Expert Panel on Detection, Evaluation, and Treatment of High Blood Cholesterol in Adults (Adult Treatment Panel III) full report: manuscript version. Available at: http://www.nhlbi.nih.gov/guidelines/cholesterol/atp3_rpt.htm. Pages 111-118. Accessed June 1, 2002.

43. Wilson PW, D'Agostino RB, Levy D, et al: Prediction of coronary heart disease using risk factor categories. *Circulation* 1998;97:1837-1847.

44. Grundy SM, Pasternak R, Greenland P, et al: Assessment of cardiovascular risk by use of multiple-risk-factor equations: a statement for healthcare professionals from the American Heart Association and the American College of Cardiology. *Circulation* 1999;100:1481-1492.

45. Wood D: Established and emerging cardiovascular risk factors. Recommendation of the Joint European Societies Task Force London, UK. *Eur Heart J* 1998;19:1434-1503.

46. Hennekens CH: Increasing burden of cardiovascular disease: current knowledge and future directions for research on risk factors. *Circulation* 1998;97:1095-1102.

47. Highlights of the Report of the Expert Panel on Blood Cholesterol Levels in Children and Adolescents. National Cholesterol Education Program Expert Panel on Blood Cholesterol Levels in Children and Adolescents. *Am Fam Physician* 1992;45:2127-2136.

48. Berenson GS, Srinivasan SR, Bao W, et al: Association between multiple cardiovascular disease risk factors and atheroscle-

rosis in children and young adults. The Bogalusa Heart Study. *N Engl J Med* 1998;338:1650-1656.

49. Goldstein JC, Brown MB: Familial hypercholesterolemia. In: Scriver CS, Beaudat AL, Sly WS, eds. *Metabolic basis of inherited disease*, New York, McGraw-Hill, 1989, pp 1215-1251.

50. National High Blood Pressure Education Program Working Group on High Blood Pressure in Children and Adolescents: The fourth report on the diagnosis, evaluation, and treatment of high blood pressure in children and adolescents. *Pediatrics* 2004;114:555-576.

51. American Heart Association: Cholesterol and atherosclerosis in children. AHA Scientific Position. Available at: http://www.americanheart.org/presenter.jhtml?identifier=4499. Accessed May 11, 2005.

52. Williams CL, Hayman LL, Daniels SR, et al: Cardiovascular health in childhood: A statement for health professionals from the Committee on Atherosclerosis, Hypertension, and Obesity in the Young (AHOY) of the Council on Cardiovascular Disease in the Young, American Heart Association. *Circulation* 2002;106:143-160.

CHAPTER 2

Screening for Cardiac and Vascular Disease

Atherosclerotic vascular disease (ASVD) is the leading cause of death and disability in the United States, accounting for more than 1 million deaths annually.[1] Coronary heart disease (CHD) accounts for most of these deaths. Many of these patients die without prior symptoms. Research has shown that lifestyle changes and medical therapy can reduce the risk of developing ASVD or slow the atherosclerotic process.[2] By properly identifying and managing your patients' risk factors, you can play an essential role in improving their overall cardiovascular health. The challenge is to find those at high risk for ASVD, to focus our efforts on helping them to reduce their risk, and to screen for significant atherosclerotic plaque before patients develop an acute vascular event.

Atherosclerosis is a slow, complex type of vascular disease that is largely preventable. Typically starting in childhood, it continues to progress as people age. Pathologic studies conducted at autopsy, following the unexpected deaths of children and young adults, have shown a positive and significant correlation between the presence and extent of atherosclerotic lesions and established risk factors such as dyslipidemia, hypertension, obesity, and tobacco use.[1] Eight percent of 10- to 15-year-old children and 33% of US teens aged 16 to 19 have significant coronary atheromas.[3] Research indicates that

90% of patients who have atherosclerosis have identifiable risk factors (Chapter 1).

This chapter focuses on screening strategies for patients at risk for cardiovascular disease (CVD) events. Noninvasive imaging tests are available that can assess ASVD and CVD risk, including exercise electrocardiogram (ECG) testing (with and without imaging), B-mode ultrasound, carotid intimal medial thickness (CIMT), electron-beam computed tomography (EBCT), magnetic resonance coronary angiography, and ankle-brachial index. These tests may be useful if they change the intensity of risk factor management of the patient.

Atherosclerosis

Atherosclerosis results from an excessive inflammatory and fibroproliferative response to numerous vascular insults caused by risk factors such as the constituents of tobacco smoke, oxidized low-density lipoprotein (LDL), and very-low-density lipoprotein. Deposits of lipids, cellular waste products, calcium, and other substances accumulate in the arterial wall (endothelial lining) over many years, altering the normal homeostatic properties of the endothelium[2,4] and forming plaques. Although these plaques can grow large enough to appreciably reduce arterial blood flow, approximately 70% of acute CVD events (eg, myocardial infarction [MI], acute coronary syndrome) occur from atherosclerotic plaque rupture of lesions that have stenosed the artery less than 50%.[5] The rupture of the plaque causes a thrombus to form on the surface and leads to an acute vascular occlusion and to ischemia. Plaques most vulnerable to rupture and acute events are those most amenable to risk factor treatment, such as cholesterol treatment, because they have large lipid cores and inflammatory cells.[6]

Atherosclerosis Begins in Childhood

Obesity, elevated blood pressure, tobacco use, dyslipidemia, and increased body mass index in childhood and adolescence are significant risk predictors for coronary artery atherosclerosis.[1] Many epidemiologic studies have revealed a disturbing increase in the prevalence of obesity beginning in childhood, with at least 22% of children ages 6 to 17 diagnosed as overweight.[1] There is substantial scientific documentation that the behaviors associated with CVD risk factors are acquired in childhood.[1] These behaviors include dietary habits, physical activity behaviors, and tobacco use. There is also increasing evidence documenting the safety and success of intervention to reduce risk factors in childhood. These studies include the Dietary Intervention Study in Children trial, which demonstrated the safety and efficacy of a low-fat diet in children with hypercholesterolemia, and the Child and Adolescent Trial for Cardiovascular Health Study, which increased physical activity levels in children by using elementary school-based programs.[1] Therefore, interventions to reduce CVD risk need to start in childhood.

Identifying children and adolescents at high risk for CVD is an important first step in CHD prevention. Table 2-1 presents the American Heart Association (AHA) general and risk-factor-specific guidelines for identifying pediatric patients at high risk for future CVD.

Screening for CVD

Although pathologic studies have documented that levels of traditional risk factors are associated with the extent and severity of atherosclerosis, the amount of atherosclerosis at every level of risk factor exposure varies. This variation in disease may be caused by many factors, including genetic susceptibility; combinations and interactions with other risk factors, including life habits; duration of exposure to the specific level of risk factors; and other factors, such as biologic and laboratory variability.

Because of this variation, subclinical disease measurements, representing the end result of risk exposures, may help to improve risk prediction for CHD.[4] Many noninvasive tests can potentially directly or indirectly measure and monitor atherosclerosis in asymptomatic persons. These tests include carotid artery duplex scanning, EBCT, ultrasound-based endothelial function studies, and magnetic resonance imaging (MRI) techniques.

Additionally, high sensitivity testing for C-reactive protein (high-sensitivity CRP or hs-CRP) may be a measure of the extent of atherosclerosis and may be considered another potential marker for atherosclerosis disease risk.[7] Chapter 12 examines hs-CRP and other emerging cardiovascular risk factors.

B-Mode Ultrasound/ Carotid Intimal Medial Thickness

B-mode ultrasound is a noninvasive technique for visualizing the lumen and wall of selected arteries—including the carotid, aorta, and femoral arteries—that is relatively inexpensive and safe. Several independent laboratories have validated B-mode ultrasound for measuring intimal medial thickness (IMT), and its reliability has been established in single- and multicenter studies.[8] Ultrasound transducers of 8 MHz or more are capable of identifying the two arterial interfaces (lumen-intima and media-adventitia) needed for measuring IMT, which is an operational measurement of atherosclerosis based on data documenting that the intima and media are involved in atherogenesis and the anatomical progression of lesions.[3] Therefore, it is possible to measure early changes in developing arterial atherosclerosis. The correlation of CIMT with coronary artery disease (CAD) and clinical CVD events has been demonstrated in many prospective studies.[9]

Unlike EBCT, which is limited to plaque that contains calcium, CIMT can provide an evaluation of early changes in the artery—intimal thickening—and the presence of early plaque that is rich in lipids and therefore more vulnerable to rupture. The correlation of atherosclerosis in

Table 2-1: Guidelines for Identification of Children and Adolescents at High Risk of CVD[1*]

Assessment

Goals for Pediatric Care Providers

- Timed, targeted risk factor assessment
- Appropriate interpretation of results and communication to families

Goals for Parents

- Recognition of risk factor significance for development of CVD, especially family history

Specific Risk Assessment: Levels of Concern

Lipids and Lipoprotein

- Total cholesterol >170 mg/dL is borderline; >200 mg/dL is elevated
- LDL-C >110 mg/dL is borderline; >130 mg/dL is elevated.
- Triglycerides >150 mg/dL
- HDL-C <35 mg/dL

Recommendations

- Family history: Update regularly (parents, grandparents, aunts, and uncles) with regard to obesity, hypertension, dyslipidemia, diabetes, cigarette smoking, and cardiovascular disease before age 55 for men and age 65 for women.

- Height, weight, BMI: Assess at every examination.
- Blood pressure: Measure at every examination after age 3; chart for age/sex/height.
- Diet and physical activity: Assess at every visit.
- Cigarette smoking: Evaluate starting at 9 to 10 years of age.

- Perform targeted screening of fasting lipids in children >2 years of age with a family history of dyslipidemia or premature CVD.
- For children in whom family history is unknown and other risk factors are present, assess lipids and lipoproteins.
- If averaged results of three fasting lipid profiles are above cut points, follow AHA guidelines for CVD risk reduction and intervention for children and adolescents.

(continued on next page)

Table 2-1: Guidelines for Identification of Children and Adolescents at High Risk of CVD[1*] *(continued)*

Assessment

Specific Risk Assessment: Levels of Concern *(continued)*

Blood Pressure

- Systolic and diastolic blood pressure >90th percentile for age, sex, and height

Body Size

- BMI >85th percentile is at risk of overweight; 95th percentile is overweight

*See Chapter 12 for these guidelines.

BMI = body mass index; CVD = cardiovascular disease; HDL-C = high-density-lipoprotein cholesterol; LDL-C = low-density-lipoprotein cholesterol.

the carotid arteries to atherosclerosis in the coronary arteries is high, making CIMT an excellent screening test of overall risk of atherosclerosis and CVD risk.

As demonstrated in many clinical studies, the severity of CIMT is an independent predictor of transient cerebral ischemia, stroke, and coronary events such as MI.[4]

Recommendations

- Know appropriate blood pressure measurement techniques, including appropriate cuff size.
- Interpret blood pressure measurements on the basis of age, sex, and height. (Blood pressure percentiles are available at http://www.nhlbi.nih.gov/health/prof/heart/hbp/hbp_ped.htm.)
- Body size should be charted by BMI. (Norms for BMI percentiles are available at http://www.cdc.gov/growthcharts.)
- The 95th percentile can be approximated by the age (in years) +13 for boys and the age (in years) +14 for girls after age 9 years.

Cross-sectional associations have been demonstrated between common CIMT and cardiovascular risk factors,[10-12] and cross-sectional studies have associated CVD with common CIMT.[11-14] CIMT is also a viable predictor of the presence of coronary atherosclerosis and its clinical sequelae.[15-19] Medial thickness, or smooth muscle hypertrophy, is associated with hypertension even when there is no atherosclerotic plaque.[3]

Many clinical intervention or prevention trials have illustrated the ability of carotid B-mode ultrasound imaging to monitor changes in CIMT over time.[20-22] Increases in intimal thickness, known as fibromuscular hyperplasia, are associated with aging.

The screening examination is performed bilaterally on three extracranial carotid artery segments: (1) the distal straight 1 cm of the common carotid arteries; (2) the carotid bifurcations; and (3) the proximal 1 cm of the internal carotid arteries.

Circumferential longitudinal scans can identify increased carotid IMT on the near and far walls of each segment. There is no radiation exposure.

The lack of established valid and reliable protocols for sonographers to monitor IMT over time in clinical practice is a barrier to routinely using IMT for serial assessment of plaque progression/regression in medical practice. If these technical issues can be resolved by using standardized protocols for scanning and monitoring IMT, B-mode ultrasound would be useful in the follow-up of patients treated for plaque progression or regression.[3] Although several reports have indicated the possibility, it is not known whether B-mode ultrasound can provide information about individual plaques that are susceptible to rupture, causing thrombosis and/or embolization. Further research is needed to determine if this is a role for B-mode ultrasound.[3]

Electron-beam Computed Tomography

Calcification within the wall of the coronary artery is a recognized marker of atherosclerosis.[23] EBCT and helical computed tomography (CT) are highly sensitive methods of detecting coronary calcium[24] and are being extensively evaluated as noninvasive means of defining coronary atherosclerotic disease and identifying asymptomatic patients at risk for CAD. There is insufficient evidence, however, that calcium screening alone is appropriate for the general population or routine clinical use.[3,23]

EBCT uses an electron sweep of stationary tungsten target rings to generate x-ray images that can detect small amounts of calcium with great accuracy.[24] Helical CT uses a continuously rotating x-ray source. Both techniques allow for quantification of calcium area and density, and both are relatively expensive.[3] Both types involve a significant radiation exposure, equivalent to 30 to 80 chest x-rays (EBCT 30 to 50, helical CT 60 to 80).

Because the severity of coronary atherosclerosis is associated with risk of coronary events, it would seem likely that coronary calcium scores correlate with risk for coronary events. However, patients with low or intermediate calcium scores can still have coronary events if they have coronary risk factors. Therefore, coronary artery calcium screening does not identify all lesions or fully predict risk. This uncertainty needs to be weighed against the costs of measurement and the risk that results might lead to inappropriate and invasive coronary evaluation.[3] For this reason, the AHA (Prevention Conference V, Writing Group III) determined that coronary calcium measurement should not be recommended for routine risk assessment in asymptomatic populations until there is more definitive information about the additive value of calcium scores in asymptomatic persons.[9] Further study is needed to determine the extent to which coronary calcium scores predict coronary events independent of the traditional and emerging coronary risk factors.

Selected use of coronary calcium scores in a patient with intermediate coronary disease risk may be appropriate.[3] A recently published study by Greenland et al found that a high coronary calcium score (greater than 300 or the highest quartile) added incremental predictive risk to patients at intermediate risk of future CVD events as calculated by a Framingham risk score.[25] Tests that can identify atherosclerosis without calcium, such as MRI and ultrafast CT, are now under development and may have greater use in the long term.

Magnetic Resonance Imaging

Clinicians have become increasingly aware that the composition of atherosclerotic plaque is important as a major risk factor for acute coronary conditions. Although current imaging techniques, such as angiography, are useful for evaluating luminal narrowing and the consequences of reduced blood flow, they are poor for evaluating the vessel wall and characterizing the plaque.[3] MRI has been shown to characterize tissue noninvasively in many different study systems.[26-28]

A recent study of patients with plaques in the thoracic aorta showed that plaque composition and size are accurately characterized and measured with MRI when compared with transesophageal echocardiography.[29] Carotid and aortic atherosclerotic assessment with MRI may lead to its use as a screening tool for predicting future cardiovascular events and evaluating therapeutic interventions.[3] A goal for MRI is imaging plaque in vivo in coronary arteries. Studies in an in vivo pig model[30,31] and normal human subjects suggest that the MRI technique may eventually be applicable for this purpose.

MRI is a promising research tool, but it is not yet appropriate for use in identifying patients at high risk for CAD. More studies of MRI in CHD risk prediction are needed, particularly regarding which patients will benefit from screening.

Endothelial Function Studies

Endothelial cells play an essential role in inhibiting the development of atherosclerosis and its thrombotic consequences. Endothelial cell production of nitric oxide vasodilates arteries; inhibits monocyte, leukocyte, and platelet adhesion to the vessel wall; decreases permeability to LDL; and inhibits smooth muscle cell proliferation.

High-resolution ultrasound techniques can study endothelial cells noninvasively by measuring endothelium-dependent vasodilator responses to various stimuli and can be used in clinical and population-based studies.[3] Although assessing endothelial function in this way is a promising technique that may represent an independent measure of CVD risk, additional prospective research is needed to demonstrate that it can really add to standard CVD risk prediction. Standardization and improvement of the measurement technique are also needed before endothelial function studies can become part of a routine clinical assessment of CVD risk.[3]

Ankle-Brachial Index

Ankle-brachial index, a simple and inexpensive test that can be performed in any clinical practice, is highly prognostic for ASVD. It requires only a blood pressure cuff and a Doppler sensor. Systolic blood pressure is measured in both arms and in one leg (placing the cuff on or below the calf and the probe over the posterior tibial or dorsalis pedis artery in the leg). The ankle pressure divided by the brachial pressure should be greater than 0.9. A ratio less than 0.9 indicates peripheral arterial disease (PAD), and the lower the value, the greater the obstruction. PAD detected by the ankle-brachial index highly correlates with CHD and future risk for CVD events. This test can identify vascular disease and is an important screening tool for PAD and risk (sensitivity is approximately 90% and specificity is 98%).[32]

Exercise Testing

Exercise, a common physiologic stress, can uncover cardiovascular abnormalities that are not present at rest and can be used to determine the adequacy of cardiac function. Exercise testing, a cardiovascular stress test that uses a treadmill or stationary bicycle combined with ECG and blood pressure monitoring, is widely available and relatively inexpensive.[33] It allows assessment of exercise capacity and correlation of symptoms with ECG changes

Table 2-2: Absolute and Relative Contraindications to Exercise Testing[29]

Absolute

- Acute myocardial infarction (within 2 days)
- High-risk unstable angina
- Uncontrolled cardiac arrhythmias causing symptoms of hemodynamic compromise
- Active endocarditis
- Symptomatic severe aortic stenosis
- Decompensated symptomatic heart failure
- Acute pulmonary embolus or pulmonary infarction
- Acute noncardiac disorder that may affect exercise performance or be aggravated by exercise (eg, infection, renal failure, thyrotoxicosis)
- Acute myocarditis or pericarditis
- Physical disability that would preclude safe and adequate test performance
- Inability to obtain consent

Relative

- Left main coronary stenosis or its equivalent
- Moderate stenotic valvular heart disease
- Electrolyte abnormalities
- Tachyarrhythmias or bradyarrhythmias
- Atrial fibrillation with uncontrolled ventricular rate
- Hypertrophic cardiomyopathy
- Mental impairment leading to inability to cooperate
- High-degree atrioventricular block

associated with myocardial ischemia. Contraindications to exercise testing are listed in Table 2-2. Exercise testing provides the highest level of incremental diagnostic and prognostic information for patients with an intermediate probability of CHD (Figure 2-1).[33] One important objective of stress testing is to identify individuals with a high risk for severe (left main or three-vessel) CHD.[34]

According to AHA guidelines, exercise testing in patients with coronary risk factors such as hypercholesterolemia and high blood pressure may be helpful, especially if the patient is experiencing symptoms suggesting CHD (Table 2-3). Detecting myocardial ischemia or other abnormal end points can lead to further diagnostic studies and appropriate management strategies.[35] Using exercise testing nonselectively in apparently healthy patients is not recommended because of the poor predictive value of minimum (1 mm) ST segment depression. This abnormal response may lead to psychological and vocational disability and unnecessary medical expense and risk. When dealing with asymptomatic patients, only combinations of other abnormal responses (such as abnormal heart rate recovery) and at least 2 mm or more ST depression should be considered predictors of increased risk of cardiovascular events.[35]

In prognostic evaluation of subjects with CAD, substantial evidence supports the use of exercise testing as the first noninvasive step following the history, physical examination, and resting ECG. Exercise test results improve the selection of subjects who should undergo further evaluation, such as coronary angiography. The exercise test is a reasonable first choice for prognostic assessment because it can be performed in the physician's office and provides valuable information about activity levels, response to therapy, and disability. Additionally, because of its widespread use, the exercise test can have a substantial impact on the cost-effective delivery of cardiovascular care.[35]

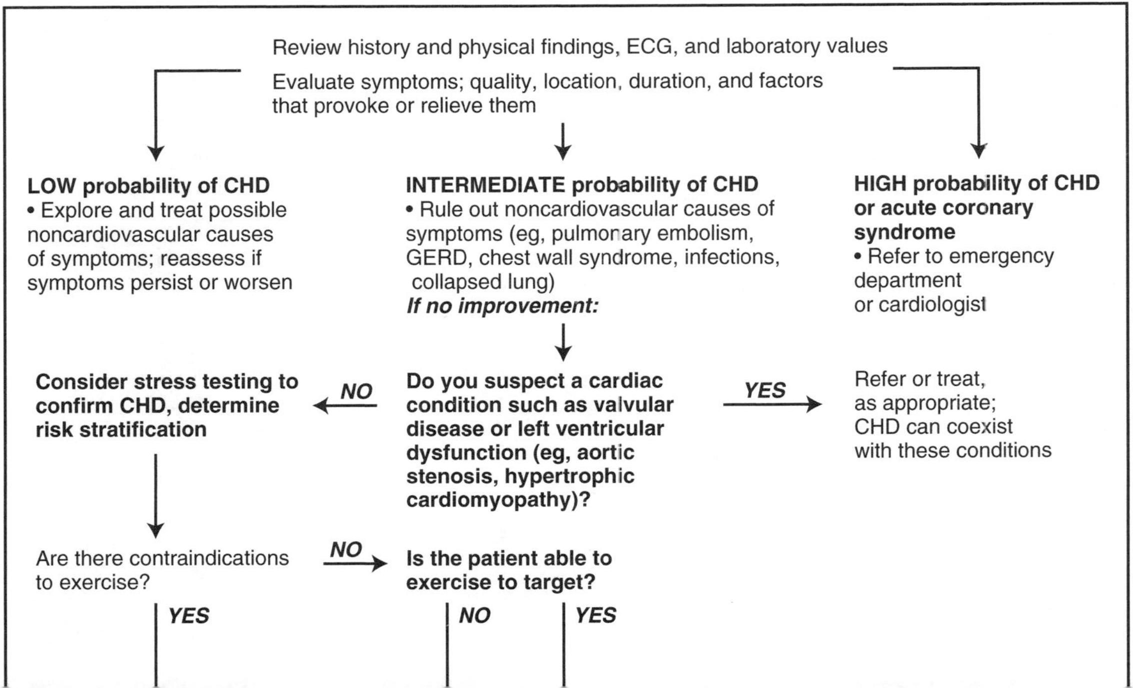
Review history and physical findings, ECG, and laboratory values
Evaluate symptoms; quality, location, duration, and factors that provoke or relieve them
LOW probability of CHD
• Explore and treat possible noncardiovascular causes of symptoms; reassess if symptoms persist or worsen
INTERMEDIATE probability of CHD
• Rule out noncardiovascular causes of symptoms (eg, pulmonary embolism, GERD, chest wall syndrome, infections, collapsed lung)
If no improvement:
HIGH probability of CHD or acute coronary syndrome
• Refer to emergency department or cardiologist
Do you suspect a cardiac condition such as valvular disease or left ventricular dysfunction (eg, aortic stenosis, hypertrophic cardiomyopathy)?
YES
Refer or treat, as appropriate; CHD can coexist with these conditions
NO
Consider stress testing to confirm CHD, determine risk stratification
Are there contraindications to exercise?
NO
Is the patient able to exercise to target?
YES
NO
YES

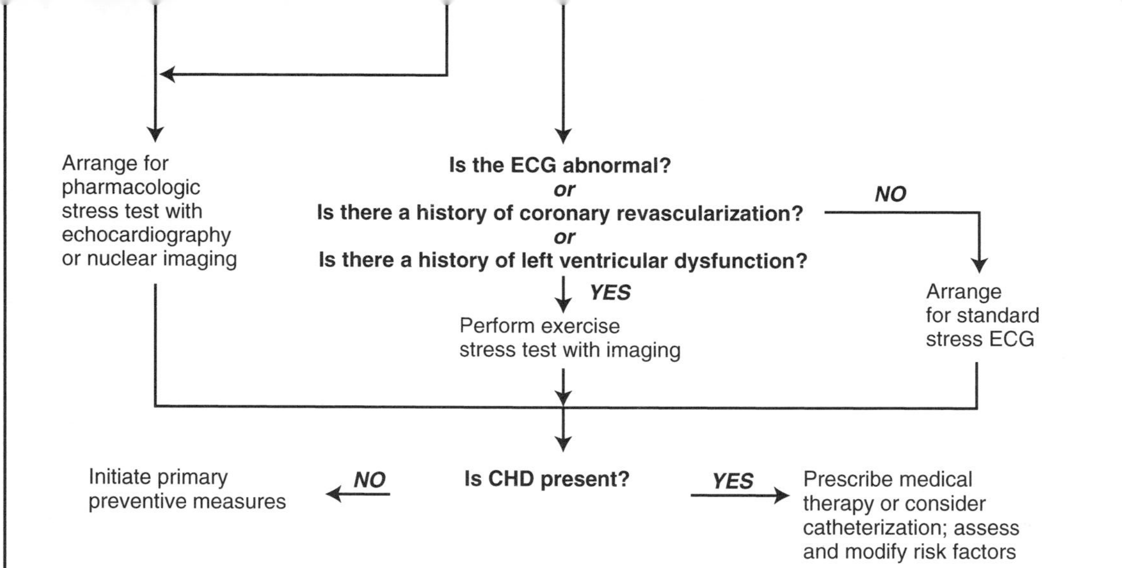

ECG = electrocardiogram; CHD = coronary heart disease; MI = myocardial infarction

Hayes et al, *J Fam Pract* 2003;52:544-551.

Figure 2-1: Evaluating chest symptoms and stratifying risk for coronary heart disease.

Table 2-3: Characteristics of Atypical (Noncardiac) vs Typical Cardiac Symptoms

Characteristics	Atypical/Noncardiac
Quality	Sharp, stabbing, positional
Location	Highly localized, below the epigastrium, above the mandible
Provoked by	'Nothing,' body movement, cough, deep inspiration, heart palpitations
Relieved by	'Nothing,' position change, analgesics, heat, antacids
Duration	'Seconds' (fleeting), or hours, days
Associated symptoms	Reflux/heartburn

When considering the use of exercise testing in individual patients, the following factors, based on the ACC/AHA guidelines for exercise testing, are important:

- The quality, expertise, and experience of the professional and technical staff performing and interpreting the study
- The sensitivity, specificity, and accuracy of the technique
- The cost and accuracy of the technique compared with those of more expensive imaging procedures
- The effect of positive or negative results on clinical decision making
- The potential psychological benefits of patient reassurance.

Candidates for exercise treadmill testing include patients with stable symptoms who can be expected to exercise to an adequate workload. A brief history and physical exami-

Typical/Cardiac
Squeezing, ache, pressure, fullness, burning, heavy, suffocating, 'discomfort'
Diffuse area–substernal chest, jaw, back, arms
Exertion, emotional stress, cold air
Rest; nitroglycerin
30 seconds to 5 minutes
Dyspnea, diaphoresis, nausea, fatigue

nation should be performed to rule out contraindications to testing or to detect important clinical signs such as cardiac murmur, gallop sounds, pulmonary bronchospasm, or rales.

Patients should have an ECG before referral for ECG stress testing. The following abnormalities will not allow interpretation of the ECG during exercise and will identify patients who may benefit from exercise tests with imaging:[34] left bundle branch block, left ventricular hypertrophy, digoxin use, and other ST-T wave changes resulting in noninterpretable stress ECGs.

Exercise testing with ECG monitoring only is reasonable, despite less sensitivity and positive predictive value, in patients with a low pretest probability of cardiac disease, or for those who are being assessed for physiologic reasons (eg, blood pressure response, exercise capacity, exercise prescription). Exercise testing with imaging (eg, echocardiography, radionuclear imaging) is recommended for those with a moderate pretest risk of CHD.[34] Patients with a high pretest probability of CHD who are being considered for possible revascularization should have a cardiac angiogram to avoid false-negative exercise test results.

Whenever possible, exercise, rather than pharmacologic agents, should be used to test for ischemia because of the additional information obtained from exercise hemodynamics, functional capacity, exercise responses, and other exercise data. Some patients referred for exercise treadmill testing are unable to reach either adequate exercise levels or the target heart rate because of comorbid conditions,[36] including degenerative joint disease, obesity, pulmonary disease, peripheral vascular disease, central nervous system disorders, physical deconditioning, and chronotropic incompetence.

Some patients have psychological or other problems that may affect their suitability for stress testing. These patients should be considered for pharmacologic stress testing.[34]

Consider withdrawing medications when exercise testing is performed for diagnostic purposes. Some drugs interfere with exercise responses and complicate the test interpretation. Medications such as β-blockers, calcium channel blockers, and nitrates will treat ischemia and mask ischemic changes during exercise. β-Blockers should be withdrawn carefully (ie, tapered) to avoid a rebound phenomenon or acute effect.[37] Medications may be held for exercise tests, or continued, depending on the reason for the exercise test. It is important to ask whether the provider wants to know how the patient is doing on or off the medication (eg, patients with known cardiac disease are often tested on their medication). A purely diagnostic test is usually performed with cardiac medications withheld.

Good clinical judgment is critical in deciding indications and contraindications for exercise testing.[37] Although exercise testing is considered a safe procedure, there are rare reports of acute MIs, deaths, and other complications. Surveys confirm that up to 10 MIs or deaths, or both, can be expected per 20,000 tests.[35,38] Table 2-2 lists absolute and relative contraindications to exercise testing. Absolute contraindications are definitive, but relative contraindications can be superseded if benefits outweigh the risks of exercise. In some cases, even submaximal testing can provide valuable information.[35]

Good physician-patient communication about the risks and benefits of exercise testing is critical. Exercise testing should be performed under the supervision of a physician who is properly trained to conduct exercise tests and in an exercise laboratory that is properly equipped. The degree of supervision needed depends on the clinical status of the patient being tested, which can be determined by asking pertinent questions about the patient's medical history, performing a brief physical examination, and reviewing the standard 12-lead ECG performed immediately before testing. For testing an apparently healthy younger patient, it may be appropriate to assign a properly trained nonphysician, such as a nurse or exercise physiologist, to directly monitor the test.

The patient's blood pressure, ECG, and physical status should be monitored throughout exercise and recovery. A physician should interpret data derived from testing and suggest further evaluation or therapy if warranted. Additionally, a physician or senior medical professional who conducts the test must be trained in advanced CPR, and a defibrillator and appropriate medications should be immediately available.[35] Detailed information on conducting exercise testing is widely available.[33-35,37]

Pharmacologic Stress Testing

Patients who are not expected to achieve an adequate exercise capacity should undergo pharmacologic stress testing using adenosine (Adenoscan®), dipyridamole (Persantine®), or dobutamine (Dobutrex®). In some cases, atrial pacing, using a swallowed esophageal electrode, is also used. Pharmacologic stress agents are sometimes combined with low-level exercise protocols, which may reduce the noncardiac side effects and improve image quality.[39]

Adenosine is the pharmacologic agent used most commonly in nuclear perfusion stress testing. An intravenous infusion of adenosine produces coronary vasodilation, which is quickly assuaged when the infusion is terminated.[34] Side effects, including flushing, palpitations, and chest pain, are short lived. Dipyridamole is used less frequently because of its prolonged side effects and reports of lower specificity.[40] Dobutamine, a β-adrenergic agonist that increases heart rate and contractility in a dose-related fashion when infused intravenously, is used most commonly in echocardiographic imaging. It can also be used with nuclear imaging when adenosine is contraindicated because of severe pulmonary or cerebrovascular disease.[34] Side effects include transient arrhythmias, hypertension or hypotension, tremor, and chest pain.

Stress Imaging Modalities

For patients with an abnormal resting ECG, evidence of left ventricular dysfunction, or a previous coronary revascularization, stress imaging with either echocardiography or nuclear perfusion scanning is appropriate.[34] Echocardiography visualizes the heart directly in real time using ultrasound. The test provides convenient assessment of the cardiac chambers, myocardium, valves, pericardium, and great vessels. It can also identify mechanical complications of acute MI, differentiate causes of reduced cardiac output and blood pressure, and help guide therapy. Interpretation of stress echocardiograms is based on analysis of segmental wall motion before and after stress. Considerable expertise in echocardiography is needed to rapidly acquire diagnostic images.

The accuracy of stress echocardiography is similar to that of nuclear stress testing.[34] There is also information to suggest that exercise echocardiography may be a particularly useful screening test for women at intermediate risk of CHD.[34]

Nuclear imaging has greatly advanced the ability to detect and assess the extent of CHD. It uses radiotracers (thallium-201, technetium-99m tetrofosmin [Myoview™], or technetium-99m sestamibi [Cardiolite®]) to evaluate myocardial perfusion and function.[34] Stress myocardial perfusion imaging has a sensitivity of >90% for detecting patients at risk of cardiac death or MI.[36] To detect ischemia or infarction, a radioisotope is injected at rest and after stress to produce images of myocardial regional uptake, which is proportional to regional blood flow. Normally, with maximal exercise or pharmacologic stress, myocardial blood flow is greatly increased above the resting condition. If a fixed coronary stenosis is present, myocardial perfusion in the area supplied by the stenotic vessel cannot be increased. This creates a flow differential and uneven distribution of the tracer.[34] Although images can be obtained in most patients using current nuclear imaging techniques, artifacts caused by breast and diaphragmatic tissue can lead to false-positive interpretation, particularly when examining women and using thallium.[34]

NMR Spectroscopy

Nuclear magnetic resonance (NMR) spectroscopy is a novel method to assess CHD risk. Traditional cholesterol tests measure the amount of cholesterol present in LDL particles, but not the number of particles in the serum.[41] Recent studies have shown that measuring the number and, to a lesser extent, size of the LDL particles, in addition to the amount of cholesterol contained in those particles, more accurately represents a patient's CHD risk than a traditional cholesterol assay.[41-43]

NMR allows clinicians to directly measure the lipoprotein content in serum.[43] A new test called *NMR LipoProfile®* uses NMR spectroscopy to directly measure the number of LDL particles and their sizes, along with VLDLs and HDLs.[41] While this test may be helpful in assessing CHD risk in certain patient groups, more research is needed to determine if it is viable alternative or adjunct to traditional cholesterol tests and if it should be used routinely when screening for CHD.

References

1. Kavey RE, Daniels SR, Lauer RM, et al: American Heart Association guidelines for primary prevention of atherosclerotic cardiovascular disease beginning in childhood. *Circulation* 2003;107:1562-1566.

2. Schauer JE, Stein JH, McBride PE: Atherosclerotic vascular disease prevention: advances in risk factor management. *Family Practice Recertification* 1998;20:13-20.

3. Berenson GS, Srinivason SR, Bao W, et al: Association between multiple cardiovascular risk factors and atherosclerosis in children and young adults. The Bogalusa Heart Study. *N Engl J Med* 1998;338:1650-1656.

4. Greenland P, Abrams J, Aurigemma GP, et al: Prevention Conference V: beyond secondary prevention: identifying the high-risk patient for primary prevention: non-invasive tests of atherosclerotic burden: Writing Group III. *Circulation* 2000;101:e16-e22.

5. Falk E, Shah PK, Fuster V: Coronary plaque disruption. *Circulation* 1995;92:657-671.

6. Naghavi M, Libby P, Folk E, et al: From vulnerable plaque to vulnerable patient: a call for new definitions and risk management strategies. Part I. *Circulation* 2003;108:1664-1672.

7. Ross R: Atherosclerosis–an inflammatory disease. *N Engl J Med* 1999;340:115-126.

8. Chambless LE, Zhong MM, Arnett D, et al: Variability in B-mode ultrasound measurements in the Atherosclerosis Risk in Communities (ARIC) study. *Ultrasound Med Biol* 1996;22:545-554.

9. Smith S, Greenland P, Grundy SM: AHA Conference Proceedings. Prevention Conference V: beyond secondary prevention: identifying high-risk patient for secondary prevention. Executive summary. American Heart Association. *Circulation* 2000;101:111-116.

10. Poli A, Tremoli E, Colombo A, et al: Ultrasonographic measurement of the common carotid artery wall thickness in hyper-

cholesterolemic patients. A new model for the quantitation and follow-up of preclinical atherosclerosis in living human subjects. *Atherosclerosis* 1988;70:253-261.

11. O'Leary DH, Polak JF, Kronmal RA, et al: Distribution and correlates of sonographically detected carotid artery disease in the Cardiovascular Health Study: The CHS Collaborative Research Group. *Stroke* 1992;23:1752-1760.

12. Mannami T, Konishi M, Baba S, et al: Prevalence of asymptomatic carotid atherosclerotic lesions detected by high-resolution ultrasonography and its relation to cardiovascular risk factors in the general population of a Japanese city: the Suita study. *Stroke* 1997;28:518-525.

13. Bots ML, Breslau PJ, Briet E, et al: Cardiovascular determinants of carotid artery disease. The Rotterdam Elderly Study. *Hypertension* 1992;19:717-720.

14. Burke GL, Evans GW, Riley WA, et al: Arterial wall thickness is associated with prevalent cardiovascular disease in middle-aged adults. The Atherosclerosis Risk in Communities (ARIC) Study. *Stroke* 1995;26:386-391.

15. Salonen JT, Salonen R: Ultrasonographically assessed carotid morphology and the risk of coronary heart disease. *Arterioscler Thromb* 1991;11:1245-1249.

16. Bots ML, Hoes AW, Koudstaal PJ, et al: Common carotid intima-media thickness and risk of stroke and myocardial infarction: the Rotterdam Study. *Circulation* 1997;96:1432-1437.

17. Chambless LE, Heiss G, Folsom AR, et al: Association of coronary heart disease incidence with carotid arterial wall thickness and major risk factors: the Atherosclerosis Risk in Communities (ARIC) Study, 1987-1993. *Am J Epidemiol* 1997;146:483-494.

18. Hodis HN, Mack WJ, LaBree L: The role of carotid arterial intima-media thickness in predicting clinical coronary events. *Ann Intern Med* 1998;128:262-269.

19. O'Leary DH, Polak JF, Kronmal RA, et al: Carotid-artery intima and media thickness as a risk factor for myocardial infarction and stroke in older adults. Cardiovascular Health Study Collaborative Research Group. *N Engl J Med* 1999;340:14-22.

20. Blankenhorn DH, Selzer RH, Crawford DW, et al: Beneficial effects of colestipol-niacin therapy in the common carotid artery. Two- and four-year reduction of intima-media thickness measured by ultrasound. *Circulation* 1993;88:20-28.

21. Furberg CD, Adams HP Jr, Applegate WB, et al: Effect of lovastatin on early carotid atherosclerosis and cardiovascular events. Asymptomatic Carotid Artery Progression Study (ACAPS) Research Group. *Circulation* 1994;90:1679-1687.

22. Hodis HN, Mack WJ, LaBree L, et al: Reduction in carotid arterial wall thickness using lovastatin and dietary therapy: a randomized controlled clinical trial. *Ann Intern Med* 1996;124:548-556.

23. Wexler L, Brundage B, Crouse J, et al: Coronary artery calcification: pathophysiology, epidemiology, imaging methods, and clinical implications. A statement for health professionals from the American Heart Association. Writing group. *Circulation* 1996;94:1175-1192.

24. Stanford W, Thompson BH, Weiss RM: Coronary artery calcification: clinical significance and current methods of detection. *AJR Am J Roentgenol* 1993;161:1139-1146.

25. Greenland P, LaBree L, Azem SP, et al: Coronary artery calcium score combined with Framingham score for risk prediction in asymptomatic individuals. *JAMA* 2004;291:210-215.

26. Fuster V, Fayad ZA, Badimon JJ: Acute coronary syndromes: biology. *Lancet* 1999;353(suppl 2):S115-S119.

27. Shinnar M, Fayad ZA, Fallon JT, et al: Magnetic resonance imaging of the vessel wall in carotids and coronaries. In: Fuster V, ed. *The Vulnerable Atherosclerotic Plaque: Understanding, Identification, and Modification.* Armonk, NY: Futura Publishing, 1999, pp 155-162.

28. Fayad ZA, Fuster V: Characterization of atherosclerotic plaques by magnetic resonance imaging. *Ann NY Acad Sci* 2000;902:173-186.

29. Fayad ZA, Nahar T, Badimon JJ, et al: In-vivo MR characterization of plaques in the thoracic aorta. *Circulation* 1998;98(suppl):I-515.

30. Shinnar M, Gallo R, Fayad ZA, et al: In vivo magnetic resonance imaging of post angioplasty coronary vessel wall lesion in pigs. *J Am Coll Cardiol* 1998;33:339A.

31. Worsthley SG, Heft G, Fayad ZA, et al: High-resolution exvivo MR imaging of in-situ coronary wall components in porcine model of atherosclerosis. *Soc Magn Reson* 1999;102.

32. Pearson TA: New tools for coronary risk assessment. What are their advantages and limitations? *Circulation* 2002;105: 886-892.

33. Gibbons RJ, Balady GJ, Bricker JT, et al: ACC/AHA 2002 guideline update for exercise testing: summary article: a report of the American College of Cardiology/American Heart Association Task Force on Practice Guidelines (Committee to update the 1997 Exercise Testing Guidelines). *Circulation* 2002;106:1883-1892.

34. Hayes SN, McBride P: Diagnosing coronary heart disease: when to use stress imaging studies. *J Fam Pract* 2003;52:544-551.

35. Fletcher GF, Balady G, Froelicher VF, et al: Exercise standards. A statement for healthcare professionals from the American Heart Association. Writing Group. *Circulation* 1995;91:580-615.

36. Bar Harbor Invitation Meeting 2000. *J Nucl Cardiol* 2001;8: 224-316.

37. Schlant RC, Blomqvist CG, Brandenburg RO, et al: Guidelines for exercise testing. A report of the Joint American College of Cardiology/American Heart Association Task Force on Assessment of Cardiovascular Procedures (Subcommittee on Exercise Testing). *Circulation* 1986;74:653A-667A.

38. Gordon NF, Kohl HW: Exercise testing and sudden cardiac death. *J Cardiopulm Rehabil* 1993;13:381-386.

39. Thomas GS, Prill NV, Majmundar H, et al: Treadmill exercise during adenosine infusion is safe, results in fewer adverse reactions, and improves myocardial perfusion image quality. *J Nucl Cardiol* 2000;7:439-446.

40. Li T, Ahlberg A, Hachamovitch R, et al: Comparison of adenosine and dipyridamole in detecting coronary artery disease using Tc-99m sestamibi single-photon emission computed tomography imaging: a randomized, prospective clinical study. *J Am Coll Cardiol* 2003;41(suppl A):461A.

41. LipoScience: Clinical basis for considering diagnostic alternatives to cholesterol testing in high-risk patients. Available at www.lipoprofile.com. Accessed October 21, 2005.

42. Blake GJ, Otvos JD, Rifai N, et al: Low-density lipoprotein particle concentration and size as determined by nuclear magnetic resonance spectroscopy as predictors of cardiovascular disease in women. *Circulation* 2002;106:1930-1937.

43. Otvos JD, Jeyarajah EJ, Cromwell WC: Measurement issues related to lipoprotein heterogeneity. *Am J Cardiol* 2002; 90(suppl):22i-29i.

CHAPTER 3

Peripheral Arterial Disease

Peripheral arterial disease (PAD) is an indication of critical arterial disease and is most commonly caused by atherosclerosis of the peripheral arterial system. Patients with PAD have three times the risk of all-cause mortality and six times the risk of death from cardiovascular disease (CVD) compared with those without PAD, yet PAD is the most commonly underdiagnosed and undertreated form of atherosclerosis.[1] There is considerable overlap among cerebral, coronary, and peripheral atherosclerotic disease.[2] The presence of PAD indicates a high concordance with CVD; in fact, the major cause of death of PAD patients is CVD. An estimated 40% of patients with CVD have symptomatic PAD. Patients with more severe PAD have a greater than 60% incidence of significant CVD (more than 70% stenosis of at least one coronary artery), and almost one third have severe, correctable, triple-vessel CVD with depressed left ventricular function.[3,4] The overall mortality rate is about 30% at 5 years and 70% at 15 years.[5]

More than 12 million people in the United States have PAD. It affects 10% of men 65 years of age or older and increases to 20% of men and women who are 75 years of age or older.[6] The annual incidence of PAD is one to three persons per 1,000. Despite the high prevalence of PAD, only 20% of patients with PAD have been told that they have the disease.[7]

New office strategies are available to improve the diagnosis and management of PAD in medical practice. Evidence indicates that risk factor modification, exercise, and medical

Table 3-1: The Fontaine Classification of PAD

- Fontaine I = asymptomatic
- Fontaine IIa and IIb = mild (IIa) and moderate-to-severe (IIb) intermittent claudication
- Fontaine III = ischemic rest pain
- Fontaine IV = ulcerations and gangrene[11]

management can significantly improve outcomes for PAD patients.[1] Despite this evidence, a number of studies have shown that patients with PAD are not getting proper medical care.[1,3,8,9] For example, in one study of 349 consecutive patients with PAD, only 46% of those with concomitant hypercholesterolemia were on lipid-lowering therapy, compared with 58% of CVD patients with hypercholesterolemia.[8] The same study found that 71% of the CVD patients exercised compared with only 50% of the PAD patients, and that while 74% of the CVD patients were told to exercise, only 46% of the PAD patients were counseled to do so.[8]

Defining PAD

Lower extremity occlusive PAD can be defined based on either anatomic or functional factors. Anatomically, PAD is defined as atherosclerotic arterial disease. Functionally, it is defined as arterial narrowing, causing a mismatch between oxygen supply and demand. This results in symptoms of intermittent claudication, exercise limitations, or tissue loss. These two definitions help divide PAD into asymptomatic and symptomatic disease states.[10] For every symptomatic patient with PAD, there are an estimated one to six asymptomatic patients.[11,12]

Symptoms of PAD

Claudication—which is painful cramping in the leg or hip, particularly when walking—is the most common

Table 3-2: Asymptomatic vs Symptomatic Peripheral Vascular Disease

	Asymptomatic	Symptomatic
Ankle-brachial index	<0.9	<0.9
Frequency	1-6 times more common	4.5% (≥55 years)
Functional capacity	Reduced	Reduced
Classification	Fontaine I	Fontaine IIa or higher
	Rutherford 0	Rutherford I or higher

symptom of PAD. It occurs when insufficient blood flows to the leg muscles. Other symptoms may include numbness, tingling, or weakness in the legs; burning or aching pain in feet or toes when resting; sores on legs or feet that will not heal; cold legs or feet; color change on the skin of legs or feet; and loss of hair on the legs.

A patient with severe atherosclerosis, with claudication symptoms at rest or with minimal exertion, accompanied by ischemic ulcers or gangrene, is said to have *critical limb ischemia.*[1] Unfortunately, PAD often goes undiagnosed because many people either do not experience symptoms in the early stages or they erroneously think that the symptoms are a normal part of aging.

PAD Clinical Classifications

Two major classifications have been developed to provide clinical information about PAD patients and their disease status. These criteria are based on the degree of PAD, ranging from asymptomatic to ischemic ulceration, gan-

Table 3-3: Risk Factors for PAD

Positive Risk Factors	*Negative Risk Factors*
• Advancing age	• Regular physical activity
• Smoking	• Moderate alcohol intake
• Diabetes (level of glycemic control) and impaired glucose tolerance	• High HDL-C
• Hypertension	
• Fibrinogen	
• Hyperlipidemia (elevated LDL-C, high TG, elevated Lp[a])	
• Homocysteinemia	

LDL-C = low-density lipoprotein cholesterol
HDL-C = high-density lipoprotein cholesterol
Lp(a) = lipoprotein(a)
TG = triglycerides

grene, and tissue loss. The Fontaine classification uses four stages (Table 3-1).

The Rutherford classification is similar. It uses four grades—0 to III—as well as six categories of claudication, with grade I having three subcategories, and it divides tissue loss into two categories, minor and major.[11] Table 3-2 compares asymptomatic and symptomatic PAD.

Risk Factors for PAD

In most patients, PAD is a disease of atherosclerosis. In general, the risk factors for PAD are the same as those for CVD (Table 3-3). Age is a consistent risk factor for PAD.[6,11]

The incidence of symptomatic PAD in individuals more than 70 years of age is approximately 5%, while asymptomatic disease is several times higher.[6,13] The strongest associations with PAD are with smoking and diabetes. The severity of PAD is directly proportional to the number of cigarettes smoked. On average, PAD is diagnosed 10 years earlier in smokers than in nonsmokers and is three times more prevalent in smokers.[11] Intermittent claudication is 3.4 times more common in men with diabetes and 5.7 times more frequent in women with diabetes.[11] Hypertension is also closely linked to PAD, both as a risk factor for, or a result of, PAD. Moderate alcohol intake and exercise are both negative risk factors for PAD.[14]

Diagnosing PAD

Obtaining a focused history and conducting a careful physical examination, aided by noninvasive and invasive studies, are the first steps in diagnosing PAD. The classic sign of intermittent claudication is pain that is evoked by exercise and relieved by rest. Most patients describe the pain as dull, aching, cramping, or heavy.[15]

Differential diagnosis. Patients can be incorrectly diagnosed as having PAD, and may have other problems, which is called *pseudoclaudication.* The most common pathology that mimics PAD is spinal stenosis (lumbar) or lumbar radiculopathy. In this condition, the symptoms can occur with standing and vary with exertion, and relief may require extended rest (10 minutes or more) as well as a change in body position. Spinal stenosis is a common comorbid condition in elderly people. Compared with intermittent claudication, the pain associated with spinal stenosis is more variable in onset. It may occur with prolonged standing and is relieved gradually by leaning forward and bending the lumbar spine.[10]

Other common causes to consider in a differential diagnosis for intermittent claudication include a history of deep venous thrombosis; chronic compartment syndrome, which

Table 3-4: Differential Diagnosis for Intermittent Claudication[3,8,11,16]

Common

- Spinal stenosis
- Venous claudication
- Chronic deep venous thrombosis causing venous claudication
- Chronic compartment syndrome
- Osteoarthritis
- Rheumatologic/connective-tissue diseases

Less Common

- Spinal cord tumor
- Arteriovenous fistulas
- Lower-pressure hydrocephalus
- Vasculopathies

is usually seen in athletes; osteoarthritis of the hip; and some less common conditions, such as rheumatologic and connective-tissue diseases. Other less common conditions that may mimic PAD include spinal cord tumor, arteriovenous fistulas, lower-pressure hydrocephalus, or vasculopathies (Table 3-4).

History. It is especially important to assess all patients with known atherosclerosis, diabetes, or multiple risk factors for PAD. These patients are most at risk for developing PAD or subsequent CVD events. History questionnaires have proven useful in clinical studies to screen for peripheral vascular disease. A modified version of the WHO/Rose questionnaire, which was developed to detect symptomatic PAD for patients with intermittent claudication, can be helpful in obtaining an accurate history. This new version, known as the Edinburgh modification, has higher sensitivity and specificity, and is easier to administer.[15] The Edinburgh modification of the WHO/Rose questionnaire consists of six questions and includes a diagram to indicate the location of the pain. The sensitivity of this modified questionnaire is 91.3% (compared with 60% to 68% for the previous version) and the specificity is 99.3% (compared with 90% to 100%).[15]

The primary criteria that identify claudication are: (1) exercise-induced calf pain; (2) pain not present at rest; (3) pain that requires stopping an activity; and (4) pain that stops with rest in less than 10 minutes

Physical examination. The physical examination of a patient with suspected PAD should focus on the arterial system. Begin by auscultating the carotid arteries for bruits, and palpating the arteries carefully so that they do not shed any fragments of a plaque. After conducting a thorough cardiovascular examination, evaluate the abdomen for bruits, evaluate the renal system, and palpate the aorta if possible. Complete the vascular examination by palpating the femoral, popliteal, posterior tibialis, and dorsalis pedis pulses and grading them for flow. The peripheral pulses should be graded as 0 to 2 (normal = 2, diminished = 1, and absent = 0). An abnormal posterior tibialis pulse is 71.2% sensitive and 91.3% specific for PAD, compared with an abnormal dorsalis pedis pulse, which is only 50% sensitive and 73.1% specific.[17]

The feet and lower extremities should also be inspected for ulcers, fissures, calluses, tinea, or tendinous xanthomas.[7] The dorsalis pedis pulse is congenitally absent in about 10% of the population, and the posterior tibialis pulse is congenitally absent in less than 1% of the population.[13,15] The absence of these pulses is more common in whites than in blacks.[13]

Diagnostic Tests for PAD

In addition to the screening tests examined in Chapter 2, several noninvasive measurements are particularly valu-

Table 3-5: Interpretation of Ankle-brachial Index (ABI)

ABI Score	
>1.30	Noncompressible
0.91 - 1.30	Normal
0.41 - 0.90	Mild-to-moderate PAD
<0.40	Severe PAD

able in diagnosing and managing PAD. They include a simple, but important, easily performed office test to screen for PAD—the ankle-brachial blood pressure index (ABI). Other tests to confirm and anatomically locate the atherosclerotic blockages include segmental limb systolic pressure measurements, arterial plethysmography/pulse volume recordings, magnetic resonance angiography (MRA), and computed tomography (CT) angiography. The tests are described below, with an emphasis on the ABI for use in office practice.

Ankle-brachial Blood Pressure Index

The ABI is a simple, inexpensive diagnostic test for PAD of the lower extremities The ABI also has a high predictive value for CVD morbidity and mortality. Normally, systolic blood pressure (BP) is higher in the lower extremities than in the upper extremities. When the ankle systolic BP is divided by the brachial systolic BP, the ABI is usually between 1.0 and 1.3. With PAD, the ankle systolic BP falls below the brachial systolic BP. An ABI of less than 0.90 is considered diagnostic of PAD.[1]

The ABI can be easily ascertained in the clinical setting. The equipment, which is inexpensive, consists of an ordinary blood pressure cuff and a Doppler ultrasonic sensor.[18-20] To conduct the test, a blood pressure cuff and Doppler detector are first used to measure the systolic BP in the brachial artery of both arms. The blood pressure cuff is then applied to the lower leg below the calf and just above the ankle, and the Doppler probe is used to determine systolic BP at the left and right posterior tibial arterics, and/or thc dorsalis pedis arteries, if necessary. Pressure in both arms and legs should be measured to calculate an ABI for each leg. The ABI equals the ratio of the higher of the two systolic pressures in the leg, and the brachial artery pressures.

An ABI less than 0.90 in either leg is considered evidence of PAD, and the lower the ABI value, the more severe the obstruction[21] (Table 3-5). Properly performed and conducted by a well-trained operator, the test-retest reliability is excellent and the validity of the test for 50% or greater stenosis in leg arteries is high (sensitivity 90% and specificity 98%).[18,19]

In population studies, individuals with a low ABI have been found to have a much higher prevalence of CVD than those with a normal ABI.[21] Patients with a low ABI but no known CVD at baseline were found to have total mortality more than three times higher and CVD mortality more than six times higher at 10 years than those with a normal ABI.[22] These data confirm that atherosclerosis is a systemic disease and that an abnormal ABI test often indicates significant atherosclerosis in other vasculature. In its Prevention V Scientific Statement, the American Heart Association concluded that ABI might be useful in assessing CVD risk in selected populations, especially in persons more than 50 years of age, or in those who might be at intermediate or higher risk for CVD based on traditional risk factor assessment. Those who are found to have an abnormal ABI can be raised to a higher risk category.[21]

Assessing hospitalized patients with CVD yields a high proportion of PAD patients. A recent investigation of lower extremity PAD in 100 hospitalized patients with CVD found that 37 patients had PAD, based on ABI measurements,[23] and only three had known prior PAD. This suggests that ABI should be used routinely to screen CVD patients for PAD.[23]

For patients with exercise-induced claudication but normal or borderline ABI measurements, ABI testing immediately after exercise may be diagnostic. Patients can walk on treadmills using predetermined protocols (eg, 1.5 to 2 mph at 10% grade for 4 to 6 minutes or until pain occurs). ABI testing is performed with the patient in a supine position immediately after stopping the exercise. The ABI of patients with PAD will drop significantly, while those with other causes of leg pain will maintain a normal ABI. Toe-raises, or pedal plantarflexion protocols, are alternatives to treadmill walking.[1]

Other PAD Testing

Additional testing is often used to identify the peripheral arterial segment that is narrowed, for both diagnostic and potential revascularization purposes. The testing mechanisms for the arterial segments that are affected include:

- Segmental limb systolic pressure measurements: blood pressure cuffs are typically placed at the thigh, calf, ankle, foot, and toe. Combining segmental limb pressures with an ABI can help localize the area of stenosis.
- Segmental plethysmography (or pulse volume recording) measures the changes in the volume of each leg, in different segments of the leg, with each cardiac cycle. When used in combination with segmental systolic pressure measurements, segmental plethysmography can be up to 95% accurate in detecting and localizing angiographic disease[24].
- Other noninvasive imaging methods—including duplex ultrasound, MRA, and CT angiography—can help to further define the anatomy and distinguish between tightly localized disease and well-collateralized long occlusions[10].
- Catheter-based, invasive angiography is still considered the gold standard for testing before revascularization or for definitive diagnosis.

Treating PAD

Treatment options for PAD fall into four categories: (1) risk factor modification; (2) exercise and cardiovascular rehabilitation; (3) pharmacologic intervention; and (4) invasive strategies. Clinicians must speak with all patients who have atherosclerotic occlusive PAD about their diagnosis and make sure they are aware of the related morbidity and mortality, especially from cardiovascular diseases. Patients are usually not aware of the significant CVD risk related to PAD.

Because patients with PAD require aggressive risk factor modification, it is necessary to conduct a systematic review of their risk factors and make appropriate interventions. Modifiable risk factors such as hypertension, hyperlipidemia, sedentary lifestyle, smoking status, diabetes, and glycemic control all must be evaluated. A smoking cessation program is an essential component of PAD treatment. Smoking cessation reduces the likelihood of amputation and may increase a patient's ABI and walking distance.[25-27]

In addition to modifying risk factors, a regular exercise program is key to the treatment of PAD. Exercise is highly effective for PAD patients and can result in increased walk time and a better quality of life. Exercise rehabilitation programs, which include both supervised exercise and risk-factor treatment, are effective and generally reimbursable using Current Procedural Terminology code (93668) for PAD patients. Exercise rehabilitation uses claudication symptoms to guide treatment. Patients are told to walk until claudication develops, stop until the pain disappears, and then begin walking again. Regular exercise has been shown to increase the initial claudication distance by an average of 179% and the maximal walking distance to 122%.[11] Aerobic exercise using their legs three times weekly for up to 30 minutes each time should be a minimal goal of PAD patients. Exercise programs need to continue for effects to endure long-term. PAD patients, as is true of all patients, should make regular exercise a lifelong habit.

Medications for PAD Patients

Hypertension in patients with PAD should be preferentially treated with β-blockers, angiotensin-converting enzyme (ACE) inhibitors, or calcium channel blockers. β-Blockers reduce the risk of associated CVD events and, contrary to a common misperception, have not been shown to worsen PAD in patients with mild to moderate PAD.[28] ACE inhibitors in patients with PAD resulted in reductions in CVD events beyond usual blood pressure (BP) treatment effects.[29] Calcium channel blockers may improve symptoms of hypertensive PAD patients. Chapter 11 examines hypertension, including treatment recommendations.

Cholesterol-lowering medications have been shown to reduce new PAD and preexisting PAD by 40%.[30] Statins have been shown to improve walking distance in hypercholesterolemic PAD patients in just 6 months of high-dose therapy.[31] Regression or stabilization of femoral atherosclerosis has been demonstrated in three different trials of cholesterol-lowering agents.[32-34]

In addition to the drugs necessary to modify risk factors, such as antihypertensives and cholesterol-lowering medications, pharmacologic therapy for PAD includes antiplatelet agents and agents that increase the distance to claudication. Aspirin therapy is indicated as an antiplatelet agent for patients with known PAD. Antiplatelet agents reduce the risk of CVD events by 25% for patients with atherosclerosis.[35] Clopidogrel (Plavix®) may be prescribed as an antiplatelet agent. In the CAPRIE trial, comparing clopidogrel 75 mg daily to aspirin 325 mg daily in CVD patients, those randomized to receive clopidogrel demonstrated a small but significantly different reduction in the end points of ischemic stroke, myocardial infarction, or vascular death (CVD event 4.9% on aspirin vs 3.7% on clopidogrel).[2] Although patients generally tolerate clopidogrel well, rare patients can develop neutropenia or thrombotic thrombocytopenic purpura (TTP) while taking this agent.[2,36,37]

Although cilostazol (Pletal®) and pentoxifylline (Trental®) are both designed to limit symptoms of intermittent claudication, the efficacy of pentoxifylline has been questioned. In a clinical trial comparing cilostazol, pentoxifylline, and placebo among patients with stable, moderate-to-severe symptoms of intermittent claudication, patients in the cilostazol group showed significant improvement in walking distance compared with patients in the pentoxifylline and placebo groups.[38] Other studies involving pentoxifylline have had conflicting results, and a recently published clinical trial with a high withdrawal rate did not strongly support use of pentoxifylline.[5,11] Cilostazol, a phosphodiesterase inhibitor, has improved walking distance in four randomized, controlled clinical trials versus placebo, but had a moderate withdrawal rate.[5] Cilostazol is contraindicated in patients with a low left ventricular ejection fraction or subjective congestive heart failure.[39]

Invasive interventions may be needed for some patients with PAD who fail to improve or who deteriorate despite aggressive risk factor modification, exercise programs, and pharmacologic interventions. Therapeutic options include percutaneous and surgical revascularization.[23] There are limited data examining the benefits of revascularization on walking distance or long-term CVD outcomes.[5]

References

1. Mohler ER: Peripheral arterial disease: identification and implications. *Arch Intern Med* 2003;163:2306-2314.

2. CAPRIE Steering Committee: A randomised, blinded trial of clopidogrel versus aspirin in patients at risk of ischaemic events (CAPRIE). *Lancet* 1996;348:1329-1339.

3. Murphy JG, ed: *Mayo Clinic Cardiology Review*, Chapter 59, Philadelphia, Lippincott Williams & Wilkins, 2000, pp 1013-1024.

4. Hertzer NR: Clinical experience with preoperative coronary angiography. *J Vasc Surg* 1985;2:510-514.

5. Anand SS, Creager MA: Peripheral arterial disease. *Am Family Phys* 2002;65:2321-2322.

6. Criqui MH, Fronek A, Barrett-Connor E, et al: The prevalence of peripheral arterial disease in a defined population. *Circulation* 1985;71:510-515.

7. McDermott MM, Fried L, Simonsick E, et al: Asymptomatic peripheral arterial disease is independently associated with impaired lower extremity functioning: The women's health and aging study. *Circulation* 2000;101:1007-1012.

8. McDermott MM, Mehta S, Ahn H, et al: Atherosclerotic risk factors are less intensively treated in patients with peripheral arterial disease than in patients with coronary artery disease. *J Gen Intern Med* 1997;12:209-215.

9. Hirsch AT, Criqui MH, Treat-Jacobson D, et al: Peripheral arterial disease detection, awareness, and treatment in primary care. *JAMA* 2001;286:1317-1324.

10. Dieter RS, Chu WW, Pacanowski JP Jr, et al: The significance of lower extremity peripheral arterial disease. *Clin Cardiol* 2002;25:3-10.

11. TASC Working Group: Management of peripheral arterial disease. *J Vasc Surg* 2000;31(suppl 1):S1-S296.

12. Schroll M, Munick O: Estimation of peripheral arteriosclerotic disease by ankle blood pressure in a population study of 60-year-old men and women. *J Chron Dis* 1981;34:261-269.

13. McDaniel MD, Cronenwett JL: Basic data related to the natural history of intermittent claudication. *Ann Vasc Surg* 1989;3:273-277.

14. Djousse L, Levy D, Murabito JM, et al: Alcohol consumption and risk of intermittent claudication in the Framingham Heart Study. *Circulation* 2000;102:3092-3097.

15. Leng GC, Fowkes FGR: The Edinburgh Claudication Questionnaire: an improved version of the WHO/Rose Questionnaire for use in epidemiological surveys. *J Clin Epidemiol* 1992;45:1101-1109.

16. Ludbrook J, Clarke AM, McKenzie JK: Significance of absent ankle pulses. *Br Med J* 1962;5294:1724-1726.

17. Criqui MH, Fronek A, Klauber MR, et al: The sensitivity, specificity, and predictive value of traditional clinical evaluation of peripheral arterial disease: results from noninvasive testing in a defined population. *Circulation* 1985;71:516-522.

18. Yao ST, Hobbs JT, Irvine WT: Ankle systolic pressure measurements in arterial disease affecting the lower extremities. *Br J Surg* 1969;56:676-679.

19. Ouriel K, McDonnell AE, Metz CE, et al: Critical evaluation of stress testing in the diagnosis of peripheral vascular disease. *Surgery* 1982;91:686-693.

20. Orchard TJ, Strandness DE Jr: Assessment of peripheral vascular disease in diabetes. Report and recommendations of an international workshop sponsored by the American Diabetes Association and the American Heart Association. September 18-20, 1992, New Orleans, Louisiana. *Circulation* 1993;88:819-828.

21. Greenland P, Abrams J, Aurigemma GP, et al: Prevention Conference V. Beyond secondary prevention: identifying the high-risk patient for primary prevention non-invasive tests of atherosclerotic burden: Writing Group III. *Circulation* 2000;101:e16-e22.

22. Criqui MH, Langer RD, Fronek A, et al: Mortality over a period of 10 years in patients with peripheral arterial disease. *N Engl J Med* 1992;326:381-386.

23. Dieter RS, Tomasson J, Gudjonsson T, et al: Lower extremity peripheral arterial disease in hospitalized patients with coronary artery disease. *Vasc Med* 2003;8:233-236.

24. Rutherford RB, Lowenstein DH, Klein MF: Combining segmental systolic pressures and plethysmography to diagnose arterial occlusive disease of the legs. *Am J Surg* 1979;138:211-218.

25. Jonason T, Bergstrom R: Cessation of smoking in patients with intermittent claudication. Effects on the risk of peripheral vascular complications, myocardial infarction and mortality. *Acta Med Scand* 1987;221:253-260.

26. Lassila R, Lepantalo M: Cigarette smoking and the outcome after lower limb arterial surgery. *Acta Chir Scand* 1988;154:635-640.

27. Quick CR, Cotton LT: The measured effect of stopping smoking on intermittent claudication. *Br J Surg* 1982;69(suppl):S24-26.

28. Heintzen MP, Strauer BE: Peripheral vascular effects of beta-blockers. *Eur Heart J* 1994;15(suppl C):2-7.

29. Yusuf S, Sleight P, Bosch J, et al: Effects of an angiotensin-converting enzyme inhibitor, ramipril, on cardiovascular events in high-risk patients. The Heart Outcomes Prevention Evaluation Study Investigators, *N Engl J Med* 2000;342:145-153.

30. Pedersen TR, Kjekshus J, Pyorala K, et al: Effects of simvastatin on ischemic signs and symptoms in the Scandinavian simvastatin survival study (4S). *Am J Cardiol* 1998;81:333-335.

31. Mondillo S, Ballo P, Barbati R, et al: Effects of simvastatin on walking performance and symptoms of intermittent claudication in hypercholesterolemic patients with peripheral vascular disease. *Am J Med* 2003;114:359-364.

32. Blankenhorn DH, Azen SP, Crawford DW, et al: Effects of colestipol-niacin therapy on human femoral atherosclerosis. *Circulation* 1991;83:438-447.

33. Lewis B: Randomised controlled trial of the treatment of hyperlipidaemia on progression of atherosclerosis. *Acta Medica Scand* 1985;701(suppl):53-57.

34. de Groot E, Jukema JW, Montauban van Swijndregt AD, et al: B-mode ultrasound assessment of pravastatin treatment effect on carotid and femoral artery walls and its correlations with coronary arteriographic findings: a report of the Regression Growth Evaluation Study (REGRESS). *J Am Coll Cardiol* 1998;31:1561-1567.

35. Antithrombotic Trialists' Collaboration: Collaborative meta-analysis of randomised trials of antiplatelet therapy for prevention of death, myocardial infarction, and stroke in high-risk patients. *BMJ* 2002;324:71-86.

36. Dieter RS: Unstable angina pectoris. *N Engl J Med* 2000; 342:1677-1678.

37. Bennett CL, Connors JM, Carwile JM, et al: Thrombotic thrombocytopenic purpura associated with clopidogrel. *N Engl J Med* 2000;342:1773-1777.

38. Dawson DL, Cutler BS, Hiatt WR, et al: A comparison of cilostazol and pentoxifylline for treating intermittent claudication. *Am J Med* 2000;109:523-530.

39. LaPerna L: Diagnosis and medical management of patients with intermittent claudication. *J Ann Osteopath Assoc* 2000;100:S10-S14.

CHAPTER 4

Family History

A family history of coronary artery disease (CAD) increases the risk of cardiovascular disease (CVD) 2 to 11 times for first-degree family members—parents, their siblings, and their children.[1] CVD is so strongly clustered in families that about 5% of families account for 50% to 60% of all cases of CAD occurring before age 60 (premature CAD).[2] Although more than 70% of unaffected first-degree relatives have one or more risk factors for CVD, most of them are unaware of their personal risk factors.[3] Research suggests that, although much of the risk for CVD is related to genetic, environmental, or behavioral risks transmitted through families, some risk factors remain unexplained or independent of known family history.[2-7] However, 58% of those with CAD do not have a family history of it.[4]

A case-controlled study by Eaton et al confirmed that family history of CVD is a powerful predictor of future heart disease, especially if a first-degree relative developed heart disease before the age of 60 or if more than one family member was affected.[4] In addition, the study indicated that family history was also a strong marker for multiple risk factors in those with CVD, and it remained an independent predictor of CVD even when controlling for traditional CVD risk factors (see Chapter 1) and newly recognized risk factors, such as lipoprotein (a), homocysteine, and fibrinogen (see Chapter 12).[4]

Current studies to determine why CAD is transmitted through the family are increasingly based on epidemiology, biochemistry, and molecular biology, and many new risk factors are being discovered that will need to be studied in high-risk families. Identifying known and emerging risk factors is important to developing a strategy for preventing CAD, but it is equally important to prevent the acquisition of negative behaviors that can be influenced by the family, such as smoking, a sedentary lifestyle, poor eating habits, and increased susceptibility to stress.[8]

Assessing High-Risk Families

A careful assessment of families with premature CAD or risk factors usually reveals that several members are at risk.[8] Studies have found that as many as 70% of siblings of a person with CAD have risk factors requiring attention.[3] Screening parents or children for abnormal lipoprotein levels often identifies common genetic dyslipidemias, such as familial hypercholesterolemia or familial combined hyperlipidemia.[9,10] Studies have also shown that behaviors such as smoking may increase genetically transmitted risk, and that risk factors may act synergistically.[11-13] The evidence that risk factors can cluster among families and can be genetically transmitted positively establishes the need for risk assessment among the family members of patients who have CAD or other identified risk factors.[14,15]

A recent study by Sdringola et al suggests that as many as half of the children and siblings of individuals with diseased coronary arteries may have signs of atherosclerosis, even though they have no symptoms of heart or vessel disease.[7] The study involved 90 people, including 18 with CAD and 32 of their immediate family members (children or siblings) who had no symptoms of heart disease; a group of 30 individuals who had heart disease risk factors but no family history of disease; and 10 volunteer control subjects with no risk factors and no family history of heart or vessel disease. All participants were given dipyridamole, a drug that mimics the way exercise increases blood flow in the heart muscle, and then underwent

Table 4-1: Risk of CAD for Men and Women With Different Definitions of Positive Family History

Relative Risk

Positive Family History (number of relatives with CAD according to age at disease onset)	**Percentage of General Population with Positive Family History**
One (any age)	38
One (younger than 55)	13
Two (any age)	8
Two (younger than 55)	2

Used with permission from Williams R: Genes at the heart of early coronary disease: practical aspects. *Cardiac Impulse* 1988;9:1-14.

CAD = coronary artery disease

positron emission tomography imaging. In response to the drug, 50% of individuals who had no symptoms but had a parent or sibling with heart disease had abnormal blood flow in their hearts, which indicated early atherosclerosis. In addition, their defects were larger than in both the control group and the group with comparable risk factors but no family history.[7]

Having a clear definition of what constitutes a 'positive' family history can help you decide how aggressive to be in identifying families that are most in need of intervention. Several studies have identified the following factors that help clarify the definition:[11,16,17]

- number of first-degree family members with documented CVD

Men 20 to 39 Years	Women 40 to 49 Years	Men 40 to 45 Years	Women 50 to 59 Years
2.9	1.7	1.8	1.2
3.9	2.5	1.9	1.2
5.9	4.8	3.3	1.6
12.7	12.0	4.5	3.7

- age at disease onset
- sex relative to that of other family members with CAD.

In general, the best single definition of a positive family history for CAD is having two or more first-degree relatives with onset of the disease before age 55 (Table 4-1).

Other factors that indicate the need to screen other family members include:[8]

- early onset of CVD in one or more family members
- unexplained premature deaths in family members
- possible genetic risk factors (lipoprotein (a), homocysteine, other).

Although it is debatable whether a family history of CAD is an independent risk factor for CVD, other modifiable risk factors, such as smoking or a poor diet, have a synergistic effect with family history risk. The overall risk of heart disease can be effectively lowered by behavior changes or treatment.[8]

A Practical Approach to Risk Reduction

Physicians' offices are ideal places to single out high-risk families and develop strategies to reduce their risks.[8] Family physicians, in particular, can play a critical role in identifying, clarifying, and counseling about family risk. Because they may have access to several family members, they can obtain more accurate histories, can screen more members, and, when warranted, can counsel the entire family. The following practical approaches help providers recognize high-risk families:

- Routinely document and periodically update the family history of patients' first-degree relatives.[8]
- Ask the age at onset of the disease in the affected family member(s) to determine whether the CVD was premature.
- Ask about known risk factors in the affected family member. Such knowledge can point to potentially inherited factors and help determine whether the patient's relatives are similarly at risk.
- Remember that family history is only one predictor of CVD; other risk factors and overall risk are still predictive.
- Consider treatment of risk factors regardless of a history of CVD in the family. The absence of a family history of CVD does not mean the patient will not develop it.
- Screen first-degree relatives (including siblings and children) of those with premature CVD (less than age 60) for risk factors, including a full lipoprotein evaluation.

One effective approach to family risk assessment for heart disease prevention is to base it on one of three levels of family care,[18] depending on the patient's needs, the family's availability, and your time and expertise

Table 4-2: A Practical Approach for Risk Reduction Intervention

- Start the assessment early by having patients fill out medical forms delivered by mail or handed out in the waiting room.
- Include family members in assessment and plans. Obtain a complete family history, including age at onset of disease, environment, and nutritional and exercise habits.
- Personalize intervention based on risk.
- Emphasize a simple message to change a single risk or behavior.
- If a patient has difficulty maintaining changes, or if treatment fails, assess family environment or dynamics.
- Organize office systems for follow-up and education, using office personnel to help with history taking, counseling, and patient monitoring.

(Table 4-2). Level one is the assessment of individual family members, beginning with a medical history questionnaire that can be filled out in conjunction with their first office visit. Level two is the evaluation of a patient within the context of the family, and includes an assessment of family systems and function in the diagnosis and treatment plan.[18] Level three is an evaluation through a family visit or conference, which is useful when a family genetic or environmental problem is identified. For example, when family members are clearly at risk for hypercholesterolemia, a family visit allows all members to be tested and efficiently educated about nutrition and lifestyle. Likewise, when a member who smokes creates

Table 4-3: Guidelines for Assessing Family Heart Disease Risk During Office Visits

First Visit

- Obtain brief family history of first-degree relatives.
- Measure blood pressure and weight, and obtain smoking and cardiac symptom history and total cholesterol level (may be nonfasting).
- If heart disease risk factors are present, personalize the message for reducing risk.
- Schedule follow-up visit.

Second Visit

- Obtain complete family history (eg, ask about details of CVD history and family risk factors).
- If family history is unclear, ask patient to get more history about relatives.
- For patients with total cholesterol levels of more than 200 mg/dL, family history of CVD, atherosclerosis, or multiple risk factors, obtain a complete fasting lipoprotein profile.

CVD = cardiovascular disease

an environmental problem that increases risk, a family visit provides an opportunity to discuss the risks associated with smoking, including passive smoking.

Accurately Assessing Risk

A family history focused on CAD can provide diagnostic information that can be used to guide evaluation and treatment. Although identifying families with more than one affected member is most beneficial, identify-

Second Visit *(continued)*

- Set goals for risk reduction and provide resources for behavior change.
- Schedule a follow-up visit based on prevention goals and plans.

Third Visit

- Explain results of overall risk assessment.
- Assess social and cultural variables associated with behavior change requirements.
- Specify goals, plans, and follow-up.
- Consider a family screening session or conference to discuss plans.

ing even one patient who has a first-degree relative with premature CVD provides ready access to a family for whom risk assessment is likely to be beneficial. To promote efficient risk assessment and recommendations for behavioral change, schedule several office visits for family members, either individually or as a group (Table 4-3).

History taking among high-risk patients should elicit enough details to allow an accurate assessment of risk.

Asking about the age at onset of angina pectoris, the first myocardial infarction (MI), coronary artery bypass surgery, or other atherosclerosis complications among family members is essential. For example, a history of sudden death at age 70 is less important than if the same person had a first MI at age 50, followed by bypass surgery and other problems before dying at age 70. When it is unclear if a family member died of CVD, it may be helpful to obtain information about that person's symptoms and preexisting medical conditions, or an autopsy report. Often, just asking family members to briefly describe what they remember about the circumstances of the patient's death can provide insights that may help determine if the cause of death suggests a need for family risk assessment.

Whether or not CVD can be identified as the cause, the sudden death of two family members in their 40s is likely enough to have been related to CAD to justify careful family screening. Similarly, testing other first-degree relatives is indicated when premature CAD, or an identifiable genetic risk factor such as familial hypercholesterolemia is detected in even one family member.[8]

A more detailed family history is usually needed only to clarify borderline family histories, to identify lipoprotein genetic histories, or to increase the potential impact of counseling. To better assess families with unusual lipoprotein disorders, a history that includes information about second-degree relatives (grandparents, aunts, uncles, nieces, nephews, and grandchildren) may be helpful. For example, familial combined dyslipidemias, which are characterized by multiple abnormal lipoprotein phenotypes in families, can often be identified by creating a family tree that indicates genetic transmission of these phenotypes in a family affected by CAD.[8]

Family Information

Because it can be difficult to obtain an accurate family history when members do not live together, you can obtain further information by reviewing medical records, requesting that patients question family members about risks, or asking relatives to undergo testing for risk factors.

A patient found to have CAD or inheritable risk factors should be encouraged to notify first-degree relatives of the need to be evaluated. Evaluation can increase awareness of risk in families and can provide reassurance to those members who do not have risk factors.

Family Behavior and Social History

Obtaining a social history of the family can help guide counseling for CVD prevention. For example, when counseling about nutrition, understanding the dietary patterns of the family may be essential to producing changes in behavior. Who shops for and cooks the food? How many meals are eaten outside the home? What are the patient's and the family members' food preferences?

The answers to these questions can be helpful in making recommendations aimed at changing behavior. It is usually counterproductive for one family member to eat differently than the others, especially when they all can benefit from reducing calories, saturated fat, or cholesterol. Providing family nutritional counseling often makes buying and preparing meals easier, and avoids the need to repeat advice for several family members.

If family members smoke, it is critical that they not smoke near other family members, to reduce exposure to tobacco smoke and to demonstrate concern. Use of other forms of tobacco increases risk for the individual concerned, and sets a poor example for other family members. All of this needs to be discussed in the context of medical visits.

Screening Tests for CVD Risk Assessment

Several screening tests are suggested to assess risk for CAD (Table 4-4). The National Cholesterol Education Pro-

Table 4-4: Recommended Screening Tests for CVD Assessment

Test	Guidelines
Blood pressure and weight	All patients at each visit
Lipoprotein profile	High-risk persons—those with atherosclerosis, family risk, elevated cholesterol levels, or several risk factors
Fasting glucose level	Person suspected of being glucose intolerant
Thyroid function	Persons with hypercholesterolemia, to rule out secondary causes, if indicated
Exercise stress test	Symptomatic persons, persons at high risk for silent ischemia, and sedentary persons aged 50 years or more with two or more CVD risk factors, for evaluation and exercise prescription.

CVD = cardiovascular disease

gram Expert Panel on Detection, Evaluation, and Treatment of High Blood Cholesterol in Adults (NCEP ATP III) recommends that all adults aged 20 years and older, and children from high-risk families, have a fasting lipoprotein profile every 5 years.[19] However, for an initial risk assessment, a nonfasting total cholesterol and high-density lipoprotein (HDL) cholesterol test is reliable and can provide important information if the person is in the office in a nonfasting state.[19] When screening a person in a high-risk family, obtain a complete fasting lipoprotein profile, including levels of total cholesterol, triglycerides, HDL cholesterol, and estimated low-density lipoprotein (LDL) cholesterol. See Chapter 10 for more information on screening for and treating dyslipidemias.

Blood pressure measurements should be obtained for all family members. High blood pressure has been shown to occur early among members of families with premature CAD. Hypertension has also been shown to be associated with other risk factors, such as central body fat deposition and low levels of HDL cholesterol.[20,21] See Chapter 11 for more information on screening for and treating hypertension.

Current recommendations about testing children are controversial. The American Academy of Pediatrics suggests measuring cholesterol levels for children with family histories of CAD or genetic cholesterol disorders,[22] but other investigators have found that this practice would overlook many children with total cholesterol levels higher than 200 mg/dL.[23] Children with risk factors have been found to develop early atheromatous fatty streaks, and children at extremely high risk have developed premature atherosclerosis.[24] Although clinical trials studying the benefits of cholesterol and blood pressure reduction have been limited primarily to adults, common sense dictates that providing nutritional and exercise information is important for children because of the high rate of childhood obesity. People establish eating patterns early in life, and families can benefit from sound advice about nutrition and activity level indicated by family history and the judgment of their family physician.[8] See Chapter 13 for information about risk reduction in children and other special populations.

Exercise stress testing can identify myocardial ischemia and is recommended for persons who have symptoms. However, it is not recommended for asymptomatic individuals because there is a low prevalence of CAD among this group, testing is expensive, and it has poor predictive value.[25] For individuals 40 years of age and older who are beginning a vigorous exercise program, stress testing may be useful for assessing functional capacity and estimating the likelihood of CAD. It can also help you tailor exercise prescriptions, and may motivate at-risk sedentary patients to change their lifestyles. See Chapter 2 for more information on exercise stress testing and other screening tests and tools for detecting cardiovascular and vascular disease.

Working With Families

Working with the entire family provides an opportunity for comprehensive assessment and risk reduction. The benefits of primary and secondary prevention of CAD are enhanced when you understand a family's risk factors, behaviors, and environment. Following are some additional benefits of working with the entire family.

- Relatives of a family member with CAD are often not aware of their own risks or risk factors. You can alert them to the importance of risk detection and counseling.
- You can discuss individual risk factors for each person being counseled and relate the risk to the family member with atherosclerosis.
- Including other family members when smoking cessation is discussed provides helpful information on the smoking status of all family members, offers the opportunity to encourage positive reinforcement for the at-risk family member, and may also encourage others who smoke to quit.
- Discussing family activities may encourage the whole family to adopt positive health habits and behaviors, such as exercise and eating a healthy diet.

Having an office visit with multiple family members to discuss risk reduction can be valuable in CVD prevention. Although time consuming, family visits provide an efficient way to assess and educate many people at once, and are often desired by families with a history of chronic disease.[26] When a visit is scheduled for a patient who is at high risk or has had a previous episode of CAD, it is a good idea to ask other family members to accompany the patient. A person with CAD is more likely to return to work and remain active if family members accompany him or her during office visits.[27] This is helpful because family members often have not been assessed for CAD and may have misconceptions about their own risks.[3] Also, family members who are now asymptomatic but who may have undetected risk factors, can be screened, counseled, or scheduled for a follow-up visit. Further, family conferences can solve a particular problem—such as a patient's failure to adhere to nutritional or exercise recommendations because of family issues—by channeling a family's tendency to 'nag' in ways that provide positive reinforcement for changing behavior.

An Important Opportunity

Knowing that CVD risk factors account for a considerable portion of family history risk is vital to your practice, your patients, and their families. Often patients, and even their physicians, view a family history of premature CVD as a death sentence and consider family history a risk factor that cannot be modified. This is an inaccurate perception. Although dyslipidemia, diabetes, and hypertension are familial risk factors that might be primarily genetically determined, they can be diagnosed and treated. Unhealthy lifestyles also cluster in families and can be improved with behavioral interventions.[3,8] From this point of view, family history is another risk factor that can be treated. The family with CVD offers you an important opportunity to consider the whole family as your patient and to assist in the health care of all individuals in it.[8,18]

References

1. Williams RR: Understanding genetic and environmental risk factors in susceptible persons. *West J Med* 1984;141:799-806.

2. Williams RR, Hunt SC, Barlow GK, et al: Health family trees: a tool for finding and helping young family members of coronary

and cancer prone pedigrees in Texas and Utah. *Am J Public Health* 1988;78:1283-1286.

3. Becker DM, Levine DM: Risk perception, knowledge, and lifestyles in siblings of people with premature coronary disease. *Am J Prev Med* 1987;3:45-50.

4. Eaton CB, Bostom AG, Yanek L, et al: Family history and premature coronary heart disease. *J Am Board Fam Pract* 1996;9: 312-318.

5. Hopkins PN, Williams RR, Kuida H, et al: Family history as an independent risk factor for incident coronary artery disease in a high-risk cohort in Utah. *Am J Cardiol* 1988;62:703-707.

6. Perkins KA: Family history of coronary heart disease: is it an independent risk factor? *Am J Epidemiol* 1986;124:182-194.

7. Sdringola S, Patel D, Gould KL: High prevalence of myocardial perfusion abnormalities on positron emission tomography in asymptomatic persons with a parent or sibling with coronary artery disease. *Circulation* 2001;103:496-501.

8. McBride P, Yeager D: A family approach to heart disease prevention. *Fam Pract Recert* 1989;11:69-88.

9. Rissanen AM, Nikkila EA: Coronary artery disease and its risk factors in families of young men with angina pectoris and in controls. *Br Heart J* 1977;39:875-883.

10. Newman WP 3rd, Freedman DS, Voors AW, et al: Relation of serum lipoprotein levels and systolic blood pressure to early atherosclerosis. The Bogalusa Heart Study. *N Engl J Med* 1986; 314:138-144.

11. Snowden CB, McNamara PM, Garrison RJ, et al: Predicting coronary heart disease in siblings—a multivariate assessment, the Framingham Heart Study. *Am J Epidemiol* 1982;115:217-222.

12. Hopkins PN, Williams RR, Hunt SC: Magnified risks from cigarette smoking for coronary prone families in Utah. *West J Med* 1984;141:196-202.

13. Perkins KA: The synergistic effect of smoking and serum cholesterol on coronary heart disease. *Health Psychol* 1985;4:337-360.

14. Williams RR, Hasstedt SJ, Wilson DE, et al: Evidence that men with familial hypercholesterolemia can avoid early coronary death. An analysis of 77 gene carriers in four Utah pedigrees. *JAMA* 1986;255:219-224.

15. Zinner SH, Rosner B, Oh W, et al: Significance of blood pressure in infancy. Familial aggregation and predictive effect on later blood pressure. *Hypertension* 1985;7:411-416.

16. Hunt SC, Williams RR, Barlow GK: A comparison of positive family history definitions for defining risk of future disease. *J Chronic Dis* 1986;39:809-821. Erratum in: *J Chronic Dis* 1987; 40:369.

17. Rissanen AM: Familial occurrence of coronary artery disease: effect of age at diagnosis. *Am J Cardiol* 1979;44:60-66.

18. Smilkstein G: The family in family medicine. *J Fam Pract* 1982;14:221-223.

19. Expert Panel on Detection, Evaluation, and Treatment of High Blood Cholesterol in Adults. Executive Summary of The Third Report of the National Cholesterol Education Program (NCEP) Expert Panel on Detection, Evaluation, and Treatment of High Blood Cholesterol in adults (Adult Treatment Panel III). *JAMA* 2001;285:2486-2497.

20. Williams RR, Hunt SC, Hopkins PN, et al: Familial dyslipidemic hypertension. Evidence from 58 Utah families for a syndrome present in approximately 12% of patients with essential hypertension. *JAMA* 1988;259:3579-3586.

21. Slyper A, Schectman G: Coronary artery disease risk factors from a genetic and developmental perspective. *Arch Intern Med* 1994;153:633-638.

22. American Academy of Pediatrics: Committee on Nutrition: Indications for cholesterol testing in children. *Pediatrics* 1989; 83:141-142. Erratum in: *Pediatrics* 1989;83:678.

23. Meyerson DA, Santanello NC: Pediatric lipid screening based upon criteria of high-risk family history fails to identify two-thirds of higher-risk children (abstract). *Circulation* 1988;72(suppl 2):383.

24. Solberg LA, Strong JP: Risk factors and atherosclerotic lesions. A review of autopsy studies. *Arteriosclerosis* 1983;3:187-198.

25. Hayes SN, McBride P: Diagnosing coronary heart disease: when to use stress imaging studies. *J Fam Pract* 2003;52:544-551.

26. Kushner K, Meyer D, Hansen JP: Patients' attitudes toward physician involvement in family conferences. *J Fam Pract* 1989; 28:73-78.

27. Davidson DM: The family and cardiac rehabilitation. *J Fam Pract* 1979;8:253-261.

CHAPTER 5

Nutrition and Cardiovascular Disease: Assessing Nutrition in Practice

Nutrition is a key to good health and plays an important role in cardiovascular disease (CVD) prevention. It is a primary consideration when planning a strategy for managing CVD risk factors such as hypertension, hyperlipidemia, diabetes, and obesity. The most recent version of the American Heart Association (AHA) Dietary Guidelines,[1] revised in 2000, emphasizes the importance of dietary and other lifestyle practices in reducing the risk of CVD. In these new guidelines, greater emphasis is placed on foods and an overall eating pattern, as well as on the need for all Americans to improve body weight to help control CVD risk factors. (See Chapter 8 for detailed information on the growing problems of overweight, obesity, and the metabolic syndrome.)

Most of the revised nutrition guidelines offer more individualized approaches involving medical nutrition therapy (MNT) for specific subgroups, such as individuals with diabetes, lipid disorders, and/or preexisting CVD. The four main goals of the new guidelines[2] are to help Americans (1) achieve an overall healthy eating pattern; (2) achieve and maintain an appropriate body weight; (3) achieve and maintain a desirable cholesterol profile; and (4) achieve and maintain a desirable blood pressure level.

Guidelines for the General Population

Table 5-1 lists the major AHA Dietary Guidelines that make up the AHA Eating Plan for Healthy Americans.[3] These are recommendations for adults to reduce the risk of premature CVD. These healthy eating guidelines may also reduce risk for other chronic health problems such as type 2 diabetes, osteoporosis, and some forms of cancer.[3]

Physicians should encourage patients to follow the eating plan outlined in Table 5-1 to achieve and maintain a healthy eating pattern. Patients should be motivated to apply the guidelines to their overall eating patterns over at least several days. Physicians should remind them that the AHA guidelines could do more than improve their heart health.

Nutrition Assessment

To determine what patients' nutritional needs might be, the physician should assess their dietary intake, including what they eat, when they eat, and how much they eat. The role of the family in food selection, food preparation, and providing support should also be assessed.

Some of the issues a physician should address with patients to assess their nutrition habits are listed in Table 5-2.

Practical Nutritional Assessment Tools for the Office

Many tools are available on the Internet that can help physicians and patients assess daily dietary intake. For assessing a patient's dietary intake in the office when there is little time for a history, we suggest using the following W.A.V.E. mnemonic:

- **W**eight (assess the patient's weight, body mass index, and weight changes)

Table 5-1: AHA Eating Plan for Healthy Americans

- Eat a variety of fruits and vegetables. Choose five or more servings per day.
- Eat a variety of grain products, including whole grains. Choose six or more servings per day.
- Include fat-free and low-fat milk products, fish, legumes (beans), skinless poultry, and lean meats.
- Choose fats and oils with 2 g or less saturated fat per tablespoon, such as liquid and tub margarines, canola oil, and olive oil.
- Balance the number of calories consumed with the number used each day. (To find that number, multiply weight in pounds by 15 calories. This represents the average number of calories used in 1 day, if a person is moderately active. Individuals who get little exercise should multiply their weight by 13 instead of 15, because people who are less active burn fewer calories.)
- Maintain a level of physical activity that maintains fitness and matches the number of calories consumed. Walk or do other activities for at least 30 minutes on most days. To lose weight, be active enough to use up more calories than consumed every day.

- **A**ctivity (assess current activity level and if there is a history of any regular physical activity, walking in occupation, and how much TV/video is watched)
- **V**ariety: assess using a dietary recall—is there a variety of fruits and vegetables (six to eight daily), dairy products (two to three daily), protein (two to three daily), grains (6 to 11 daily)?

- Limit intake of foods high in calories or low in nutrition, including foods like soft drinks and candy that have a lot of sugars ('simple' or refined carbohydrates).
- Limit foods high in saturated fat, trans fat, and/or cholesterol, such as full-fat milk products, fatty meats, tropical oils, partially hydrogenated vegetable oils, and egg yolks. Instead, choose foods low in saturated fat, trans fat, and cholesterol from the first four points above.
- Eat less than 6 g of salt per day (2,400 mg of sodium).
- Women should have no more than one alcoholic drink per day, and men should have no more than two. 'One drink' contains no more than 1/2 ounce of pure alcohol. Examples of one drink are 12-oz beer, 4-oz wine, 11 1/2 oz of 80-proof spirits, or 1 oz of 100-proof spirits.

AHA= American Heart Association

- **E**xcess: is there a dietary excess of calories? Fat? Saturated fat? Sugars?

Another useful office tool is called R.E.A.P. (Rapid Eating Assessment for Patients). It can be used rapidly for more detailed nutrition assessment in the office. These assessment tools and others are available at the Brown University Web site (http://bms.brown.edu/nutrition). A

Table 5-2: Nutrition Habits to Discuss With Patients

- Meals and snacking patterns
- Fat from dairy products and fatty meats, commercial snack foods and pastries, fried food, added fats and oils
- Refined carbohydrates from baked products, desserts, cookies, etc
- Fiber from fruits, vegetables, legumes, and whole grains
- Sweetened beverages and alcohol
- Major sources of sodium from processed foods, eating out, and added salt
- Portion sizes
- Frequency of eating restaurant meals, fast food, take-out food
- Over-the-counter products–vitamin/mineral supplements, herbal, and other dietary supplements

National Institutes of Health (NIH) Nutrition Academic Award funded the development of these materials.

A nutrition history form to use for patients in the office is available at: http://aafp.org/afp/990315ap/1521.html. The form was included in a journal article that appeared in *American Family Physician*.[4]

The US Department of Agriculture offers a Web-based dietary assessment tool at http://www.nal.usda.gov/fnic/etext/000108.html. Users enter a day's diet and receive a score based on the Food Guide Pyramid. Amounts of total fat, saturated fat, cholesterol, and sodium are also provided.

The following Web sites also can help with nutrition assessment: (1) for nutritional information about take-

Table 5-3: Total Fat and Saturated Fat Content of Dairy Products

	Total Fat (g)	Saturated Fat (g)
1 cup whole milk	8	4.9
1 cup 2% milk	4.9	3
1 cup 1% milk	2.4	1.5
1 oz cheddar cheese	9.4	6
1 oz farmer cheese	5	3
1/2 cup Haagen-Dazs ice cream	18	10.8
1/2 cup frozen yogurt	3	1.9

out food, fast food, and restaurant meals, go to http://www.foodfacts.info; (2) for nutritional information about dietary supplements, go to http://supplementwatch.com.

The American Diet and Vascular Disease

The AHA's revised dietary guidelines offer a framework to help you adapt specific MNT to accommodate the requirements of patients with existing CVD and those with risk factors—such as high blood pressure, cholesterol disorders, and diabetes—that put them at high risk for developing CVD.

The American diet is typically rich in saturated fatty acids. These saturated fats come primarily from animal fats (meat fat and butterfat) and tropical oils. The American diet contains about 34% total fat, 11% saturated fat, 2.6% trans fat, and 256 mg cholesterol. Patients, particularly those who are at high risk for CVD, need to be reminded that cholesterol and saturated fats are not essential nutrients. Because the body makes all it needs, we do not need to consume any to survive.

Table 5-4: Total Fat and Saturated Fat Content of Meats

	Total Fat (g)	Saturated Fat (g)
3 oz turkey breast, no skin	2.7	0.9
3 oz chicken breast, no skin	3.0	0.9
3 oz pork tenderloin	4.1	1.4
3 oz extra-lean ham	4.2	1.4
3 oz beef top round	4.3	1.5
3 oz turkey dark meat, no skin	4.3	1.4
3 oz chicken dark meat, no skin	8.8	2.4
3 oz beef T-bone steak, lean and fat	24.6	10.2
3 oz shoulder ham, lean and fat	21.4	7.7
3 oz bratwurst	25.9	9.3

Saturated fats raise blood cholesterol more than any other dietary component. For every 1% of calories as saturated fat, there is a 2.7% rise in blood cholesterol. Tables 5-3 and 5-4 list the amounts of total fat and saturated fat in commonly used dairy products and meats.

Although individual response to dietary cholesterol varies, studies estimate that there is a 10-mg/dL rise in serum cholesterol for each additional 100 mg dietary cholesterol.[1]

Table 5-5 lists the cholesterol content of some common foods.

Trans fats, which are created when vegetable oils are partially hydrogenated to a solid form, increase low-density lipoprotein cholesterol (LDL-C) and may decrease high-density lipoprotein cholesterol (HDL-C). The most significant sources of trans fat are commercial baked goods

Table 5-5: Cholesterol Content of Foods

Type of Food	Serving Size	Cholesterol (mg)
Egg yolk	1	240
Liver or kidneys	3 oz	350
Beef	3 oz	80
Chicken	3 oz	75
Fish	3 oz	65
Shrimp	3 oz	180
Whole milk	1 cup	35
Cheddar cheese	1 oz	30

(biscuits, cookies, crackers, pie crust) and commercially fried foods (french fries, etc), with margarines contributing a lesser amount.

Table 5-6 lists the trans fat content of some common food items.

Dietary LDL-Cholesterol Treatment

Physicians can help patients reduce LDL-C levels by encouraging them to follow the recommendations in Table 5-7.

There are many special diets specifically designed to help reduce saturated fat intake. As a first step, the AHA dietary recommendations for Americans suggest that the daily eating plan look approximately like this: total fat = 30% of calories or less; saturated and trans fat = 8% to 10% of calories; cholesterol = 300 mg or less per day; carbohydrate = 50% to 55% of calories; and protein = 10% to 15% of calories.

The average LDL-C reduction achieved through this type of diet—if a person has been consuming higher amounts of saturated fat, trans fat, and cholesterol—is 5% to 15%.[1,3]

Table 5-6: Trans Fat Content of Foods

Type of Food	Amount	Trans Fat (g)
Soft tub margarine	1 tablespoon	0 to 2
Stick margarine	1 tablespoon	2 to 3.5
Vegetable shortening	1 tablespoon	2 to 3
Corn chips	1 ounce	1.5
Danish pastry	average	3.0
Microwave popcorn	3 cups	3.0
Frozen fish sticks	6	3.0
Frozen fries	large (5 oz)	4.0
Frozen pot pie	1	13 to 16

Recently, the National Cholesterol Education Program decided to include more than just eating in its recommendations, by adding recommendations for regular physical activity and weight reduction (if the patient is overweight).[5] This plan, the Therapeutic Lifestyle Change (TLC) diet, is recommended for people with a diagnosis of heart disease or diabetes, and for those with cholesterol abnormalities. It is more restrictive on saturated fat and cholesterol because it is targeted primarily at reducing cholesterol levels. The TLC diet recommends limiting saturated and trans fat to 7% of calories or less, cholesterol to 200 mg per day, and adding viscous fiber (psyllium, oat bran, etc) and plant sterols/stanols if these TLC diet changes are not adequate to reduce serum lipids to target levels.

Although diet treatment does not typically reduce serum lipids as much as medication, clinical diet trials have demonstrated significant lipid reduction and, in some studies, significant regression of atherosclerotic plaque.[5] A meta-analysis of dietary trials shows that lowering cho-

Table 5-7: Recommendations for Reducing Levels of LDL-Cholesterol

- Substitute unsaturated fats for saturated fats. Monounsaturated fats are recommended over polyunsaturated fats because they are more resistant to oxidation and because polyunsaturated fats may produce a small reduction in high-density lipoprotein cholesterol (HDL-C).
- Reduce trans fats in the diet (particularly by reducing intake of processed foods).
- Reduce dietary cholesterol.
- Reduce body weight if overweight or obese.

lesterol with diet reduces CVD risk as much as lowering cholesterol with medications.[6,7] In addition, medication is more effective when patients consume a diet low in saturated fat and cholesterol.[8]

Diet modification is recommended as the initial treatment for all lipid disorders, except in the case of high triglycerides or high CVD risk, when medications should be started immediately. In most cases, a diet trial of 6 weeks to 3 months, with revisits for reinforcement, should be attempted before medication is prescribed. Research indicates that patients who receive reinforcement for behavior change within 4 to 6 weeks of the initial recommendation are most likely to sustain their new habits.[5] Physicians should see patients soon after making lifestyle recommendations to reinforce and extend them. Follow-up is the best predictor of success in behavior change.[5] Cholesterol reduction on low saturated fat, low trans fat, and low-cholesterol diets is greatest when initial LDL-C levels are high, when the saturated fat content of the original diet is high, when the patient is genetically a diet responder, and when adherence to the diet is good.

Average LDL-C and triglyceride reduction with the TLC diet is 20% to 30%.[5]

Some experts recommend low-fat diets for aggressive treatment of heart disease. These diets contain 10% fat, 15% to 20% protein, and 70% to 75% carbohydrate. The most effective low-fat diets are vegetarian or nearly vegetarian, containing only small amounts of fish, white meat of poultry, and low-fat dairy products, but generous amounts of soy, nuts, high-fiber vegetables, grains, fruits, and legumes. These diets are effective for weight loss, cholesterol reduction, and LDL-C reduction, but may reduce HDL-C and raise triglyceride levels because there is more substrate (carbohydrate) available for endogenous triglyceride production. To guarantee nutritional adequacy, a dietitian should evaluate patients following low-fat diets. Dietitians should also caution patients not to include large amounts of simple sugars or refined carbohydrates in their diets.

Diets moderate in fat (30% to 35% of calories) with an emphasis on monounsaturated fat (15% to 20%), ω-3 fats, and limited saturated fat (less than 7%), are consistent with a Mediterranean diet and have been associated with reduced risk for heart disease. The Lyon Diet Heart Study showed a 70% reduction in coronary events and cardiac death using a diet high in fruits, vegetables, fish, grains, nuts, legumes, and canola oil.[9] The Indo-Mediterranean Diet Heart Study showed an approximately 50% reduction in cardiac deaths and nonfatal myocardial infarctions using a diet rich in fruits, vegetables, whole grains, legumes, walnuts, almonds, and soybean or mustard oil.[10]

Recommendations for total fat intake should be personalized, ranging from 10% of calories to 35% of calories. LDL-C levels are independent of the total amount of dietary fat, as long as saturated and trans fats are controlled. Moderate total fat diets, with an emphasis on ω-3 fatty acids, may be most appropriate for patients with

Table 5-8: Omega-3 Fats in Fish[10]

Type of Fish	Serving Size	Omega-3 Fat (g)
Atlantic salmon (farmed)	3 ounces	1.09 to 1.83
Atlantic herring	3 ounces	1.71
Canned sardines	3 ounces	0.98 to1.70
Atlantic mackerel	3 ounces	0.34 to 1.57
Atlantic salmon (wild)	3 ounces	0.9 to 1.56
Fresh tuna	3 ounces	0.24 to 1.28
Pink salmon	3 ounces	1.09
Rainbow trout (farmed)	3 ounces	0.98
Rainbow trout (wild)	3 ounces	0.84
Sockeye or chum salmon	3 ounces	0.68
Canned white tuna	3 ounces	0.73
Canned light tuna	3 ounces	0.26
Atlantic cod	3 ounces	0.24
Wild catfish	3 ounces	0.2

moderately high triglyceride levels and low HDL-C levels, but may make weight loss more difficult because of caloric density. Low-fat diets are high in carbohydrate and generally should not be recommended for patients with the metabolic syndrome, moderately high triglycerides, and low HDL-C.

Although ω-3 fats are polyunsaturated, their benefits include reduction of platelet aggregation as well as anti-inflammatory and anti-arrhythmic effects. Omega-3 fats are found in fish and some plant foods, such as flax seed and canola oil. The AHA recommends fish consumption at least twice per week. Alpha-linolenic acid is an ω-3 fat found in plants. Table 5-8 lists the amount of ω-3 fats found in different types of fish.

Other Dietary Aids for Reducing CVD Risk

A fiber intake of 20 to 30 g/d (with 10 to 25 g of soluble fiber per day) is recommended and has been shown to reduce the risk of heart disease. Viscous, or water-soluble fiber, reduces LDL-C and blood sugar levels. In addition, because they are filling, high-fiber diets may lead to a lower calorie intake and facilitate weight loss. Insoluble fiber, such as the methylcellulose found in wheat, has not been demonstrated to lower cholesterol (unless it is substituted for a saturated fat). The recommended 20 to 30 g of fiber can be obtained from five or more servings of fruit and vegetables and at least six servings of grain products, of which at least half are whole grain (oats and barley are especially high in soluble fiber). Legumes (dried beans and peas) are also good sources of viscous fiber.

Soy protein has a cholesterol-reducing effect. Studies have shown that 25 g of soy protein per day can reduce serum cholesterol levels by 5%. Table 5-9 lists the soy-protein content of some foods.

Plant stanols/sterols (2 g per day) reduce LDL-C levels 5% to 15% by interfering with the absorption of cholesterol from the gut. They are now available as additives in certain margarines (Benecol®, Take Control®), and in a special orange juice (Heartwise®), and are likely to be added to more food products in the near future. Remember, however, that these treatments are modest and have not been tested for long-term cardiac outcomes.

Nutrition and Hypertension

The Dietary Approaches to Stop Hypertension (DASH) study demonstrated that significant reductions in systolic and diastolic blood pressure are achieved through dietary change. The original DASH diet included 8 to 10 serv-

Table 5-9: Soy Protein Content of Foods*

Food Source	Amount	Soy Protein	Isoflavones
Roasted soy beans	1/2 cup	30 g	110 mg
Soy flour	1/2 cup	15 g	85 mg
Textured soy protein	2 cups	24 g	56 mg
Soy milk	1/2 cup	3 g	12 mg
Tempeh	1/2 cup	16 g	46 mg
Tofu, firm	1/2 cup	20 g	28 mg

*Source: www.soyfoods.com

ings of fruits and/or vegetables, 2 to 3 servings of low-fat dairy products, and 3,000 mg sodium per day. This diet led to an average 11.6/5.3 mm Hg blood pressure reduction, which is equal to or greater than that of single-medication therapy.[11]

The DASH-Sodium diet added a 1,500 to 2,400 mg/d sodium limitation to the original guidelines and achieved an additional 3.5 mm Hg systolic and 2.2 mm Hg diastolic blood pressure reduction.[12] A moderate sodium restriction (2,400 mg/d) produces an average reduction of 5 mm Hg for both systolic and diastolic blood pressure. The results are greater in sodium-sensitive people (50% of hypertensive patients). The DASH diet is consistent with the AHA Eating Plan for Healthy Americans.[12] See Table 5-10 for some advantages of the DASH diet.

In the DASH-Sodium study, reducing dietary sodium to 1,600 mg a day achieved the lowest blood pressure, but a dietary sodium intake of 2,400 mg per day also reduced

Table 5-10: Advantages of the DASH Diet

- Compared to a typical American diet, the DASH diet:
  - Emphasizes more fruits, vegetables, and low-fat dairy foods
  - Contains smaller amounts of red meat, total and saturated fat, cholesterol, and sugar
  - Includes whole grains, poultry, fish, and nuts
- At 2,000 calories a day the DASH diet provides approximately:
  - 4,700 mg (120 mEq) potassium
  - 500 mg magnesium
  - 1,240 mg calcium
  - 90 g protein
  - 30 g fiber
- The calorie level of the DASH Eating Plan is adjusted to meet individual patient needs.

DASH=Dietary Approaches to Stop Hypertension study

blood pressure and may be more achievable in everyday life.[8] Blood pressure reduction occurred in all groups studied, (men, women, African Americans, and elderly people). It was achieved within weeks of starting the DASH Eating Plan, and was greatest in patients with hypertension and least in normotensive patients.[8]

Patients should be reminded that just limiting use of the saltshaker is unlikely to lower sodium intake enough to meet DASH-Sodium goals. Most restaurant and take-out foods are high in sodium. The most common high-sodium sources in the American diet are canned vegetables and soups, frozen and boxed dinners, instant and ready-to-eat cereals, chips and other snacks, and processed and lunch meats (eg, sausage, bologna).

Table 5-11: Ways to Decrease Dietary Sodium

1. Select foods with less than 300 mg of sodium per serving, as listed on the labels' Nutrition Facts.
2. Add no salt at the table.
3. Instead of salt use more spices in foods, or use lower-sodium alternatives such as Morton's Lite Salt®, herbs, or herb blends (eg, Mrs. Dash®, Vegit).
4. If salt is used in cooking, use half, or less, of the amount the recipe calls for.
5. When eating out, select fresh foods whenever possible.

Table 5-11 includes some suggestions for decreasing dietary sodium that a physician can share with patients.

Table 5-12 presents the DASH Eating Plan. Although this example is based on 2,000 calories a day, the calorie level of the DASH Eating Plan should be adjusted to meet the individual needs of patients. The number of daily servings in a food group will vary according to individual patients' daily calorie needs.[13]

Nutrition and Diabetes

Managing patients with diabetes mellitus requires a balance of medications, diet, and physical activity to maintain glucose levels as close to normal as possible. Diet therapy should be specifically prescribed and considered part of the treatment plan. See Chapter 9 for detailed information on diabetes and CVD prevention. The American Diabetes Association (ADA) has established goals for nutrition therapy that apply to all people with diabetes[14] (Table 5-13).

MNT for both type 1 and type 2 diabetes patients who need insulin is based on calorie needs and carbohydrate

Table 5-12: The DASH Eating Plan[12,13]

Food Group	Servings	Serving Size
Grains & grain products	7 to 8 daily	1 slice bread 1 cup ready-to-eat cereal* 1/2 cup cooked rice, pasta, or cereal
Vegetables	4 to 5 daily	1 cup raw leafy vegetable 1/2 cup cooked vegetable 6 ounces vegetable juice
Fruits	4 to 5 daily	1 medium fruit 1/4 cup dried fruit 1/2 cup fresh, frozen, or canned fruit 6 ounces fruit juice
Low-fat or fat-free dairy foods	2 to 3 daily	8 ounces milk 1 cup yogurt 1 1/2 ounces cheese

choices, and is reimbursable in most insurance plans. Patients on a fixed insulin dose should have consistent meal times each day and a consistent amount of carbohydrate at each meal. For patients who take multiple daily insulin

Food Group	Servings	Serving Size
Lean meats, poultry, & fish	2 or fewer daily	3 ounces cooked lean meats, skinless poultry, or fish
Nuts, seeds, & dried beans	4 to 5 per week	1/3 cup or 1 1/2 ounces nuts 1 tablespoon or 1/2 ounce seeds 1/2 cup cooked dry beans
Fats & oils**	2 to 3 daily	1 teaspoon soft margarine 1 tablespoon low-fat mayonnaise 2 tablespoons light salad dressing 1 teaspoon vegetable oil
Sweets	No more than 5 per week	1 tablespoon sugar 1 tablespoon jelly or jam 1/2 ounce jelly beans 8 ounces lemonade

* Check the Nutrition Facts Label to determine accurate serving size.
** Fat content changes serving counts for fats and oils.

injections and those who use an insulin pump, meal times and contents can be more flexible than for those on a fixed insulin dose. Diet and activity preferences should be considered when determining a patient's insulin regimen.

Table 5-13: American Diabetes Association Goals for Nutrition Therapy

- Achieve blood glucose levels as close to normal range as safely possible.
- Promote calorie levels to attain and maintain reasonable weight.
- Maintain lipid profile that reduces the risk for macrovascular disease.
- Maintain blood pressure levels that reduce the risk for vascular disease.
- Provide optimal nutrition.
- Promote physical activity.
- Alter diet to prevent and treat acute and chronic complications.

MNT for patients with diabetes who do not take insulin should be based on the individual patient's metabolic profile and on diagnoses related to the presence of symptoms associated with the metabolic syndrome. Patients with the metabolic syndrome should emphasize exercise and weight loss to reverse the syndrome, with a focus on reducing total calories, especially those of low nutritional value. (For details on the metabolic syndrome, see Chapter 8.)

Nutritional Recommendations for Patients With Diabetes

The amount of carbohydrates, including sugars and starches, included in each meal is critically important to patients with diabetes. Major carbohydrate sources include grains, breads, cereals, dry beans, starchy vegetables, fruit and fruit juice, milk and yogurt, sweets, and desserts. Sucrose and sucrose-containing foods do not have to be to-

Table 5-14: Food Sources of Fiber

Food	Soluble Fiber (g)	Total Fiber (g)
Cereal Grains (1 cup cooked)		
Barley	1	4
Oatmeal	2	4
Fruit (1 medium)		
Apple	1	4
Banana	1	3
Citrus (orange, grapefruit)	2	2-3
Pear	2	4
Beans/Lentils (1/2 cup cooked)		
Black, kidney, navy beans	2-3	5-7
Lentils	1	8
Peas, green	Less than 0.5	3
Vegetables		
Broccoli	Less than 0.5	1.5
Carrots	1	2.5
Seeds		
Psyllium seeds, ground, 1 tbsp (aka Metamucil®)	5	6

tally eliminated, but they should be included in the total carbohydrate allotment and eaten in the context of a healthy diet.

Fiber is an essential part of a healthy diet, regardless of a patient's health status. The diets of most Americans are low in fiber, with a usual daily intake of 12 to 14 g. The recommended daily amount of fiber is 25 to 35 g per day. Soluble fiber, found in foods such as oats, barley, and brown rice,

Table 5-15: Considerations About Dietary Protein for Diabetic Patients

- Dietary protein has minimal effect on plasma glucose concentration.
- Dietary protein stimulates insulin secretion as much as carbohydrate does. Protein should be limited to not more than 20% of total calories for patients with type 2 diabetes who are often already hyperinsulinemic.
- No evidence exists to support traditional advice to include a protein source with carbohydrate to prevent hypoglycemia. The peak response and the subsequent rate of glucose fall are similar with ingested dietary carbohydrate alone vs carbohydrate plus protein.
- Protein intake equal to 15% to 20% of calories is not associated with development of nephropathy.
- High-protein, low-carbohydrate diets (eg, Atkins Diet) are not recommended because of the high amounts of saturated fat and the lack of antioxidant-rich, high-fiber fruits and vegetables. In addition, the long-term safety and efficacy for patients with diabetes are not known.

and in psyllium, will reduce blood glucose and LDL-C levels for many patients. Table 5-14 lists food sources of fiber.

Glycemic Index

Should patients with diabetes use the glycemic index when planning their meals? Foods with a low glycemic index—dairy products, legumes, certain fruits, unprocessed grains—may reduce postprandial blood sugar levels and help prevent obesity and cardiovascular disease.[15,16] However, foods are generally not consumed alone, as the

Table 5-16: What Patients Should Know About Carbohydrates

- A specific number of carbohydrate choices is assigned for meals and snacks based on calorie needs.
- Most adults with moderate activity need three to five carbohydrate choices per meal.
- A carbohydrate choice is the amount of food that contains 15 g of carbohydrate.
- Food groups that contain carbohydrate are starch/bread, fruit, milk, desserts, and sweets.
- Food groups with limited or no carbohydrate are non-starchy vegetables, meat or meat substitutes, fats, and 'free foods' (ie, foods with less than 20 calories per serving). Carbohydrate choices can be excessive even in a meal that is 'healthy' and does not contain foods with added sugar.

glycemic index is measured. According to the ADA, there is not enough evidence to support the long-term benefits of a low-glycemic-index diet as the primary method for meal planning. On the other hand, a low-glycemic-index diet may be useful to 'fine tune' glycemic control.[17]

For patients with diabetes, the ratio of fat to carbohydrate in the diet should be individualized based on each patient's metabolic profile. Saturated fats should be limited to no more than 10% of calories, and the intake of trans fatty acids should be limited by using liquid oils and soft margarine and avoiding commercial foods prepared with hydrogenated fats and foods fried in restaurants. Margarines with added plant stanol/sterol esters can lower LDL-C as much as 10%, but, because they contain 40 to 80 calories per tablespoon, calories from other foods may need to be decreased to prevent weight gain.

Table 5-17: Comparison of Carbohydrate Choices* in Two Lunch Meals

Menu 1	Carbohydrates
1 cup beef stew/potatoes	2
1 slice bread/margarine	1
1 tennis-ball-sized apple	1
1 can diet soda	0
Total carbohydrates	4
Menu 2	**Carbohydrates**
1 cup pasta salad	2
1 large bagel with tuna	4
1 large apple	2
12 oz unsweetened orange juice	3
Total carbohydrates	11

* Carbohydrate choice = 15 g of carbohydrate of a given food (or 60 calories)

The ADA recommends that 15% to 20% of calories come from protein. For an 1,800-calorie diet, that is 65 to 90 g/d. Table 5-15 lists some considerations related to dietary protein and the diabetic diet.

Meal Planning for Diabetic Patients

Because diet complexity varies with the diabetes treatment regimen and the functional level of the patient, individual meal plans tailored to specific patients have replaced the standardized 'one-size-fits-all' ADA diets. All meal plans should help patients work toward decreased total and saturated fat content of their diet, with emphasis on monounsaturated fats; low-fat dairy products, low-fat meats, and non-meat protein sources; and increased fiber from fruits, vegetables, and whole grains.

Table 5-18: Estimating Portion Size

Food Item	One Portion
1 medium fruit	Tight fist (woman) Tennis ball
Fruit, pasta, potato, cooked cereal	Tight fist (woman) Tennis ball
1 medium baked potato	Computer mouse
1 cup cold cereal	Large handful
1 teaspoon margarine	Thumb tip
1 ounce cheese	Ice cube
2 oz meat, poultry, fish	Palm of woman's hand Deck of cards

It is important that patients who have diabetes understand the carbohydrate content of foods. Table 5-16 cites facts about carbohydrates that physicians should share with patients.

Table 5-17 presents a comparison of carbohydrate choices in two lunch meals.

Estimating Portion Size

It is important that all patients understand portion size. Americans have become so accustomed to the large portions offered at most restaurants and the 'super-sized' fast-food portions that they have no idea what a healthy serving size really is. As suggested in Table 5-18, visual images can help them estimate portion sizes.

The Bottom Line

An individualized approach to nutrition education that empowers the patient can be effective in helping him or her achieve a healthy diet, but change in eating habits is a long-term process that requires regular follow up to reassess progress, provide encouragement, and restructure goals.

If nutrition is a priority in national efforts to improve the health of our population, physicians need to be encouraged to implement innovative and efficient methods for nutritional counseling. They and their staffs need access to effective nutritional assessment tools and training to use these tools. In addition, procedures in primary care practice need to be examined and revised to facilitate efficient patient educational systems, targeting patients who are at highest risk and who are motivated to make changes.

References

1. Krauss RM, Eckel RH, Howard B, et al: AHA Dietary Guidelines. revision 2000: A statement for healthcare professionals from the Nutrition Committee of the American Heart Association. *Circulation* 2000;102:2284-2299.

2. Journal Report. American Heart Association dietary recommendations dish out a more individualized approach. American Heart Association. October 5, 2000. Available at www.americanheart.org/presenter.jhtml?identifier=3296. Accessed on September 24, 2003.

3. American Heart Association. Dietary Guidelines. Available at: www.americanheart.org/presenter.jhtml?identifier=1330. Accessed on September 24, 2003.

4. Hark L, Deen D Jr: Taking a nutrition history: A practical approach for family practice physicians. *Amer Fam Physician* 1999;59:1521-1528, 1531-1532.

5. Expert Panel on Detection, Evaluation, and Treatment of High Blood Cholesterol in Adults. Executive summary of The Third Report of the National Cholesterol Education Program (NCEP) Expert Panel on Detection, Evaluation, and Treatment of High Blood Cholesterol in Adults (Adult Treatment Panel III). *JAMA* 2001;285:2486-2497.

6. Superko HR, Krauss RM: Coronary artery disease regression. Convincing evidence for the benefit of aggressive lipoprotein management. *Circulation* 1994;90:1056-1069.

7. Denke MA: Cholesterol-lowering diets. A review of the evidence. *Arch Intern Med* 1995;155:17-26.

8. Hunninghake D, Stein EA, Dujovne CA, et al: The efficacy of intensive dietary therapy alone or combined with lovastatin in outpatients with hypercholesterolemia. *N Engl J Med* 1993;328:1213-1219.

9. de Lorgeril M, Salen P, Martin JL, et al: Mediterranean diet traditional risk factors, and the rate of cardiovascular complications after myocardial infarction: final report of the Lyon Diet Heart Study. *Circulation* 1999;99:779-785.

10. Singh RB, Dubnov G, Niaz MA, et al: Effect of an Indo-Mediterranean diet on progression of coronary artery disease in high-risk patients (Indo-Mediterranean Diet Heart Study): a randomized single-blind trial. *Lancet* 2002;360:1455-1461.

11. Appel LJ, Moore TJ, Obarzanek E, et al: A clinical trial of the effects of dietary patterns on blood pressure. *N Engl J Med* 1997;336:1117-1124.

12. Sacks FM, Svetkey LP, Vollmer WM, et al: Effects on blood pressure of reduced dietary sodium and the dietary approaches to stop hypertension (DASH) diet. DASH-Sodium Collaborative Research Group. *N Engl J Med* 2001;344:3-10.

13. National Institutes of Health. Facts about the DASH Eating Plan. Available at: http://www.nhlbi.nih.gov/health/public/heart/hbp/dash/index.htm.

14. Franz MJ, Bantle JP, Beebe CA, et al: Evidence-based nutrition principles and recommendations for the treatment and prevention of diabetes and related complications. *Diabetes Care* 2003;26(suppl 1):S51-S61.

15. Ludwig DS: The glycemic index: Physiological mechanisms relating to obesity, diabetes, and cardiovascular disease. *JAMA* 2002;287:2414-2423.

16. Brand-Miller J, Hayne S, Petocz P: Low-glycemic index diets in the management of diabetes: A meta-analysis of randomized controlled trials. *Diabetes Care* 2003;26:2261-2267.

17. Franz MJ: The glycemic index: not the most effective nutrition therapy intervention. *Diabetes Care* 2003;26:2466-2468.

CHAPTER 6

Physical Activity Versus a Sedentary Lifestyle

A sedentary lifestyle is a major risk factor for developing coronary artery disease, and it increases the risk of stroke. It also ranks with such other major cardiovascular risk factors as obesity, hypertension, low high-density lipoprotein (HDL) cholesterol, and diabetes mellitus. Unfortunately, most Americans get little or no physical activity in their daily lives. According to *A Report of the Surgeon General on Physical Activity and Health*, more than 60% of American adults are not regularly physically active, and 25% are not active at all.[1] The American Heart Association (AHA) reports that only 22% of American adults claim to get regular, sustained physical activity of any intensity at least 5 times per week. Table 6-1 cites some additional statistics on physical activity and cardiovascular health.

Benefits of Physical Activity

Physical activity is defined as 'bodily movement produced by skeletal muscles that requires energy expenditure and produces overall health benefits.'[2] Physical inactivity implies a level of activity that is less than that needed to maintain good health. The benefits of a physically active lifestyle have been well documented. Physical activity can reduce the risk of dying from coronary heart disease and of developing hypertension, colon cancer, and diabetes mellitus; can help reduce blood

Table 6-1: AHA Statistics on Physical Activity and Cardiovascular Health

- An estimated 300,000 deaths per year in the United States—about 12% of total deaths—are caused by poor diet and physical inactivity.
- The relative risk of coronary heart disease associated with physical inactivity ranges from 1.5 to 2.4, an increase in risk comparable to that observed for high cholesterol, hypertension, or cigarette smoking.
- Less-active persons have a 30% to 50% greater risk of developing hypertension.
- Surveys show that 30% of Americans 18 years of age or older get no exercise.
- Although 62% of adults get some exercise, they do not do it regularly or intensely enough to protect their hearts.
- Only 23% of American adults get enough leisure-time exercise to achieve cardiovascular fitness.
- The National Children and Youth Fitness Study, completed in 1987, found that at least half of youth do not engage in physical activity that promotes long-term health; less than 36% of elementary and secondary schools offer daily physical education (PE) classes; and most PE classes are unlikely to foster lifelong physical activity.

AHA = American Heart Association

pressure in some people with hypertension; can help maintain healthy bones, muscles, and joints; can reduce symptoms of anxiety and depression, and foster improvements in mood and feelings of well-being; and

Table 6-2: Health Benefits of Regular Physical Activity[3]

Health Issue	Benefits of Physical Activity
Cardiovascular health	• Improves myocardial performance • Increases peak diastolic filling • Increases heart muscle contractility • Increases aerobic capacity • Reduces systolic and diastolic blood pressure • Improves physical endurance
Obesity	• Decreases abdominal adipose tissue • Increases lean muscle mass • Reduces percentage of body fat
Lipoproteins/ glucose intolerance	• Reduces cholesterol/very low-density lipoprotein • Reduces triglycerides • Increases high-density lipoproteins • Reduces blood glucose and improves insulin sensitivity

can help control weight, develop lean muscle, and reduce body fat.

Table 6-2 illustrates some specific health benefits that result from regular physical activity.

Activity that reduces the risk factors for cardiovascular disease and confers many other health benefits does not require a structured or vigorous exercise program. Any amount of activity is better than none. People who are sedentary should start out with lower-intensity activity for shorter periods and increase to 30 minutes per day gradually over several weeks. A complete guideline issued by

Health Issue	Benefits of Physical Activity
Osteoporosis	• Slows decline in bone mineral density • Increases bone density
Psychologic well-being	• Improves perceived well-being and happiness • Increases levels of catecholamines, norepinephrine, and serotonin
Muscle weakness and functional capacity	• Reduces risk of musculoskeletal disability • Improves muscle strength and flexibility • Reduces risk of falls through increased strength • Reduces risk of fractures • Increases muscle performance, reaction time, and strength • Sustains cerebral perfusion and cognition

the AHA reviews the health benefits, risks, costs, and improved outcomes for programs designed to improve physical activity.[4] Recommendations from the National Institutes of Health (NIH) and the Centers for Disease Control and Prevention (CDC) related to physical activity and health appear in Table 6-3.

Patients can realize most of the benefits of physical activity by performing activities with moderate intensity, but they must perform them frequently to maintain the benefits. It is not necessary to achieve a high level of intensity or a certain percentage of CVD maximum to ben-

Table 6-3: Physical Activity and Health Recommendations From the NIH and CDC

- All people in the United States should increase their physical activity to a level appropriate to their capacities, needs, and interests.
- All children and adults should set a long-term goal to accumulate at least 30 minutes (or more) of moderate-intensity physical activity on most, or preferably all, days of the week.
- Intermittent or shorter bouts of activity (at least 10 minutes), including occupational and non-occupational activity, or tasks of daily living, also have cardiovascular and health benefits if performed at a level of moderate intensity with an accumulated duration of at least 30 minutes per day.
- People who already meet the recommended minimal standards may derive additional health benefits from becoming more physically active or including more vigorous activity.
- Previously sedentary people who begin physical activity programs should start with short sessions (5 to 10 minutes) of physical activity and gradually build up to the desired level.

NIH = National Institutes of Health
CDC = Centers for Disease Control and Prevention

efit from physical activity.[1,5] Any sedentary person who becomes even modestly or moderately active will significantly reduce his or her risk of CVD and of bladder, breast, colon, and prostate cancer.[6] According to the CDC, a moderate amount of physical activity is roughly equal to

Table 6-4: Moderate Amounts of Physical Activity[3]

Activity	Time Spent
Washing and waxing a car	45 to 60 minutes
Washing windows or floors	45 to 60 minutes
Playing volleyball	45 minutes
Playing touch football	30 to 45 minutes
Gardening	30 to 45 minutes
Wheeling self in wheelchair	30 to 40 minutes
Walking 1 $^{3}/_{4}$ miles	35 minutes (20 min/mile)
Shooting baskets	30 minutes
Bicycling 5 miles	30 minutes
Dancing fast (social)	30 minutes
Pushing a stroller 1 $^{1}/_{2}$ miles	30 minutes
Raking leaves	30 minutes
Walking 2 miles	30 minutes (15 min/mile)
Water aerobics	30 minutes
Swimming laps	20 minutes
Wheelchair basketball	20 minutes
Basketball (playing a game)	15 to 20 minutes
Bicycling 4 miles	15 minutes
Jumping rope	15 minutes
Running 1 $^{1}/_{2}$ miles	15 minutes (10 min/mile)
Shoveling snow	15 minutes
Stair walking	15 minutes

activity that uses 150 calories (kcal) of energy per day, or about 1,000 calories per week. Because the amount of activity is a function of duration, intensity, and frequency, the same amount can be obtained in longer sessions of moderately intense activity (eg, brisk walking), as in

Table 6-5: Types of Physical Exercise

Type of Exercise	Purpose
Cardiorespiratory endurance	Increases heart rate and breathing for extended periods. Improves the health of the head, lungs, and circulatory system. Helps prevent or delay some diseases.
Resistance exercise	Muscle strength and endurance exercise make individuals strong enough to do both the things they need to do and the things they like to do.
Balance exercise	Helps prevent falls, which are a major cause of disability for older adults
Stretching	Helps keep the body limber and flexible. Can help prevent injuries. Gives more freedom of movement.

shorter sessions of more strenuous activities (eg, running). Patients who have led a sedentary lifestyle can achieve significant health-related benefits from moderate-intensity activities. In addition, they are more likely to continue moderate-intensity activities than high-intensity activities.[1] Participants in a lifestyle change group that encouraged lifestyle physical activity, compared to a group randomized to a higher-intensity, supervised exercise program, had significant and comparable improvements in physical activity and cardiorespiratory fitness over a 2-

Recommendations
The goal for cardiovascular endurance exercise (eg, walking, jogging, swimming, bicycling) is to build up to at least 30 minutes of endurance exercise on most, or all, days of the week.[8]
Should be performed for all major muscle groups at least twice a week.[8]
Can be incorporated into strength training exercises. Any of the lower-body exercises for strength that require standing are also balance exercises.[8] T'ai chi is a practical way to maintain and improve balance.[9]
Should be performed regularly before and after exercise. Yoga, which involves stretching, meditation, and 'care breathing,' can be safely practiced by people of all ages.[9]

year period.[7] Table 6-4 lists some moderate activities and the time required to achieve health benefits.

Types of Exercise

Exercise is physical activity defined as 'a planned, structured, and repetitive bodily movement done to improve or maintain one or more components of physical fitness.'[2] The CDC, the AHA, the National Institute on Aging, and many other health-care organizations agree that people of all ages should be encouraged to develop

Table 6-6: Sample Activity Log

Date	Type of Exercise/ Activity	Total Minutes	How I Felt

and maintain a practice of regular physical activity that is performed daily, or on most days of the week.

Fitness includes four major components: (1) cardiorespiratory (aerobic) endurance; (2) muscle strength and endurance; (3) balance; and (4) flexibility.

Table 6-5 defines the types of exercise, explains their purpose, and offers some related recommendations for achieving each component of fitness.

Evaluating Exercise

It is important to ask your patients about their level of physical activity. The most important questions to ask are: 'Are you physically active?' or 'Do you exercise regularly?' Perceptions of appropriate physical activity can vary, based on an individual's gender, age, weight, marital status, family roles and responsibilities, disability, and social class.[2] To get a more complete picture of a patient's level of physical activity, ask questions about his or her job and what it entails, and about normal daily routine, hobbies, family responsibilities, and physical problems or symptoms that may affect level or type of physical activity. Providing a complete exercise prescription, including the four components of fitness—strength, endurance, flexibility, and balance—requires more time and expertise. Referral to an exercise physiologist or trainer may be necessary.

To help determine a patient's true physical activity level from walking, you might suggest that he or she purchase and wear a pedometer, an easy way to keep track of every step taken each day. The recommended goal is 6,000 to 10,000 steps per day. Another idea is to have the patient maintain an activity log for a designated period (eg, 4 to 6 weeks). Table 6-6 illustrates a simple activity log that the AHA recommends. Self-monitoring motivates patients, and providing their own feedback helps, too.

Improving Physical Activity in the Community

Working with and encouraging individual patients is the physician's obvious task. However, you can also promote healthy behavior in your community. The best way to help people maintain their health is to reach them before they need medical attention. Table 6-7 lists some steps you can take to encourage people to increase their physical activity before they become your patients.

Prescribing Exercise

According to the *NIH Consensus Statement on Physical Activity and Cardiovascular Health*, preliminary evidence suggests that health-care providers can play a key

Table 6-7: Steps to Improve Physical Activity in the Community

1. Encourage people to reduce time spent in front of video screens (television, movies, computers, video games). The amount of time spent in front of video screens is directly associated with obesity and lack of fitness, especially in children and adolescents.
2. Work closely with schools to maintain physical education programs and activities for all children—physical education is decreasing in US schools.
3. Encourage communities to create environments that are more conducive to activity, such as sidewalks, parks, bike trails, safety strategies, and community action plans.
4. Work with national groups, including YWCA and YMCA, Boys and Girls Clubs, and other health and fitness centers to encourage membership and use of the facilities.
5. Encourage health care professionals to set the example of regular physical activity and to routinely recommend physical activity to patients.
6. Encourage families to set a goal to be physically active and physically fit and to exercise, with parents setting the example for their children.

role in promoting physical activity as a risk-reduction behavior for their patients. Authors of the report state, 'It is highly probable that people will be more likely to increase their physical activity if their health-care provider counsels them to do so.'[2] Clinicians can do this by learning to recognize stages of behavior change, communicating the need for increased activity, assisting patients in initiating activity, and following up appropriately.

Communicating with your patients is a critical factor in increasing compliance, whether it is with taking medications appropriately or adapting to lifestyle recommendations. Patients frequently find it difficult to follow recommended lifestyle changes, such as stopping smoking, improving their nutrition, and increasing their daily activity level. If a patient does not tell a physician about a change in lifestyle behavior or about problems with following through on recommendations, these issues are not addressed. Both the patient and the physician need a cue if preventive strategies are to be successfully incorporated into clinical practice. Therefore, it is essential that you mention important lifestyle recommendations to your patients, and offer guidelines and tips to enhance their compliance. The CDC offers guidelines for prescribing increased physical activity. Although you may need to further refine their guidelines, as listed in Table 6-8, for specific individuals and population groups, physical activity is more likely to be initiated and maintained if the patient follows them.

As stated earlier, physical activity does not need to be strenuous to provide health benefits. It is important to tell your patients that moderate amounts of physical activity can be achieved in ways that can fit into their daily lives without requiring the large blocks of time needed for some formal exercise programs. Patients who resist the idea of a formal exercise program may be encouraged to know that just 30 minutes of brisk walking each day provides important long-term health benefits. In addition, making small changes in their lives, such as taking a 10- to 15-minute walk during their lunch hour, taking stairs instead of escalators and elevators, and parking farther from a store or office building, can add more activity to their daily routine. In short, the appropriate activity for an individual patient is determined by individual preference and what

Table 6-8: Factors That Make Patients Likely to Initiate and Maintain Physical Activity

- They perceive a net benefit.
- They choose an enjoyable activity.
- They feel competent doing the activity.
- They feel safe doing the activity.
- They can easily access the activity on a regular basis.
- They can fit the activity into their daily schedule.
- They feel that the activity does not generate financial or social costs that they are unwilling to bear.
- They experience a minimum of negative consequences, such as injury, loss of time, negative peer pressure, and problems with self identity.
- They can successfully address issues of competing time demands.
- They recognize the need to balance the use of labor-saving devices (eg, power lawnmowers, golf carts, automobiles) and sedentary activities (eg, watching television, using computers) with activities that involve a higher level of physical exertion.

the patient is likely to sustain. Remind patients that a brisk 10-minute walk 3 times a day, or a 15-minute walk twice a day, amounts to 30 minutes of moderate exercise.[1] This may give them the incentive they need to begin increasing their daily activity.

For some patients, it may be advisable, or even necessary, for you to prescribe an individualized exercise plan.

The AHA suggests that the health-care provider indicate the type of exercise to be done; specify and gradually increase frequency, duration, and intensity of the exercise; ensure that the patient can recognize and deal with abnormal physical responses to exercise; have the patient document exercise; and enhance the patient's adherence to the exercise goals by identifying barriers to exercise and reinforcers for complying with the goals.

Motivating the Patient

Your frequent and continual encouragement can go a long way toward keeping a patient motivated to develop and maintain a daily routine of physical activity. Table 6-9 provides tips for success that you could share with your patients.

In addition to these suggestions, advise patients who may be planning to invest in exercise equipment that they should buy only high-quality equipment and should try it out before purchasing it.

Exercise and Cardiovascular Disease

Strong evidence suggests that regular physical exercise, particularly if provided as part of a cardiac rehabilitation program, significantly improves health outcomes for patients with CVD.[10] Randomized controlled trials of exercise in post-myocardial infarction patients found reductions in total mortality and CVD mortality.[10] Trials of lifestyle treatment and exercise progression have demonstrated atherosclerosis regression in coronary and peripheral arteries and decreased CVD events.[11-13]

Unfortunately, fewer than 30% of cardiac patients are referred to cardiac rehabilitation following an acute CVD event.[10] Cardiac rehabilitation, including exercise and secondary prevention disease management, is indicated for patients with recent myocardial infarction, coronary artery bypass surgery, cardiac valve repair, congestive heart failure, and new-onset angina. Exercise improves CVD

Table 6-9: American Heart Association Tips for Physical Activity Success

- Choose activities that are fun, not exhausting.
- Add variety so that exercise doesn't become boring or routine.
- Wear comfortable, properly fitted footwear and comfortable, loose-fitting clothing that is appropriate for the weather and the activity.
- Find a convenient time and place to do activities. Try to make it a habit, but be flexible. If you miss an exercise opportunity, work activity into your day in another way.
- Use music to keep yourself entertained.
- Surround yourself with supportive people.
- Find a companion to exercise with you, if it will help you stay on a regular schedule and add to your enjoyment.

outcomes in these patients, including reducing total mortality, recurrent cardiovascular events, cardiovascular mortality, and hospitalizations, and significantly improves exercise capacity and symptoms.[10]

Cardiac patients can resume physical work, sexual activity, and other activities based on their monitored performance during stress testing and monitoring after their CVD diagnosis. Difficulties with sexual intercourse are rare, and if a patient has accomplished >4 metabolic equivalents (METs) in stress testing, he or she has exceeded the maximal METs usually required for sexual activity and can safely resume sexual intercourse.[14] Maximal stress testing is indicated at 6 or more weeks after the cardiac event

- Don't overdo it. Do low-to-moderate-level activities, especially at first. You can slowly increase the duration and intensity of your activities as you become more fit.
- Keep a record of your activities and reward yourself at special milestones. Nothing motivates like success!
- Pick rhythmic, repetitive activities that challenge the circulatory system, and exercise at an intensity appropriate for you.
- If you decide walking is a great activity, choose a place that has a smooth, soft surface, does not intersect with traffic, and is well lighted and safe.
- Take time to warm up and cool down while exercising, and make sure you stretch slowly. Remember that muscular adaptation and elasticity generally slow with age.

to stratify risk in stable patients, based on their current disease state, and to assess risk in higher-risk patients.

Practice Tools

The demands of maintaining a busy medical practice can make it difficult to find the time to personally provide all of the information, support, and motivation your patients may need to comply with your recommendations for increasing their physical activity. Familiarize yourself with resources in your community that can help individuals reach their exercise goals, and provide a list of these resources to your patients. The AHA Web site (www.americanheart.org) is a good source for information on physical activity and exercise, as well as other cardiovascular risk-reduction topics, that can be downloaded, printed, and distributed to your patients. Examples include: 'Why Should I Be Physically Active?', 'How Can Physical Activity Become a Way of Life?', and 'How Can I Keep Track of Exercise and Eating?'

Fact sheets on the importance of physical activity are also available from the CDC (www.cdc.gov), the American College of Sports Medicine (www.acsm.org), the American Diabetes Association (www.diabetes.org), and other health-care organizations. Other print and online resources on this subject are listed in Appendix B.

References

1. Physical Activity and Health: A Report of the Surgeon General At-A-Glance. National Center for Chronic Disease Prevention and Health Promotion. Available at http://www.cdc.gov/nccdphp/sgr/ataglan.htm. Accessed October 13 and December 9, 2003.

2. Physical activity and cardiovascular health. *NIH Consens Statement* 1995;13:1-33.

3. National Blueprint: Increasing Physical Activity Among Adults Age 50 and Older. Robert Wood Johnson Foundation. Available at www.agingblueprint.org. Accessed January 24, 2006.

4. Thompson PD, Buchner D, Pina IL, et al: Exercise and physical activity in the prevention and treatment of atherosclerotic cardiovascular disease: a statement from the Council on Clinical Cardiology (Subcommittee on Exercise, Rehabilitation, and Prevention) and the Council on Nutrition, Physical Activity, and Metabolism (Subcommittee on Physical Activity). *Circulation* 2003;107:3109-3116.

5. Blair SN, Jackson AS: Physical fitness and activity as separate heart disease risk factors: a meta-analysis. *Med Sci Sports Exerc* 2001;33:762-764.

6. Blair SN, Kohl HW 3rd, Paffenbarger RS Jr, et al: Physical fitness and all-cause mortality. A prospective study of healthy men and women. *JAMA* 1989;262:2395-2401.

7. Dunn AL, Marcus BH, Kampert JB, et al: Comparison of lifestyle and structured interventions to increase physical activity and cardiorespiratory fitness: a randomized trial. *JAMA* 1999;281:327-334.

8. Exercise: A guide from the National Institute on Aging. National Institutes of Health and National Institute on Aging, NIH Publication No. 01-4258, April 2004. Available at www.nih.gov/nia. Accessed January 23, 2006.

9. How to Choose a Healthy Exercise. The American Federation for Aging Research. Available at http://www.infoaging.org/l-exer-4-healthy.html. Accessed January 24, 2006.

10. Ades PA: Cardiac rehabilitation and secondary prevention of coronary heart disease. *N Engl J Med* 2001;345:892-902.

11. Schuler G, Hambrecht R, Schlierf G, et al: Regular physical exercise and low fat diet. Effects on progression of coronary heart disease. *Circulation* 1992;86:1-11.

12. Ornish D, Scherwitz LW, Billings JH, et al: Intensive lifestyle changes for reversal of coronary heart disease. *JAMA* 1998;280: 2001-2007.

13. Haskell WL, Alderman EL, Fair JM, et al: Effects of intensive multiple risk factor reduction on coronary atherosclerosis and clinical cardiac events in men and women with coronary heart disease. The Stanford Coronary Risk Intervention Project (SCRIP). *Circulation* 1994;89:975-990.

14. DeBusk RF: Sexual activity in patients with angina. *JAMA* 2003;290:3129-3132.

CHAPTER 7

Tobacco Screening and Intervention

The evidence that cigarette smoking is a major risk factor for all forms of coronary artery disease (CAD) is indisputable.[1-3] More than half of all smoking-related deaths in America each year are caused by heart disease, stroke, or other cardiovascular disease.[1-2] Smoking as few as one to four cigarettes per day or being exposed to secondhand smoke increases the risk of subsequent myocardial infarction (MI).[2] Smoking promotes atherosclerosis; triggers coronary thrombosis, coronary artery spasm, and cardiac arrhythmias; and reduces the blood's capacity to deliver oxygen.[1] In fact, cigarette smoking is the most significant preventable contributor to premature death, disability, and unnecessary health expense in the United States.[2-4]

Tobacco use is responsible for more than 430,000 deaths each year, and the cost to society of tobacco death and disease is nearly $100 billion.[5,6] The National Cancer Institute (NCI) estimates that environmental tobacco smoke causes 35,000 to 62,000 heart disease deaths in nonsmokers each year. Even a few cigarettes' worth of passive smoke exposure per day increases the risk of coronary heart disease (CHD) by 20% to 30%.[7] Although the overall prevalence of smoking has declined during the past 30 years, 25% of all American adults still smoke, and 3,000 children and adolescents become regular tobacco users every day.[5,6] In a 2003 update of heart disease and stroke statistics, the American Heart Association (AHA) reported

Table 7-1: Key Steps in Promoting Tobacco Use Cessation

- *Ask* about tobacco use at every visit.
- *Advise* patients who use tobacco to quit.
- *Assess* interest in cessation.
- *Assist* in cessation: counseling and pharmacotherapy.
- *Arrange* follow-up—the best predictor of success.

that 38.5% of male students and 29.5% of female students in grades 9 to 12 reported using tobacco in 2001. Slightly more than 22% of male students and 8.5% of female students reported using cigars, and 14.8% of male students and 1.9% of female students reported using smokeless tobacco. In addition, about 5 million American men and women use chewing tobacco.[8]

Smoking cessation can reduce the risk of heart disease and the risk of mortality from CHD for individuals with symptomatic CAD. For example, Framingham Heart Study participants who stopped smoking by the age of 65 years reduced their risk of initial or recurrent serious coronary events by 50% compared to those who continued to smoke.[9] The AHA estimates that the risk of heart disease is cut in half 1 year after quitting smoking; after 5 to 15 years, the risk is similar to that of a person who never smoked.[8] A recent HMO study found that for post-MI patients, the risk declined to equal that of nonsmokers as early as 3 years after smoking cessation.[10] A recent systematic review found that smoking cessation in patients with CHD had a reduction in mortality of 36% compared to those who continued to smoke, regardless of age, gender, or type of cardiac event.[11]

Table 7-2: Assist the Patient in Quitting[5,6]

Action	Strategies for Implementation
Help patients with a quit plan	• Encourage patients to *set a quit date*–ideally within 2 weeks. • Suggest that patients tell family, friends, and coworkers about quitting and request their understanding and support. • Tell patients to *anticipate* challenges to their planned quit attempt, including nicotine withdrawal symptoms, particularly during the critical first few weeks. • Instruct patients to *remove* tobacco products from their environment. Suggest that they avoid smoking in places where they spend a lot of time (eg, work, home, car) before quitting.
Provide practical counseling and problem-solving training	• *Abstinence.* Remind patients that total abstinence is essential. 'Avoid even a single puff after the quit date.' • *Past quit experience.* Review past attempts to quit and identify what helped during the quit attempt and what factors contributed to the relapse. • *Alcohol.* Because alcohol can cause relapse, recommend that patients consider limiting or abstaining from alcohol while attempting to quit.

Action	Strategies for Implementation
Provide practical counseling and problem-solving training *(continued)*	• *Other smokers in the household*: Because quitting is more difficult when there is another smoker in the household, a patient should encourage housemates to quit, too, or ask them to not smoke in his or her presence.
Provide social support	• Provide a supportive clinical environment while in their quit attempt. You can say, 'My office staff and I are available to assist you.'
Help patients obtain extra-treatment social support	• Help patients develop social support outside of the treatment setting for their attempt to quit smoking. For example, you might suggest, 'Ask your spouse/partner, friends, and coworkers to support you in your quit attempt.'
Recommend the use of approved pharmacotherapy to all who are attempting cessation, except when contraindicated.	• Explain that there are safe, effective medications that can increase smoking cessation success and reduce withdrawal symptoms.

(continued on next page)

Table 7-2: Assist the Patient in Quitting[5,6] *(continued)*

Action	Strategies for Implementation
Provide leads to online programs and materials: • American Lung Association Freedom from Smoking program: http://www.ffsonline.org • American Cancer Society: http://www.cancer.org • American Heart Association: http://www.americanheart.org • QuitNet®: http://www.quitnet.com—a program that involves support, expert help, and more	• *Sources*. Federal agencies, such as the AHRQ and NCI; professional organizations, such as ACS, AHA, and ALA. • *Type*. Appropriate to patient's age, culture, race, and education level. • *Location*. Readily available in the waiting area and in the examination room.

AHRQ = Agency for Healthcare Research and Quality; NCI = National Cancer Institute; ACS = American Cancer Society; AHA = American Heart Association; ALA = American Lung Association.

Effective smoking cessation treatments are now available, and every patient who smokes should be offered one or more of them.[5,6] Smoking cessation interventions are proven to be cost-effective, costing less than some routine preventive medical practices, such as periodic mammography. The average per-smoker cost of effective cessation treatment is less than $200.[5,6]

As a clinician, you have the opportunity and the responsibility to help patients stop using tobacco and to ensure that nonusers continue to resist smoking by informing them about the health risks associated with tobacco use. Health-care providers should also serve as good role models by refraining from the use of tobacco products. In addition, all health-care professionals should advocate insurance coverage of smoking cessation treatments. Table 7-1 lists the key steps in promoting cessation. Tables 7-2 and 7-3 will help you implement general tobacco cessation guidelines.

Clinical Assessment

The first and most important step in treating tobacco use and dependence is to ask your patients about their tobacco-use status. This should be done for every patient aged 12 years or older at every visit when vital signs are taken. By doing this, you can identify the three main groups of patients and tailor your treatment strategy accordingly. The three groups are:

1. Smokers who are willing to try quitting
2. Smokers who are not yet ready to try quitting
3. Former smokers who may be at risk for relapsing.

One strategy for implementing an office-wide system for identifying tobacco users (recommended by the Agency for Healthcare Research and Quality [AHRQ] smoking cessation guidelines) is to expand the vital signs to include tobacco use. Adding tobacco as a vital sign has resulted in a doubling of smoking cessation success in primary care.[5,6] See Figure 7-1 for a sample vital signs record.

Repeated assessment is not needed for adult patients who have never used tobacco or those who have not used it for many years. This information should be clearly documented in the medical record. For nonsmokers, you might consider placing 'nonsmoker' stickers on appropriate pa-

Table 7-3: The '4 Rs'[5,6]

Relevance	Motivational information given to a patient has the greatest impact if it is relevant to the patient's health, health concerns, family situation (eg, children in the home), age, gender, and other important characteristics (eg, prior quitting experience).
Risk	Ask the patient to identify the potential negative consequences of smoking and highlight those that seem most relevant to him or her. Examples of consequences include: • Acute risks: shortness of breath, exacerbation of asthma, impotence, infertility • Long-term risks: heart attacks, strokes, lung and other cancers, chronic obstructive pulmonary disease • Risk of secondhand smoke: increased risk of lung cancer in spouse and children; increased risk of sudden infant death syndrome, upper respiratory infection, asthma, and ear infection in children

tient charts or indicating tobacco-use status using electronic medical records or computer reminder systems.

Once you have asked your patients about tobacco use, you need to assess their willingness to make an attempt at quitting. See Table 7-4 for the kinds of issues you may face and Table 7-5 for some guidelines in assisting patients to quit.

Guidelines and methods are also available to improve organizational systems to reduce smoking in larger populations of patients.[12] Families and employers, as well as individuals, should be assisted in reducing expo-

Reward	Ask the patient to identify the potential benefits of quitting tobacco use and highlight those that seem most relevant. Examples of rewards include: • Save money • Improve taste of food • Improve sense of smell • Improve smell of home, car, and breath • Improve chances of having healthy babies and children • Improve sports performance • Improve self-esteem • Eliminate worry about quitting • Conquer addiction • Set a good example for children • No longer expose others to smoke
Repetition	The motivational intervention should be repeated every time an unmotivated patient visits your office or clinic.

sure to environmental tobacco smoke and educated about its importance.[13]

Behavioral Interventions

Table 7-2 outlines action steps and implementation strategies to share with patients who are willing to attempt to quit smoking.

Motivating the Unwilling Patient

Patients who indicate that they are not ready to make an attempt to quit smoking may be concerned about the negative effects of quitting, such as nicotine withdrawal symp-

Blood pressure ____________________

Pulse rate ____________________

Temperature ____________________

Height __________ **Weight** __________

Body mass index ____________________

Waist circumference at iliac crest ____________________

Tobacco use: *(Circle one)*

Current   Former   Never   Exposure

Interested in quitting?   Yes   No

Recommendation or follow-up ____________________

____

____

____

____

____

Figure 7-1: Sample of a vital signs record for patients.

toms or weight gain, or they may be demoralized by past failures to quit. It is best to avoid confronting these patients. However, you need to let them know that quitting is important and that you want to help them when they are ready. Providing a brochure describing the benefits of tobacco cessation may help some individuals; others may respond to the motivational interventions suggested in Table 7-3.

Motivating Adolescent Tobacco Users

Direct patient interventions with appropriately targeted messages have proven effective in influencing adolescents

Table 7-4: Issues a Practitioner May Face in Helping a Patient to Quit Smoking

- If the patient is willing to try quitting, how and when will you provide assistance?
- If the patient is willing to undergo intensive treatment, can you provide it, or will you refer the patient to an intensive intervention program?
- If the patient clearly states that he or she is not willing to try quitting at present, are you prepared to provide a motivational intervention?
- If the patient is an adolescent, pregnant, or a racial or ethnic minority, is your office prepared to offer additional information?

to consider smoking cessation. Table 7-6 lists some brief messages you may wish to use when talking to teens.

Motivating Pregnant Women to Quit

Smoking during pregnancy presents risks to the mother and the fetus. It has been shown to cause such adverse fetal outcomes as stillbirth, spontaneous abortion, decreased fetal growth, premature birth, low birth weight, placental abruption, sudden infant death syndrome, cleft palates and lips, and childhood cancers.

Many women are motivated to quit smoking during pregnancy. You can take advantage of this motivation by reinforcing the knowledge that cessation will reduce the fetal health risks described above. Although quitting smoking before conception or early in pregnancy is most beneficial, health benefits result from abstinence at any time. You should continue to encourage pregnant smokers to quit, and offer to help them quit, throughout their pregnancy. Table 7-7 outlines the AHRQ clinical practice guidelines for helping pregnant women quit smoking.

Table 7-5: Key Clinical Guidelines for Successful Cessation

- Pharmacotherapy should be considered for all cessation attempts unless there are special circumstances (eg, pregnancy, contraindications, less than 10 cigarettes per day).
- Any of the pharmacotherapies can be used: bupropion, nicotine patch, nicotine inhaler, nicotine gum, nicotine nasal spray.
- Bupropion may be especially useful if the patient has a history of depression or of weight gain on previous attempts.
- Pharmacotherapies may be combined and may be used for 6 months or longer if the patient has a history of relapse or significant nicotine addiction.
- Counseling and follow-up, along with pharmacotherapy, significantly increase success of cessation attempts.

Pharmacologic Intervention

Pharmacotherapy can improve the chances that patients will be successful in their efforts to quit smoking. The AHRQ guidelines recommend that clinicians offer pharmacotherapy to all smokers who are motivated to try quitting, unless specific contraindications exist. A patient may be an appropriate candidate for pharmacologic support if evidence of nicotine addiction exists, if he or she is in the action stage of quitting, and if he or she has expressed interest in using medication as an aid during nicotine withdrawal. (See Table 7-8 for the Fagerstrom Test for Nicotine Dependence.) Remember that the integration of behavioral therapy and pharmacotherapy has the highest success rate.[5,6,14] Pharmacotherapy will be most success-

Table 7-6: Messages for Teens

- Tobacco causes yellow teeth and fingers, bad breath, smelly clothes, and wrinkled skin.
- Cigarettes contain 4,000 chemicals, of which 400 are toxic and 40 cause cancer.
- Eating healthy foods and exercising are better ways to lose weight than smoking.
- Smoking a pack of cigarettes a day costs more than $23 a week—more than the cost of a compact disc.
- 'It's not cool.' Most people—three of four adults and more teens—don't smoke.
- Increasingly, cities and states are passing laws that forbid smoking in restaurants and other public places.

ful when the patient is motivated to quit within the month; agrees to quit using tobacco products when he or she begins nicotine replacement therapy (NRT); agrees to participate in a follow-up program; and previous quit attempts have failed because of withdrawal symptoms.

The AHRQ Guidelines for Treating Tobacco Use and Dependence identified five first-line pharmacotherapies that reliably increase long-term smoking abstinence rates. They also cited two second-line therapies—clonidine (Catapres®) and nortriptyline (Aventyl®, Pamelor®)—that are efficacious and may be considered if first-line pharmacotherapies are not effective. The first-line therapies are bupropion SR (Wellbutrin®, Zyban®), nicotine patch, nicotine gum, nicotine inhaler, and nicotine nasal spray.

Over-the-counter nicotine patches and gum are available and have proven to be effective. Their use should be encouraged.

Table 7-7: Clinical Practice When Assisting a Pregnant Patient in Smoking Cessation[5,6]

Clinical Practice	Rationale
Assess pregnant woman's tobacco-use status using a multiple-choice question to improve disclosure	Many pregnant women deny smoking, and the multiple-choice question format improves disclosure. For example: Which of the following statements best describes your cigarette smoking: • I smoke regularly now—about the same as before finding out I was pregnant. • I smoke regularly now, but I have cut down since I found out I was pregnant. • I smoke every once in a while. • I have quit smoking since finding out I was pregnant. • I wasn't smoking around the time I found out I was pregnant, and I do not now smoke cigarettes.
Congratulate those smokers who have quit on their own.	To encourage continued abstinence.
Motivate quit attempts by providing educational messages about the impact of smoking on the woman's and the fetus's health.	These messages are associated with higher quit rates.

Clinical Practice	Rationale
Give clear, strong advice to quit as soon as possible.	Quitting early in pregnancy provides the greatest benefit to the fetus.
Suggest the use of problem-solving methods and provide social support and pregnancy-specific self-help materials.	Reinforces pregnancy-specific benefits and ways to achieve cessation.
Arrange for follow-up assessments throughout pregnancy, including further encouragement of cessation.	The woman and her fetus will benefit even when quitting occurs late in pregnancy.
In the early post-partum period, assess for relapse and use relapse prevention strategies, recognizing that patients may minimize or deny tobacco use.	Postpartum relapse rates are high even if a woman maintains abstinence throughout pregnancy. Relapse may start during pregnancy.

Table 7-8: Fagerstrom Test for Nicotine Dependence
How soon after you wake up do you smoke your first cigarette?
Do you find it difficult to refrain from smoking in places where it is forbidden, such as the grocery store, restaurants, or movie theater?
Which cigarette would you hate to give up?
How many cigarettes do you smoke per day?
Do you smoke more frequently during the first hour after waking than during the rest of the day?
Do you smoke when you are so ill that you are in bed most of the day?
Scoring: 0-4 = low; 5 = medium; 6-7 = high; >8 = very high nicotine dependence Patients who score high or very high are potential candidates for pharmacologic therapy.

Bupropion SR

Sustained-release bupropion, which was initially marketed as an anxiolytic, is a highly effective aid in smoking cessation, even in nondepressed patients. It helps reduce nicotine withdrawal symptoms and cravings through neurochemical pathways. In a recent clinical trial, bupropion SR (150 to 300 mg/d) had cessation rates at 1 year of

Score			
0	**1**	**2**	**3**
>1 hr	30 min-1 hr	6-30 min	≤5 min
No	Yes		
Any other	1st in AM		
<10	11-20	21-30	>31
No	Yes		
No	Yes		

23%, compared to 13% for placebo.[15] It has proven highly effective in clinical trials, doubling abstinence rates compared to placebo and reducing or delaying risk of smoking relapse.[16] Bupropion combined with a nicotine patch showed even greater efficacy. Bupropion may reduce the weight gain associated with smoking cessation, is well tolerated with few side effects, and is equally ef-

Table 7-9: Pharmacologic Therapy for Smoking Cessation

Therapy	Dose	Max Dose
Nicotine gum		
Nicorette®	2 mg/piece	30 pieces/d
Nicorette® DS	4 mg/piece	20 pieces/d
Generic	2 mg, 4 mg	20-30 pieces/d
Nicotine lozenge		
Commit®	2 mg/lozenge	30 lozenges/d
	4 mg/lozenge	20 lozenges/d

MI = myocardial infarction,
TMJ = temporomandibular joint

Instructions	Contraindications
Chew slowly for 30 min and intermittently place between cheek and gum	• Active TMJ • Angina, arrhythmias, immediately post MI • Continued use of tobacco products • Gastric ulcer • Hypersensitivity to nicotine • Uncontrolled hypertension
Dissolve in mouth over 20-30 min Do not chew/bite/swallow Avoid food or drink for 15 min before and after lozenge	• Hyperthyroidism • Unstable CAD • Arrhythmias • Hypersensitivity to nicotine • Uncontrolled hypertension • Use cautiously with acute MI and with severely impaired renal or liver function

(continued on next page)

Dosage regimens should be appropriately adjusted for prescription vs OTC and for smokers who smoke more or less than 10 cigarettes a day.

UW Tobacco Cessation Guidelines. Available at: http://www.ctri.wisc.edu/HC.Providers/healthcare.htm.

Table 7-9: Pharmacologic Therapy for Smoking Cessation *(continued)*

Therapy	Dose	Max Dose
Nicotine transdermal patch		
Habitrol® Nicoderm CQ®	Adults: 21 mg/d x 4-6 weeks *then* 14 mg/d x 2-4 weeks *then* 7 mg/d x 2-4 weeks Adolescents (or <10 cigarettes/d): 7 mg/d x 6-8 weeks	1 patch/d
Nicotrol®	15 mg/d x 4-6 weeks	1 patch/d
ProStep®	22 mg/d x 4-8 weeks *then* 11 mg/d x 2-4 weeks	1 patch/d
Generic	7 mg, 14 mg, 21 mg	1 patch/d

fective in men, women, and various ethnic groups. The most common side effects are insomnia (30% to 40%), dry mouth (5% to 15%), and other minor adverse effects. A history of seizures is a contraindication to using bupropion. Table 7-9 lists treatment recommendations.

Instructions	Contraindications
Apply patch on awakening No smoking while on the patch Apply to a hairless area between neck and waist	• Angina, arrhythmias, immediately post MI • Continued use of tobacco products • Hypersensitivity to nicotine

(continued on next page)

MI = myocardial infarction

Dosage regimens should be appropriately adjusted for prescription vs OTC and for smokers who smoke more or less than 10 cigarettes a day.

UW Tobacco Cessation Guidelines. Available at: http://www.ctri.wisc.edu/HC.Providers/healthcare.htm.

Start bupropion SR at 150 mg per day for 3 days, then 150 mg b.i.d. for 8 to 12 weeks. The target quit date is usually 1 week after starting treatment. If after 4 weeks, the patient has not been able to stop smoking, continued therapy with bupropion SR may not be helpful. Other treat-

Table 7-9: Pharmacologic Therapy for Smoking Cessation *(continued)*

Therapy	Dose	Max Dose
Nicotine nasal spray* Nicotrol® NS	0.5 mg/nostril	5/hr or 40/d
Nicotine inhaler Nicotrol® Inhaler	6-16 cartridges/d x 12 weeks, then gradually reduce (if needed) x 6-12 weeks	16 cartridges/d
Bupropion Zyban®	150 mg/d x 3 weeks *then* 150 mg b.i.d. x 7-12 weeks	300 mg/d

MAOI = monoamine oxidase inhibitor

*Absorbed through the nasal mucosa; drug reaches the brain faster. This advantage makes the potential for dependence highest among nasal spray users; therefore, it is not used for more than 6 months.

Instructions	Contraindications
Potential for addiction Use 6 months or less	• See contraindications for nicotine transdermal patch
Inhale or puff through the mouth May inhale for up to 20 min Use 6 months or less	• See contraindications for nicotine transdermal patch
	• Administration with an MAOI, Wellbutrin®, Wellbutrin SR®, or any medication that contains bupropion • Current or prior diagnosis of bulimia or anorexia nervosa • Demonstrated allergic reaction to bupropion or other ingredients in formulation • Seizure disorder

Dosage regimens should be appropriately adjusted for prescription vs OTC and for smokers who smoke more or less than 10 cigarettes a day.

UW Tobacco Cessation Guidelines. Available at: http://www.ctri.wisc.edu/HC.Providers/healthcare.htm.

Table 7-10: Characteristics of Nicotine Replacement Products

- Nicotine patches are simpler to use than other forms of nicotine replacement and have fewer adherence problems. They generally have higher compliance rates than other nicotine replacement products, but combining a patch with other nicotine products may have higher cessation efficacy.[20] Patients should be instructed about appropriate use, including not smoking while using the patch, the appropriate dose, side effects, and follow-up.
- Nicotine spray is especially useful in heavily addicted smokers because of the speed of its delivery, the greater capacity for self-titration of dose, and the rapid increase in plasma nicotine concentration. Dosing should be individualized based on each patient's degree of nicotine dependence and the occurrence of symptoms of nicotine excess.
- Nicotine gum (4 mg) produces greater relief of symptoms for highly dependent smokers. Patients should be educated about the appropriate use of the gum, including chewing technique, avoiding acidic beverages for 15 minutes before and after chewing, and using enough gum to achieve benefit. The 4-mg gum has greater efficacy than the 2-mg gum.

ment options should be considered, such as intensive behavioral therapy or adding NRT. Treatment with bupropion SR for up to 12 months may be necessary to reduce risk of relapse in patients with a history of relapse.

Nicotine Replacement

The goal of NRT is to diminish physical withdrawal symptoms and cravings after smoking cessation. NRT reduces anxiety, irritability, and restlessness and improves cessation success rates by approximately twofold compared to placebo.[17] Clearly, the cardiotoxic effects of smoking are related to carbon monoxide and other adulterants, not to nicotine. Therefore, NRT is safe and does not increase cardiovascular events, even in high-risk patients.[18,19] Patients should be warned not to use tobacco products while undergoing NRT because of the risk of nicotine toxicity. Because NRT can be habit-forming, it is also important to counsel patients on how and when to stop the medication at the end of the effective dosing period. Table 7-10 gives details about available nicotine replacement products. For treatment recommendations on these products, see Table 7-9.

Special Precautions

Remind patients using the nicotine patch not to smoke while wearing the patch because of the risk of nicotine overdose. Symptoms of acute nicotine overdose include nausea, lightheadedness, upset stomach, and rapid heart rate. Table 7-11 lists other precautions related to using NRT.

Preventing Relapse

The greatest risk to smokers who are trying to stop smoking is relapse. More than 90% of those who attempt to stop smoking relapse on most attempts. This rate can be reduced with behavioral and pharmacologic therapy and with close follow-up, but most smokers will relapse on their first attempts to stop smoking. All former smokers are at risk of relapse, but some groups of patients are at higher risk than are others. Some predictors of relapse include high levels of nicotine dependence, high score on the Fagerstrom Test for Nicotine Dependence (Table 7-8), psychiatric comorbidity, and low levels of motivation to quit.

Table 7-11: Precautions for Nicotine Replacement Therapy

- The nicotine patch should be used for pregnant women only if the increased benefits of smoking cessation outweigh the risks of nicotine replacement and potential concurrent smoking.
- Although not an independent risk factor for acute myocardial infarction, the risks and benefits of nicotine replacement should be weighed in the following groups:
  - Patients in the immediate (within 4 weeks) postmyocardial infarction period
  - Patients with serious arrhythmias
  - Patients with severe or worsening angina pectoris
- Up to 50% of patients using the nicotine patch will have a mild and self-limiting local skin reaction that can worsen over the course of the therapy. Hydrocortisone (5%) or triamcinolone (0.5%) and patch rotation may reduce local reactions. Fewer than 5% of patients require discontinuation of patch treatment.
- The safety and efficacy of nicotine replacement in adolescent smokers have not been extensively evaluated. However, because nicotine itself has not been shown to be carcinogenic, delivering nicotine via patch or gum, which lack the carcinogens and toxins of cigarettes, is safer than continuing to smoke.
- The safety and efficacy of bupropion in the adolescent smoking population have not been established.
- Used and unused nicotine delivery systems should be kept out of the reach of children and pets. The amounts of nicotine that are tolerated by adult smokers can produce symptoms of poisoning and be potentially fatal to children.

Table 7-12: Topics to Discuss With a Patient Who Recently Quit Smoking

- The benefits, including potential health benefits, the patient may derive from smoking cessation
- Any success the patient has had in quitting (eg, duration of abstinence, reduction in withdrawal)
- The problems encountered or anticipated threats to maintaining abstinence (eg, depression, weight gain, alcohol, other tobacco users in the household)

When you encounter a patient who has recently quit smoking, reinforce the patient's decision to quit, review the benefits of quitting, and help him or her resolve any residual problems that might arise from quitting. Although relapse most often occurs early in the quitting process, patients may relapse months or even years after the quit date. Relapse interventions are especially important soon after quitting. They can be delivered during scheduled office visits, via telephone calls, or any time you encounter a former smoker. According to AHRQ guidelines, relapse prevention can be divided into two categories: minimal practice interventions and prescriptive interventions.

Minimal practice interventions should be part of every encounter with a patient who has recently quit smoking. Every ex-tobacco user should receive congratulations on any success and strong encouragement to remain abstinent. When encountering a recent quitter, it is a good idea to use open-ended questions designed to initiate patient problem solving. For example, you might ask, 'How has stopping tobacco use helped you?' You should also encourage the patient to actively discuss the topics listed in Table 7-12.

Table 7-13: Components of Prescriptive Relapse Prevention[5,6]

Problems	Responses
Lack of support for cessation	• Schedule follow-up visits or telephone calls with the patient. • Help the patient identify sources of support within his or her environment. • Refer the patient to an appropriate organization that offers cessation counseling or support.
Negative mood or depression	• If significant, provide counseling, prescribe appropriate medications, or refer the patient to a specialist.
Strong or prolonged withdrawal symptoms	• If the patient reports prolonged craving or other withdrawal symptoms, consider extending the use of an approved pharmacotherapy or adding or combining pharmacologic medications to reduce strong withdrawal symptoms.

Problems	Responses
Weight gain	• Recommend starting or increasing physical activity; discourage strict dieting. • Reassure the patient that some weight gain after quitting is common and appears to be self-limiting. • Emphasize the importance of a healthy diet. • Maintain the patient on pharmacotherapy known to delay weight gain (eg, bupropion SR or NRT, especially nicotine gum). • Refer the patient to a specialist or program.
Flagging motivation or feelings	• Reassure the patient that these feelings of deprivation are common. • Recommend rewarding activities. • Probe to ensure that the patient is not engaged in periodic tobacco use. • Emphasize that beginning to smoke (even a puff) will increase urges and make quitting more difficult.

NRT = nicotine replacement therapy

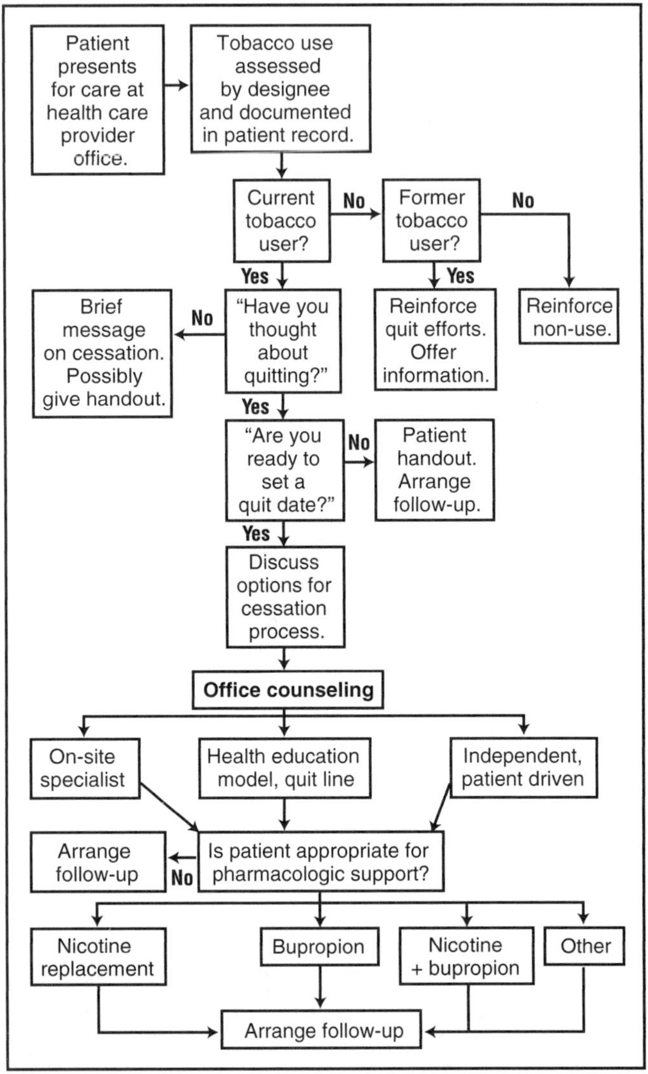

Figure 7-2: Adult and adolescent tobacco cessation clinical practice guidelines.[21]

Prescriptive relapse preventions are individualized based on information obtained about problems the patient has encountered in maintaining abstinence. Table 7-13 lists some specific problems patients may report and suggested responses.

Algorithm

Figure 7-2 summarizes the clinical practice guidelines presented in this chapter in a practical algorithm.

References

1. Goldstein M, Niaura R: Smoking. In Topol E, Califf R, Isner J, et al, eds: *Textbook of Cardiovascular Medicine*. Philadelphia, Lippincott Williams & Wilkins, 1998.

2. US Department of Health and Human Services: The Health Benefit of Smoking Cessation, a report of the Surgeon General. DHHS Publication no. (CDC) 90-8416. Rockville, MD, US Department of Health and Human Services, Public Health Service, Centers for Disease Control, 1990.

3. US Department of Health and Human Services: The Health Consequences of Smoking: Cardiovascular Disease. A report of the Surgeon General. Rockville, MD, US Department of Health and Human Services, 1983.

4. US Department of Health and Human Services: The Health Consequences of Smoking: Nicotine Addiction. A report of the Surgeon General. DHHS Publication no. (CDC) 88-8406. Rockville, MD, US Department of Health and Human Services, Public Health Service, Centers for Disease Control, 1988.

5. Fiore MC, Bailey WC, Cohen SJ, et al: Treating tobacco use and dependence. Clinical practice guideline. Rockville, MD: US Department of Health and Human Services. Public Health Service, June, 2000.

6. A clinical practice guideline for treating tobacco use and dependence: a US Public Health Service report. The Tobacco Use and Dependence Clinical Practice Guideline Panel, Staff and Consortium Representatives. *JAMA* 2000;283:3244-3254.

7. He J, Vupputuri S, Allen K, et al: Passive smoking and the risk of coronary heart disease—a meta-analysis of epidemiologic studies. *N Engl J Med* 1999;340:920-926.

8. Cigarette smoking among adults—United States, 2000. *MMWR Morb Mortal Wkly Rep* 2002;51:642-645.

9. Kannel W, McGee D, Castelli W: Latest perspectives on cigarette smoking and cardiovascular disease: the Framingham Study. *J Cardiac Rehabil* 1984;4:267-277.

10. Rea TD, Heckbert SR, Kaplan RC, et al: Smoking status and risk for recurrent coronary events after myocardial infarction. *Ann Intern Med* 2002;137:494-500.

11. Critchley JA, Capewell S: Mortality risk reduction associated with smoking cessation in patients with coronary heart disease: a systematic review. *JAMA* 2003;290:86-97.

12. US Public Health Service. Treating tobacco use and dependence—a systems approach. A guide for health care administrators, insurers, managed care organizations, and purchasers. November 2000. Accessed June 2003. Available at: http://www.surgeongeneral.gov/tobacco/systems.htm.

13. Hopkins DP, Briss PA, Ricard CJ, et al: Reviews of evidence regarding interventions to reduce tobacco use and exposure to environmental tobacco smoke. *Am J Prev Med* 2001; 20(suppl 2):16-66.

14. Mallin R: Smoking cessation: integration of behavioral and drug therapies. *Am Fam Physician* 2002;65:1107-1114.

15. Hurt RD, Sachs DP, Glover ED, et al: A comparison of sustained-release bupropion and placebo for smoking cessation. *N Engl J Med* 1997;337:1195-1202.

16. Hays JT, Ebbert JO: Bupropion sustained release for treatment of tobacco dependence. *Mayo Clin Proc* 2003;78:1020-1024.

17. Lancaster T, Stead L, Silagy C, et al: Effectiveness of interventions to help people stop smoking: findings from the Cochrane Library. *BMJ* 2000;321:355-358.

18. Joseph AM, Norman SM, Ferry LH, et al: The safety of transdermal nicotine as an aid to smoking cessation in patients with cardiac disease. *N Engl J Med* 1996;335:1792-1798.

19. Benowitz NL, Gourlay SG: Cardiovascular toxicity of nicotine: implications for nicotine replacement therapy. *J Am Coll Cardiol* 1997;29:1422-1431.

20. Rigotti NA: Clinical practice. Treatment of tobacco use and dependence. *N Engl J Med* 2002;346:506-512.

21. UW Health Tobacco Cessation Task Force: UW Health Tobacco Cessation Guidelines. Madison, WI, University of Wisconsin Medical Foundation, 2002.

CHAPTER 8

Overweight, Obesity, and the Metabolic Syndrome

Obesity is a major public health problem in the United States. It is strongly linked to cardiovascular disease (CVD), peripheral vascular disease, stroke, hypertension, and type 2 diabetes mellitus. In addition, obesity is associated with other chronic diseases, including sleep apnea, osteoarthritis, degenerative joint disease, gastroesophageal reflux disease, low back pain, depression, stress incontinence, and cancer.

The rates of overweight and obesity in the United States have risen dramatically in the last 20 years. In the 1970s, one in four adults was overweight; by the 1990s, that figure had increased to two of every three adults. Data from the 1999-2000 National Health and Nutrition Survey, the Centers for Disease Control and Prevention (CDC), and the National Center for Health Statistics indicate that approximately 130 million US adults older than 20 years—64.7 million men and 64.6 million women—are overweight or obese (Figure 8-1).[1] Overweight is defined as having a body mass index (BMI) of at least 25.0 kg/m^2. More than 30% of the adult population (26.4 million men and 34.8 million women) have a BMI of at least 30.0 kg/m^2, which is considered obese.[1]

Severe obesity (>100 lb or >45 kg overweight) quadrupled in prevalence from 1986 to 2000, to a current rate of 1 in 50 US adults.[2] The prevalence of a BMI greater than 50 increased by a factor of 5, from about 1 in 2,000 adults to 1 in 400.

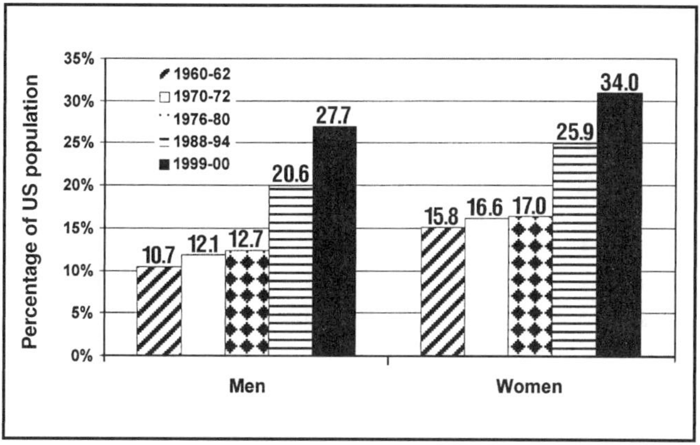

Figure 8-1: Age-adjusted prevalence of obesity in Americans aged 20 to 74 years by sex and survey. American Heart Association: Statistical Fact Sheet—Risk Factors. Overweight and obesity, 2001.

The growing number of overweight children and adolescents is even more alarming. According to American Heart Association (AHA) statistics, obesity rates have doubled in children (aged 6 to 11 years) and tripled in adolescents (aged 12 to 19 years) in the past 20 years. One in seven young people is obese, and one in three is overweight. An estimated 25% of children 5 to 10 years of age have high cholesterol, high blood pressure, or other early warning signs of heart disease. More than 80% of obese children will become obese adults and will be at risk for earlier onset of diabetes, coronary heart disease (CHD), and other complications of obesity. Type 2 diabetes in adolescents has increased 10-fold in the past decade. As a result, the lifetime risk of developing diabetes mellitus for a person born in the year 2000 is approximately 33% for men and 38% for women.[3] The life expectancy of individuals with diabetes is significantly reduced by approximately 12 to 14 life-years and 19 to 22 quality-adjusted life-years.

Obesity not only places individuals at higher risk for heart disease, but also aggravates known CHD risk factors. For example, it raises blood pressure, blood cholesterol, and triglyceride levels; lowers high-density lipoprotein (HDL) cholesterol; and can induce diabetes. The AHA therefore recognizes obesity as a major risk factor for CHD.

The Metabolic Syndrome

Health professionals need to be aware of the metabolic syndrome, a common syndrome that affects approximately 24% of US adults older than 30 years and more than 40% of US adults older than 60 years.[4] The metabolic syndrome, also known as insulin resistance syndrome (or, mistakenly, as syndrome X, which is used in cardiology to describe chest pain with angiographically normal coronary arteries), involves a cluster of risk factors that can lead to atherosclerosis and an increased risk for CVD and kidney disease. Central, or visceral, obesity and insulin resistance characterize the metabolic syndrome. Overweight individuals with the metabolic syndrome are at significantly greater risk of CVD than overweight individuals without it.[5]

The risk factors associated with the metabolic syndrome include hyperglycemia (fasting glucose >110 mg/dL); hyperinsulinemia; high blood pressure; abnormal low-density lipoprotein (LDL) cholesterol, high triglyceride, and low HDL levels; and abnormal lipoprotein densities. Because there is a high correlation between hypertriglyceridemia and increased abdominal visceral fat, Lemieux has proposed that the criteria for the syndrome be based on two variables called the 'hypertriglyceridemic waist': triglycerides >2.0 mmol/L (>158 mg/dL) and waist >90 cm.[6] These criteria can be used to diagnose the syndrome in most people, but recognition of the National Cholesterol Education Program Adult Treatment Panel III criteria cited in Table 8-1 is useful in reducing the risk of CVD.

The most sensitive measures of the metabolic syndrome are high triglycerides and low HDL cholesterol. Hyper-

Table 8-1: Clinical Identification of the Metabolic Syndrome

Risk Factor	Defining Level
Abdominal obesity	
Men	>102 cm (>40 in) waist circumference
Women	>88 cm (>35 in) waist circumference
Triglycerides	≥150 mg/dL
High-density lipoprotein cholesterol	
Men	<40 mg/dL
Women	<50 mg/dL
Blood pressure	≥130/85 mm Hg
Fasting glucose	≥110 mg/dL

National Cholesterol Education Program: *Detection, Evaluation, and Treatment of High Blood Cholesterol in Adults (Adult Treatment Panel III),* 2002. NIH Publication no. 02-5215.

tension and impaired fasting glucose are less sensitive, but the metabolic syndrome is almost certainly present when they are clustered with the other risk factors. All of the risk factors can be expressed in early life, can be associated with the development of obesity, and are usually evident by the third decade of life.[7] See Chapter 10 for more information on the clinical identification of the metabolic syndrome. This syndrome can even affect normal-weight individuals who have a disproportionate amount of weight in their abdomen. Approximately 5% of normal-weight adults, 22% of overweight adults, and 60% of obese adults have the metabolic syndrome.[8] Rates are far higher in minority populations.

There are several mechanisms whereby visceral obesity and insulin resistance increase the risk of CVD. Visceral adipose cells secrete fatty acids, which drain directly to the liver. This affects metabolism by reducing lipolysis and decreases insulin sensitivity. Increased levels of free fatty acids also increase triglyceride synthesis and decrease HDL cholesterol levels. Visceral adipose cells also secrete signaling proteins that alter metabolism, thus increasing production of inflammatory proteins associated with atherosclerosis; foster renal retention of sodium; and activate the sympathetic nervous system. Fibrinolysis and production of nitric oxide by vascular endothelium are reduced, while thrombotic risk and production of oxidizing lipoproteins are increased. The response of the liver to some of these signals is to release C-reactive protein, which further increases atherosclerotic risk.

Awareness of the metabolic syndrome is important, not only because of the significant risk of CVD, but also because weight loss can be beneficial in preventing or treating this syndrome to reduce the risk of further consequences. Two recent studies demonstrated that lifestyle changes in people with glucose intolerance reduced the development of diabetes mellitus by nearly 60%.[9,10] Useful patient education materials to prevent diabetes in high-risk patients are available at the National Diabetes Information Clearinghouse Web site: http://diabetes.niddk.nih.gov/index.htm.

Early intervention with vigorous lifestyle changes is critical to delaying or avoiding the multiple consequences of the metabolic syndrome. Failure to initiate these changes in a timely fashion may require the patient to take multiple medications to deal with each of the sequelae. Early recognition of the metabolic syndrome in individuals and families can lead to more comprehensive screening and earlier treatment. By recognizing how multiple risk factors can cluster and are synergistic, clinicians can direct medical therapy to those at highest risk and encourage affected patients to begin exercise programs and improve their dietary habits.[11] Table 8-2 lists steps that clinicians should follow to help their patients prevent the serious consequences associated with the metabolic syndrome.

Exercise and weight loss are highly effective in treating the metabolic syndrome, particularly in lowering diastolic blood pressure and levels of insulin and triglycerides.[12] Weight loss can prevent the development of diabetes in almost 60% of patients with glucose intolerance.[9,10] Metformin (Glucophage®) was shown to reduce the risk of developing diabetes in patients with glucose intolerance by 31%, which was only half as effective as exercise, healthy eating, and weight loss.[10] Treatment of the underlying risk factors is important to reduce CVD risk.

Treatment Approaches

Effective approaches for treating the metabolic syndrome include weight loss, decreased caloric intake, regular physical activity, pharmacologic treatment of metabolic abnormalities (eg, abnormal lipids, hypertension, diabetes), and direct treatment of insulin resistance. Newer approaches may include the thiazolidinediones and other agents that target peroxisome proliferator-activated receptor agonists, which simultaneously improve insulin resistance, glucose intolerance, elevated triglycerides, and low HDL-cholesterol levels. The usefulness of these new treatment approaches must still be assessed in outcome trials that evaluate the reduction in CVD events.

Preventing Obesity

The economic cost of obesity for individuals, families, and society as a whole is enormous. On a personal level, more than $16 million is spent on diet soda, $9 million is spent in health clubs, $600 million is spent in medically supervised programs, $5 million is spent on diet meals, $4 million is spent on exercise equipment, and $2 million

Table 8-2: AHA Recommendations for Preventing Serious Consequences of the Metabolic Syndrome

- Measure height, weight, body mass index, and waist circumference at the iliac crest as vital signs in adults. A waist circumference of >35 inches in a woman or >40 inches in a man makes the diagnosis of the metabolic syndrome highly likely.
- Monitor blood glucose, lipoproteins, and blood pressure.
- Encourage patients to achieve ideal body weight and increase physical activity, both of which are highly effective in improving insulin sensitivity, blood pressure, and lipoprotein levels.
- Treat diabetes and hyperlipidemia according to established guidelines (see Chapters 8 and 9).
- Choose drug therapy for hypertensive patients with care. Different agents have different effects on insulin sensitivity.

AHA = American Heart Association

is spent on commercial weight-reduction programs.[13] Nationally, the direct costs of CHD, type 2 diabetes mellitus, and hypertension attributed to obesity have been shown, in at least one study, to amount to $42.6 billion. The indirect costs of type 2 diabetes attributed to obesity were estimated at $30.7 billion. According to the AHA, the economic costs of weight-related disease become significant when a person's BMI is greater than 25 kg/m^2. In 1995, 5.7% ($99.2 million) of the US health expenditure was related to patients with a BMI of 29 kg/m^2.[13]

The primary challenge for the medical community is to determine how to reduce the growing prevalence of obesity and related serious health conditions in children and adults. Side effects of therapy, the tendency to regain weight once the lifestyle or pharmaceutical intervention is discontinued, and the potentially serious problems associated with surgery, which is the only permanent 'cure' for obesity, make it difficult to lose weight and maintain the loss. A preventive approach to obesity that begins in early childhood and focuses on eating and activity patterns and on health rather than appearance is clearly needed. The AHA recommends two strategies: the individual and family approach, which requires a multidisciplinary technique involving physicians, dietitians, nurses, and physical therapists; and the population approach, which should focus on areas such as the media, communities, and schools.

Most health-care professionals focus their attention on the individual approach, using the strategies examined in this chapter. It seems evident that it is time to also give serious consideration to a population approach to obesity. Unfortunately, the scientific community does not agree on feasible ways to address the problems associated with obesity. Although there is some room for optimism, the pharmacologic approach to treating obesity has had disappointing results. What the population approach requires is a systematic education of the public about the dangers of obesity. Health-care professionals need to work together with health agencies to disseminate this message to all population groups and to become involved in efforts to promote healthful behaviors, address the social factors that contribute to obesity, and initiate broad-scale attempts to modify these factors.

Assessing Obesity

Most importantly, patients and their families must recognize that they are obese and that the consequences are

$$\text{BMI} = \left(\frac{\text{Weight in pounds}}{(\text{Height in inches}) \times (\text{Height in inches})} \right) \times 703$$

$$\text{BMI} = \frac{\text{Weight in kilograms}}{(\text{Height in meters}) \times (\text{Height in meters})}$$

$$\text{BMI} = \left(\frac{\text{Weight in kilograms}}{(\text{Height in centimeters}) \times (\text{Height in centimeters})} \right) \times 10{,}000$$

Figure 8-2: Body mass index formulas for adults.

serious. Many patients do not recognize this issue, assuming that their weight is close to the societal norm and, therefore, that they are not at much increased risk. Excess body fat is generally the result of an excess intake of fat and total calories and a lack of physical activity. Although the definition of obesity, or being overweight, is still controversial, the BMI formula has become the most frequently used method for indirectly measuring body composition (Figure 8-2). This formula, which assesses body weight relative to height, is considered useful because, in most people, it has a high correlation to body fat. Online BMI calculators are available from the CDC Web site: http://www.cdc.gov/nccdphp/dnpa/bmi/calc-bmi.htm.

Although the BMI is a useful indirect measure of body composition, it does not take into account body fat distribution. Most of the comorbidities that link obesity to heart disease increase as BMI increases, but they are also related to body fat distribution. Visceral, or abdominal, obesity confers a significant risk of heart disease because of the increased risk of the metabolic syndrome. However, a BMI over 40 kg/m^2 is a highly significant risk for premature mortality. If BMI is greater than 40 kg/m^2 by age 35, the risk for premature mortality is five times greater than that of a healthy, normal-weight person. There is substantial evidence that an increased waist circumference or waist-to-hip ratio predicts comorbidities and mortality from obesity.[14,15] A waist circumference, measured at the iliac crest in exhalation, of greater than 40 inches in males or 35 inches in females is highly correlated with the metabolic syndrome (Figure 8-3).

More practical and more accurate methods of determining body composition that can be used in clinical settings include measurements of triceps and subscapular skin folds. Bioelectrical impedance, total body electrical conductivity methods, and dual-energy x-ray absorptiometry can also be used.

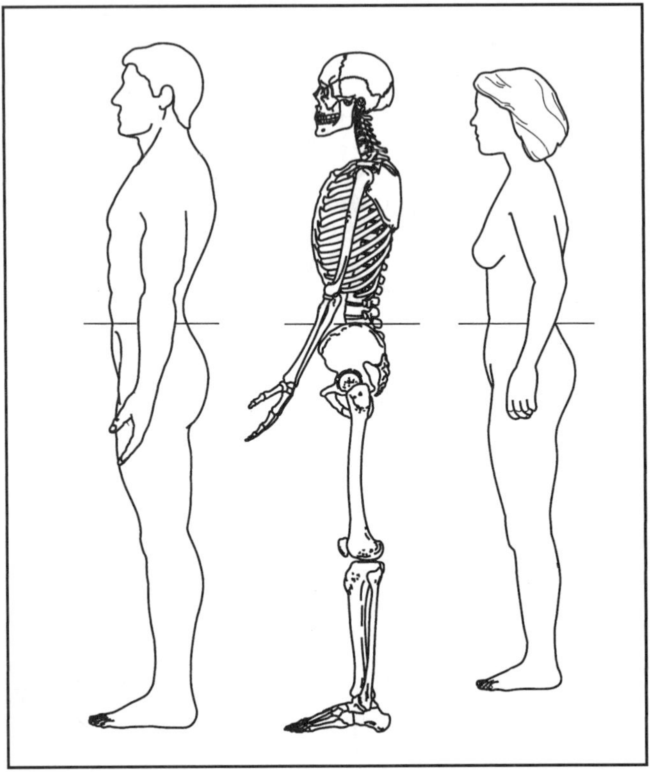

Figure 8-3: Waist measurement at the iliac crest.[16]

History

A valid and reliable measure of the patient's dietary intake is essential, one that takes into consideration the amount and types of food eaten. It can be compiled using food records, dietary recalls, and food frequency questionnaires. However, the strengths and weaknesses of these tools must be taken into account, and strategies should be developed to minimize the problems associated with them and to appropriately interpret the collected data.

An assessment of the patient's level of physical activity is also critical. Knowing the energy expended in physical activity is important to understanding why obesity occurs and how it can be treated. Approximately 40% of obesity is genetically determined. Although it is obvious that obesity can develop when there is an imbalance between energy intake and energy expenditure, the relative contributions of energy intake and energy expenditure to the development of obesity are not entirely clear. Total energy expenditure involves resting metabolic rate, which is the largest single component of energy expenditure; the thermic effect of food, which is the energy expenditure that occurs after eating; and the energy expended in physical activity, which varies according to differences in body mass. Encouraging patients to increase their energy expenditure by increasing physical activity is important in treating obesity.

Guidelines for Weight Management in Adults

Because obesity is a disorder and because recidivism is common, prevention of obesity through diet and regular physical activity is critical to maintaining cardiovascular health. The AHA has made weight loss to improve cardiovascular health a high priority and has developed guidelines for use by healthy adults. The guidelines are not recommended for people who are severely or morbidly obese, children younger than 18 years, or adults with preexisting illness or metabolic disorders. They focus on the health benefits of weight loss associated with a healthy lifestyle and emphasize the importance of weight management programs in which participants achieve and maintain realistic weight loss goals for a lifetime, based on the knowledge that even small weight losses may be associated with improvements in cardiovascular risk factors. In the Diabetes Prevention Program, modest weight loss (8 to 10 lb) and modest increases in physical activity (approximately 2.5 hours per week) resulted in substantial benefits in preventing diabetes (58% reduction).[10]

A weight management program is more likely to be effective if it is adapted to the individual characteristics of each participant. The following are some other factors to consider when deciding who should lose weight:

- People who could benefit medically should be targeted because the reduction of risk factors for heart disease, hypertension, and diabetes improves quality of life and reduces future health-care costs.
- People with a history of weight cycling should be encouraged to enroll in professionally supervised weight management programs that are based on realistic weight loss goals.
- People who want to use weight management programs just to achieve aesthetic changes should be discouraged because of the risk of weight cycling.
- People who are within 20% of their ideal body weight might be more appropriately encouraged to increase their physical activity and reduce their dietary fat intake to levels recommended for good health rather than to lose weight.
- People who are 20% heavier than their ideal body weight should be considered potential candidates for a weight loss program, especially if they are at risk for CHD, hypertension, or diabetes.
- People with abdominal obesity should be screened for unfavorable lipid profiles, high blood pressure, or abnormal glucose tolerance because abdominal obesity has been associated with increased risk for these problems.

In addition to being nutritionally sound, a good weight loss program must be based on a reduction of energy intake and an increase of energy expenditure through physical activity. Patients should be reminded that the amount and duration of physical activity are more important to weight loss than the intensity of the activity. In addition to being associated with more injuries, higher-intensity activities cannot be sustained for longer periods, resulting in fewer calories used per session. Patients should also understand that they must gradually increase physical activity to maintain

Table 8-3: AHA Guidelines for Weight Management in Adults

- Inform patient and obtain informed consent.
- Screen all patients beginning a weight management program, using an appropriate medical form to identify participants who need physician supervision.
- Have and follow guidelines that state who requires a physician evaluation before beginning the program.
- Ensure that the program is staffed by qualified personnel who have the education, training, and experience to provide necessary services.
- Identify reasonable weight loss goals, based on the reason needed (eg, reduce risk for cardiovascular disease, improve general health).
- Recommend that the patient participate in a maintenance program for at least 2 years.
- Evaluate the long-term effectiveness and safety of the program.
- Meet with the patient once a week during the initial phase, which generally lasts from 12 to 24 weeks.

AHA = American Heart Association

weight control because their energy needs will decrease as they lose weight and their resting metabolic rate declines. If they continue to consume the same amount of energy in food without increasing energy expenditure, weight loss will be slowed. In addition, fat calories are more easily and more completely stored in the body.

Table 8-4: Guide to Weight Loss Counseling

1. Assess Obesity Risk

- Height, weight, body mass index
- Waist circumference at iliac crest
- Cardiovascular disease risk factors

2. Ask About Readiness to Lose Weight

- Motivation
- Barriers and life stress
- Psychological illness history
- Prior weight loss attempts and outcomes
- Social support for weight loss

3. Advise About an Individualized Weight Loss Plan

- Mutual negotiation on plans
- Dietary plans (500 to 1,000 kcal/d deficit)
- Physical activity program (30 to 45 min/d of moderate activity on most, preferably all, days of the week)
- Behavior therapy goals (self monitoring, stimulus control, using family/social support)
- Pharmacotherapy or weight loss surgery plan?

4. Arrange for Follow-up

- Referral to weight loss program or specialist?
- Progress made or goals achieved?
- Assess setbacks and reconsider plans
- Maintain plan and follow-up

Exercise may have a preferential effect on reducing abdominal fat (visceral obesity) in people with the metabolic syndrome. In a study of patients with visceral obesity, despite only a 1.4-kg total body weight loss, a moderate-intensity exercise program resulted in a significant weight loss from visceral fat.[17] Based on several studies, it is estimated that a 5% weight loss for a 200-lb person, or 10 lb, can reduce triglycerides by 20%, raise HDL cholesterol by 15%, lower fasting glucose, and improve blood pressure by 12 mm Hg systolic and 9 mm Hg diastolic. Reducing weekly calories by just 500 to 1,000 calories per week will result in a weight loss of 1 lb per week. AHA guidelines listing the essential components of an effective weight management program for adults 18 years and older are presented in Table 8-3. According to the National Weight Loss Registry, those successful at long-term weight loss had three common long-term behaviors: eating a low-fat diet, monitoring their weight, and exercising regularly.[18] Table 8-4 contains a guide to weight loss counseling.

Diet and Nutrition

The nutritional recommendations for each patient's weight management program should be personalized to account for current eating habits, lifestyle, ethnicity and culture, energy needs, any diet prescription related to medical treatment, and potential nutrient-drug interactions. The daily energy intake prescribed should be adjusted so that the patient can achieve, but not exceed, the safe rate of weight loss. The dietary prescriptions should be consistent with the AHA dietary guidelines for healthy adults: (1) total fat intake should be less than 30% of total energy; (2) saturated fatty acid intake should be less than 10% of total energy; (3) polyunsaturated fatty acid intake should make up the rest of total fat intake, about 10% to 15% of total energy; and (4) cholesterol intake should be no more than 300 mg/d. The AHA dietary guidelines also include the recommendations for food selection listed in Table 8-5.

Table 8-5: AHA Dietary Recommendations

- No more than 5 to 8 teaspoons of fats and oils per day, including the fats used in cooking and baking and in salad dressings and spreads
- 6 oz or less of lean meat, fish, or skinless poultry
- No more than 3 or 4 egg yolks per week
- 2 to 4 servings of nonfat or low-fat milk and dairy products per day
- 5 or more servings of fruits and vegetables per day
- 6 or more servings of breads, cereals, rice, pasta, or other grains, and starchy vegetables per day

AHA = American Heart Association

Fad diets should be avoided unless there is ample scientific evidence to support their safety and efficacy with long-term outcomes, the same as for treatments of any other medical condition. Nearly always, fad diets lead to a 'yo-yo' cycle of weight loss and weight gain, resulting in the return to baseline weight, which frustrates the patient and results in reluctance to try other, rational methods. Low-carbohydrate, high-fat, high-protein diets (such as the Atkins diet) are an example. The Atkins diet has had only two recent studies of 6 and 12 months' duration, and these studies evaluated only weight loss and a few other metabolic parameters, not outcomes such as cardiovascular events.[19] The studies had 40% dropout rates and resulted in losses of 12 and 8 lb, respectively, which was only modestly greater than losses achieved through low-fat, high-nutritional-variety diets. The dropouts were not followed to determine whether they regained weight. People on diets such as the Atkins diet are eating foods that are high in saturated fats and cholesterol and low in fiber and other essential nutrients, and they may become accustomed to eating foods demonstrated to increase the progression of atherosclerosis and cardiovascular events. A scientific review of low-carbohydrate diets found that the only predictors of weight loss (which was modest) were total calories and diet duration; carbohydrate intake had no effect on the outcomes.[19] In contrast to these diets, diets that encourage variety; are high in fruits, vegetables, whole grains, and monounsaturated oils; and recommend low-fat meat and dairy products have been shown to lead to dramatic reductions in cardiovascular events for patients with CVD.[20,21]

Medical Treatment for Obesity

Medication should be considered for patients with a BMI greater than 30 kg/m^2 or with for those less-severe obesity but with comorbidities.[22,23] Only two medications are approved for medical treatment for weight loss: orlistat (Xenical®) and sibutramine (Meridia®). Topiramate (Topamax®) and zonisamide (Zonegran®) are under investigation, with promising short-term reports.[17]

Orlistat, a lipase inhibitor, works by decreasing intestinal fat absorption. This can lead to loose, greasy stools, with fecal soiling of clothes. Gastrointestinal side effects are greater if the meal contains more fat, which encourages the patient to eat less fat. In long-term clinical trials, gastrointestinal symptoms were significant during the first year but subsided during the second year.[13] Orlistat has moderate effects on weight loss, approximately 5% to 9% (10 to 12 pounds) for those who maintain treatment. Weight loss and decreased fat absorption with orlistat has been associated with improvements in the metabolic abnormalities associated with obesity, such as blood lipids, blood pressure, and glucose. It is recommended that the patient take a multivitamin daily because of the potential for fat-soluble vitamin loss. The medication dose is 120 mg three times daily. The monthly cost is approximately $100.

Sibutramine is a sympathomimetic medication that reduces food intake and increases thermogenesis. It inhibits the reuptake of norepinephrine, serotonin, and some dopamine at neuronal receptors, which likely reduces appetite. Clinical trials have demonstrated a 5% to 8% decrease in body weight for those who remain on the medication. The usual dose is 10 to 15 mg daily. It is associated with a 1- to 3-mm Hg increase in blood pressure and a 4- to 5-bpm increase in heart rate.[13] The sympathomimetic side effects make the medication contraindicated in patients with poorly controlled blood pressure, arrhythmias, congestive heart failure, prior stroke, or known CVD. Sibutramine is also not recommended for those with severe hepatic or renal dysfunction or anorexia nervosa. The price is $85 to $100 per month, depending on the dose.

Phentermine, released in the 1950s, is still used for appetite suppression and weight loss, but it has significant side effects, and its use is recommended only by weight loss specialists. Because it may be addictive, it is classified as a DEA Class IV drug and is recommended for short-term use only. It is an adrenergic-sympathomimetic stimulant that works similarly to amphetamines for weight loss. Phentermine should be avoided in patients with poorly controlled hypertension or with CVD. Phentermine was associated with cardiac valvular abnormalities when combined with fenfluramine. This combination, known as fen-phen, was removed from the market in the 1990s.

Obesity often has significant long-term metabolic consequences and should be considered a chronic disease condition. If the risks posed by obesity are serious enough to warrant the use of antiobesity drugs, it is likely that long-term use will be required. Even with current medical obesity treatments, weight loss is modest, with the best results reported as 10% to 15%.[24] The clinician should discuss the rationale for antiobesity drug use and the potential adverse effects with the patient and document the conversation in the patient's record. Cessation of medical

Table 8-6: Further Reading

- Anderson DA, Wadden TA: Treating the obese patient. Suggestions for primary care practice. *Arch Fam Med* 1999;8:156-167.
- Bravata DM, Sanders L, Huang J, et al: Efficacy and safety of low-carbohydrate diets: a systematic review. *JAMA* 2003;289:1837-1850.
- Freedman MR, King J, Kennedy E: Popular diets: a scientific review. *Obes Res* 2001;9(suppl 1): 1S-40S.
- Wadden TA, Foster GD: Behavioral treatment of obesity. *Med Clin North Am* 2000;84:441-461.
- Yanovski JA, Yanovski SZ: Treatment of pediatric and adolescent obesity. *JAMA* 2003;289:1851-1853.

therapy without significant behavioral change on the part of the patient will likely lead to a return of the lost body weight and metabolic abnormalities.

When a patient has a BMI greater than 35 kg/m^2 and comorbidities, gastrointestinal bypass surgery may be considered to reduce risk. For patients with a BMI higher than 40 kg/m^2, gastrointestinal surgery is a serious consideration, but the risk-benefit issues and prognosis should be assessed.[25] The safest and most effective surgery at present is the vertically banded gastric bypass surgery. Weight declines are approximately 40% at 1 year and 62% at 5 years.[26] Surgical complications can occur, particularly infection and deep-vein thrombosis, but morbidity is less than 10%, and mortality is less than 1%. Reoperation rates are as high as 15% to 20%, and many patients regain weight because of poor dietary compliance. Careful follow-up of patients after surgery is needed to ensure that they remain on a dietary program and that they avoid high caloric intake from liquids. Pain, dumping syndrome, and vitamin deficiencies caused by abnormal digestion are the primary side effects of surgery.[27] Monitoring of hematologic and electrolyte status, renal and liver functions, and vitamin status is recommended. Psychological issues, especially depression, must be addressed to achieve long-term success.

Newer laparoscopic techniques and gastric (appetite) pacemakers are under investigation.

Before beginning a weight management program involving more formal therapy, patients should sign a behavioral contract/consent form that describes the following:

- The number and format of contacts between the patient and the program leader;
- A reasonable weight goal;
- Estimated time frames for reaching the weight goal;
- Personal, health, and psychological benefits that can be achieved through weight loss;
- Physical and psychological risks associated with weight loss;
- The credentials of the people providing weight management supervision;
- The requirements for complying with the contractual conditions of the program; and
- The actual cost of treatment, including all products, services, supplements, and laboratory tests.

Managing Obesity in Children and Adolescents

As mentioned, there is a growing amount of evidence demonstrating an alarming increase in the prevalence of obesity beginning in childhood. The incidence of obesity in young people in the United States has tripled since 1970, from 5% to more than 15% in 2001. More than 20% of African-American and Hispanic adolescents are overweight. According to the AHA, at least 22% of 6- to 17-year-olds have diagnosable overweight. More than 80%

of obese children become obese adults.[28] There is now substantial evidence documenting that behaviors associated with risk factors for obesity, including dietary habits, physical activity behaviors, and the use of tobacco, are acquired in childhood. There is also ample evidence documenting the safety and efficacy of interventions to reduce risk factors in childhood.[29] Although there has not been (and probably never will be) a controlled trial comparing the effect of risk reductions beginning in childhood on the subsequent development of atherosclerotic disease, existing evidence indicates that primary prevention of atherosclerotic disease should begin in childhood.[29]

The AHA guidelines for cardiovascular health promotion relating to diet, smoking, and physical activity are the same for adults, children, and adolescents (see Chapters 5, 6, and 7 for details). AHA risk-factor-specific guidelines for identifying pediatric patients at high risk of future CVD are shown in Appendix A, as are goals of reducing risks in children and adolescents at high risk for future CVD and recommendations for achieving them. For more information on obesity, insulin resistance, diabetes, and cardiovascular risk in children, see the scientific statement from the AHA, endorsed by the American Diabetes Association.[30] Table 8-6 lists some other suggested references on the treatment of obesity.

References

1. American Heart Association: Statistical Fact Sheet—Risk Factors. Overweight and obesity. 2001. Available at: http://www.americanheart.org/presenter.jhtml?identifier=2016. Accessed August 28, 2003.

2. Sturm R: Increases in clinically severe obesity in the United States, 1986-2000. *Arch Intern Med* 2003;163:2146-2148.

3. Narayan KM, Boyle JP, Thompson TJ, et al: Lifetime risk for diabetes mellitus in the United States. *JAMA* 2003;290:1884-1890.

4. Brolin RE: Bariatric surgery and long-term control of morbid obesity. *JAMA* 2002;288:2793-2796.

5. Reaven GM: Importance of identifying the overweight patient who will benefit the most by losing weight. *Ann Intern Med* 2003;138:420-423.

6. Lemieux I, Pascot A, Couillard C, et al: Hypertriglyceridemic waist: a marker of the atherogenic metabolic triad (hyperinsulinemia; hyperapolipoprotein B; small, dense LDL) in men? *Circulation* 2000;102:179-184.

7. Austin MA, King MC, Vranizan KM, et al: Atherogenic lipoprotein phenotype. A proposed genetic marker for coronary heart disease risk. *Circulation* 1990;82:495-506.

8. Park YW, Zhu S, Palaniappan L, et al: The metabolic syndrome: prevalence and associated risk factor findings in the US population from the Third National Health and Nutrition Examination Survey, 1988-1994. *Arch Intern Med* 2003;163:427-436.

9. Tuomilehto J, Lindstrom J, Eriksson JG, et al: Prevention of type 2 diabetes mellitus by changes in lifestyle among subjects with impaired glucose intolerance. *N Engl J Med* 2001;344:1343-1350.

10. Knowler WC, Barrett-Connor E, Fowler SE, et al: Reduction in the incidence of type 2 diabetes with lifestyle intervention or metformin. *N Engl J Med* 2002:346:393-403.

11. McBride PE: Atherogenesis, families, and family practice: recognizing and treating an important syndrome [editorial]. *J Am Board Fam Pract* 1996;9:64-66.

12. Watkins LL, Sherwood A, Fineglos M, et al: Effects of exercise and weight loss on cardiac risk factors associated with syndrome X. *Arch Intern Med* 2003;163:1889-1895.

13. Krauss RM, Winston M, Fletcher BJ, et al: Obesity: impact on cardiovascular disease [online], 1998. Available at: http://www.americanheart.org/presenter.jhtml?identifier=1818. Accessed August 28, 2003.

14. Lapidus L, Bengtsson C, Larsson B, et al: Distribution of adipose tissue and risk of cardiovascular disease and death: a 12 year follow up of participants in the population study of women in Gothenburg, Sweden. *Br Med J (Clin Res Ed)* 1984;289:1257-1261.

15. Larsson B, Svardsudd K, Welin L, et al: Abdominal adipose tissue distribution, obesity, and risk of cardiovascular disease and death: 13 year follow up of participants in the study of men born in 1913. *Br Med J* 1984;288:1401-1404.

16. *Clinical Guidelines on the Identification, Evaluation, and Treatment of Overweight and Obesity in Adults. The Evidence Report.* NIH Publication no. 98-4083. National Heart, Lung, and Blood Institute, Bethesda, MD, 1998.

17. Irwin ML, Yasui Y, Ulrich CM, et al: Effect of exercise on total and intra-abdominal body fat in postmenopausal women: a randomized controlled trial. *JAMA* 2003;289:323-330.

18. Wing RR, Hill JO: Successful weight loss maintenance. *Annu Rev Nutr* 2001;21:323-341.

19. Foster GD, Wyatt HR, Hill JO, et al: A randomized trial of a low-carbohydrate diet for obesity. *N Engl J Med* 2003;348:2082-2090.

20. de Lorgeril M, Salen P, Martin JL, et al: Mediterranean diet, traditional risk factors, and the rate of cardiovascular complications after myocardial infarction: final report of the Lyon Diet Heart Study. *Circulation* 1999;99:779-785.

21. Singh RB, Dubnov G, Niaz MA, et al: Effect of an Indo-Mediterranean diet on progression of coronary artery disease in high risk patients (Indo-Mediterranean Diet Heart Study): a randomised single-blind trial. *Lancet* 2002;360:1455-1461.

22. Long-term pharmacotherapy in the management of obesity. National Task Force on the Prevention and Treatment of Obesity. *JAMA* 1996;276:1907-1915.

23. Guidelines for the approval and use of drugs to treat obesity. A position paper of The North American Association for the Study of Obesity. *Obes Res* 1995;3:473-478.

24. Yanovski SZ, Yanovski JA: Obesity. *N Engl J Med* 2002;346: 591-602.

25. Gastrointestinal surgery for severe obesity: National Institutes of Health Consensus Development Conference Statement. *Am J Clin Nutr* 1992;55(2 suppl):615S-619S.

26. Capella JF, Capella RF: The weight reduction operation of choice: vertical banded gastroplasty or gastric bypass? *Am J Surg* 1996;171:74-79.

27. Brolin RE: Bariatric surgery and long-term control of morbid obesity. *JAMA* 2002;288:2793-2796.

28. Whitaker RC, Wright JA, Pepe MS, et al: Predicting obesity in young adulthood from childhood and parental obesity. *N Engl J Med* 1997;337:869-873.

29. Kavey RE, Daniels SR, Lauer RM, et al: American Heart Association guidelines for primary prevention of atherosclerotic cardiovascular disease beginning in childhood. *Circulation* 2003;107:1562-1566.

30. Steinberger J, Daniels SR: Obesity, insulin resistance, diabetes, and cardiovascular risk in children: an American Heart Association scientific statement from the Atherosclerosis, Hypertension, and Obesity in the Young Committee (Council on Cardiovascular Disease in the Young) and the Diabetes Committee (Council on Nutrition, Physical Activity, and Metabolism). *Circulation* 2003;107:1448-1453.

CHAPTER 9

Diabetes Mellitus and Cardiovascular Disease Prevention

Aggressive cardiovascular disease (CVD) prevention strategies are necessary for all patients with diabetes mellitus. This is particularly true for those with type 2 diabetes because of the significant metabolic abnormalities that accompany this disease. The insulin resistance of type 2 diabetes is associated with obesity, dyslipidemia, hypertension, increased sympathetic system activity, a prothrombotic and proinflammatory state, and other risks for CVD.[1] Seven to 10 years after diagnosis, people with diabetes have the same accelerated rate of atherosclerosis, including a risk of coronary heart disease (CHD) events, as patients with a history of CVD. Patients with a history of type 2 diabetes and CHD have approximately a 50% 10-year CHD event risk.[2,3]

Approximately 17 million people in the United States have diabetes mellitus, and an estimated 95% have type 2 diabetes.[4] Based on fasting plasma glucose levels, approximately one third of all cases of type 2 diabetes (5 to 6 million people) are undiagnosed and untreated.[3] Almost 35 million Americans—20% of those in middle age and more than 35% of those in older age groups—have abnormal glucose tolerance. The incidence of diabetes is increasing in the United States, largely because of the epidemic of obesity and sedentary lifestyles. The age-adjusted prevalence of diabetes has risen markedly since 1960, when 2.6% of adults aged 45 years and older had diagnosed diabetes. By 1990, that number had grown to 7.0%.[5] By 2002, 12% of adults aged 45 to 64 years, 22% of those aged 65 to 74 years, and 19% of those older than 74 years had diabetes, according to the Centers for Disease Control and Prevention.[6]

Diabetes, particularly type 2 diabetes, has dramatically risen in children and adolescents, increasing the probability that they will develop premature CHD. The growing ethnic diversity in the United States—including groups who are more susceptible to type 2 diabetes, such as Hispanics, African Americans, Native Americans, and South Asians,[7]—is also contributing to the increasing prevalence of type 2 diabetes. It is estimated that the incidence of diabetes in the United States will double in the next decade.[8] The American Heart Association (AHA) has formally designated diabetes a major independent risk factor for coronary artery disease (CAD) based on facts such as the following: (1) the prevalence of all forms of CVD is markedly increased in people with diabetes; (2) people with type 2 diabetes are two to four times more likely to develop CHD than those without diabetes, and their prognosis for survival is worse; (3) some form of CVD is cited as the cause of death in approximately 65% of people with diabetes, and more than 80% have some complication of CHD in their lifetime;[7] (4) multivessel atherosclerosis is often present in patients with diabetes before symptoms occur and before treatment is started, and this delayed recognition often worsens the prognosis for survival; (5) patients with diabetes also have a high incidence of cardiomyopathy, and they are three times more likely to die from stroke than people without diabetes;[7] and (6) the incidence of peripheral arterial disease is twofold to fourfold higher in those with diabetes, and the risk for amputation more than 12 times higher for a diabetic patient.[8]

Screening and Assessment

New guidelines from the American Diabetes Association (ADA) allow a diagnosis of type 2 diabetes at a fasting glucose level of more than 125 mg/dL, which is lower than the level previously used. They also define glucose intolerance much more stringently (fasting glucose more than 100 mg/dL) because those with elevated fasting glucose have a high likelihood of developing diabetes mellitus.[9] The new recommendations and updated guidelines for the management of type 2 diabetes can be found on the Web at http://www.diabetes.org/diabetescare.

When assessing for diabetes, it is important to educate and involve the patient as much as possible. A survey in 2003 indicated that only 44% of adults with diabetes knew what hemoglobin A_{1c} (Hb A_{1c}) was, and 61% reported receiving some evaluation of diabetes in the previous 6 months. Among those who reported that they were aware of Hb A_{1c}, more than 50% did not know that a level of less than 7% indicated good control.

Because mortality from CVD is greater in individuals with diabetes, and because CHD risk factors are synergistic with diabetes in causing atherosclerosis, it is vital to evaluate patients with diabetes for major and predisposing risk factors and to aggressively pursue risk factor modification as a secondary prevention strategy.

Major Risk Factors

Identifying risk factors is an important first step in developing a risk-reduction plan for diabetic patients. Major risk factors for CVD in diabetic patients include cigarette smoking/tobacco use, hypertension, dyslipidemia, and hyperglycemia.

Lipoprotein analysis should clearly distinguish between elevated low-density lipoprotein cholesterol (LDL-C) concentrations and atherogenic dyslipidemia, as indicated by elevated triglycerides and low LDL-C and high-density lipoprotein cholesterol (HDL-C) levels. In patients with diabetes, because of the altered metabolism of insulin resistance, even borderline high-risk LDL-C levels (100 to 159 mg/dL) are of concern and require aggressive intervention (see Chapter 10). Also, because hyperglycemia alone is associated with increased risk for CVD, patients with other risk factors (eg, hypertension, smoking, dyslipidemia) are at further increased risk and require more aggressive intervention for all risk factors. Table 9-1 presents specific steps for evaluating major risk factors in patients with diabetes.

Predisposing Risk Factors

Predisposing risk factors can be important in individuals with diabetes, especially if they are extreme in their value, but they are not as predictive for CVD as the major risk factors. However, identification of predisposing risk factors can provide insight into the causes of major risk factors and is, therefore, an important aspect of risk assessment in patients with diabetes. Predisposing risk factors include obesity, physical inactivity, and family history of premature CVD. Abdominal obesity usually indicates the presence of insulin resistance (the metabolic syndrome).

Carefully assessing the status of each predisposing risk factor is an important first step in therapeutically modifying life habits. A positive family history of CVD or diabetes may indicate greater need for pharmacologic control of risk factors and often identifies family members who also need risk factor intervention. Table 9-2 presents specific steps for evaluating predisposing risk factors in patients with diabetes.

Emerging Risk Factors

Many new risk factors, including factors associated with metabolism, inflammation, and other aspects of atherosclerosis, are under investigation for their potential use in clinical practice. Research suggests that they have a role in the development of CHD, but they have not been definitively related to disease risk. They include high-sensitivity C-reactive protein, lipoprotein size and densities, lipoprotein (a), homocysteine, and other markers of in-

Table 9-1: Evaluation of Major Risk Factors in Diabetic Patients

Risk Factor	Evaluation
Cigarette smoking	*History:* Record current and past smoking duration (years of use) and intensity (number of cigarettes smoked per day); determine passive smoke exposure at home and at work.
Blood pressure	*History:* Record history of blood pressure (BP) and measures of treatment, including current and past antihypertensive agents. Also determine acquired factors affecting BP, such as body weight, physical activity level, sodium intake, and alcohol consumption. *Physical examination:* Define current BP from multiple measurements; measure BP supine, sitting, and standing in elderly patients; consider 24-hour automated, ambulatory BP monitoring in older patients to detect autonomic dysfunction, episodic hypertension, orthostatic hypertension, and resistant hypertension.

(continued on next page)

Table 9-1: Evaluation of Major Risk Factors in Diabetic Patients *(continued)*

Risk Factor	Evaluation
Serum lipids and lipoproteins	*History:* Assess dietary habits and alcohol intake, exercise habits, efforts to modify lifestyle habits, use of medications that influence lipoprotein levels, family history of premature vascular disease and dyslipidemia, and history of thyroid disorders or pancreatitis. *Physical examination:* Check for eruptive xanthomas and lipemia retinalis (signs of severe hypertriglyceridemia), tuberoeruptive xanthomas (sign of dysbetalipoproteinemia), xanthelasma (suggestive of hyperlipidemia), and signs of hypothyroidism. *Laboratory:* Measure fasting serum total cholesterol, triglyceride, low-density lipoprotein (LDL) cholesterol, and high-density lipoprotein cholesterol (optional: total apolipoprotein B*, lipoprotein (a), LDL size). Check thyroid, renal, and liver function.

Risk Factor	Evaluation
Albuminuria	Measure serum creatinine. Test urine, with a dipstick, for protein. If dipstick is negative, measure urine albumin-to-creatinine ratio in the first morning urine specimen.
Glycemic status	*History:* Record age of onset of hyperglycemia, course of diabetes management, family history of diabetes, and history of diabetic complications. *Physical examination:* Check cardiovascular status, retinopathy, and other diabetic complications. *Laboratory:* Fasting plasma glucose (FPG); hemoglobin A_{1c} (periodically); diabetes = FPG >126 mg/dL (x2); impaired fasting glucose = 110 to 126 mg/dL (x2).

* Total apolipoprotein B is especially useful if triglycerides are elevated but LDL cholesterol is in the normal range.

Table 9-2: Evaluation of Predisposing Risk Factors in Diabetic Patients

Risk Factor	Evaluation
Body weight and fat distribution	*History:* Assess history of body weight, age at onset of overweight, history of weight loss and weight gain. Assess eating and exercise habits, social and occupational factors affecting body weight, family support, history of body weight in family members in childhood and adulthood, and attitudes and motivation for weight control. *Physical examination:* Measure body weight (kg) and height (m); calculate body mass index (BMI) (kg/m^2); categorize body weight (BMI 25 or 29.9 = overweight; >30 = obese); measure waist circumference (abdominal obesity = >40 inches [102 cm] in men or >36 inches [88 cm] in women; borderline abdominal obesity in men, 88 to 102 cm).
Physical activity	*History:* Assess past and current levels of physical activity; ascertain activity on the job, participation in sports, regular walking, jogging, or swimming; in women, ask about activity in housework, child care; determine

Risk Factor	Evaluation
Physical activity *(continued)*	opportunities and available facilities for regular exercise. *Physical examination:* Assess level of cardiovascular fitness in cardiac rehabilitation facilities.
Family history	*History:* Assess family history for cardiovascular disease or sudden death. (Family history is positive if cardiovascular disease or sudden death occurred in first-degree male relative before age 55 years or first-degree female relative before age 65 years.) Determine presence or absence of other risk factors—high cholesterol levels, cigarette smoking, hypertension, diabetes—in first-degree relatives (biological parents, siblings, offspring). If possible, expand family tree to second-degree relatives (grandparents, uncles, aunts). Create a simple family tree. *Laboratory:* Measure glucose and lipids (cholesterol, triglycerides, and high-density lipoprotein cholesterol) in first-degree relatives.

flammation. Some are potential targets for screening and treatment, particularly in patients with diabetes, because they are associated with the abnormal metabolism found in these patients. See Chapter 12 for more details.

Clinical Evaluation

Studies have shown that patients with diabetes have an increased likelihood of sudden cardiac death and unrecognized myocardial infarction (MI).[10] The diagnosis of MI is commonly missed or delayed in patients with diabetes because the typical cardiac symptoms are often masked. Complications from acute ischemic syndromes, peripheral arterial disease, and advanced CVD are also more common in patients with diabetes than in those without.[11] Therefore, developing effective strategies for earlier detection of CVD can potentially reduce morbidity and mortality in patients with diabetes. In some patients with diabetes, detecting subclinical atherosclerosis and early clinical signs of CVD could lead to more effective primary prevention. Table 9-3 contains guidelines to primary prevention of CVD in patients with diabetes.

Table 9-4 presents a general approach to detecting clinical and subclinical CVD in hyperglycemic patients. Stress testing should be performed according to American College of Cardiology/AHA guidelines and with special considerations for exercise testing in patients with diabetes. Noninvasive evaluation of cardiac function in hyperglycemic patients who are suspected of having myocardial dysfunction may be useful in the cardiovascular management of some patients. Many patients with diabetes suffer from autonomic dysfunction that impairs their quality of life and predisposes them to life-threatening complications. Also, the finding of subclinical CVD indicates the need for more aggressive preventive measures. However, a recent report from the AHA, 'Prevention Conference VI: Diabetes and Cardiovascular Disease,' does not recommend routine noninvasive evaluation of cardiac function in asymptomatic patients. The authors' conclusion is based on the AHA recommendation that patients with diabetes belong in the same high-risk category as patients with known CVD, and therefore, "the results of noninvasive testing, whether negative or positive, would not change medical management."[11]

Evaluation of Renal Status

Chronic renal failure, a major clinical outcome in patients with diabetes, is more likely to develop in type 1 diabetes than in type 2 diabetes. However, the growing prevalence of type 2 diabetes has made this form of diabetes a major cause of end-stage renal disease (ESRD). Appropriately monitoring the renal status of diabetic patients to effectively intervene at the earliest signs of renal disease is therefore important. Because microalbuminuria indicates early diabetic nephropathy, the first step is testing for urine albumin and protein. For patients with type 1 diabetes, it is an indication of ongoing renal damage; in type 2 diabetes, it also suggests enhanced risk for CVD. The presence of macroalbuminuria, nephrotic-range proteinuria, or both predicts a decline in renal function. It may be useful to coordinate care of patients with macroalbuminuria with a nephrologist, who can help plan a strategy for preventing progression to ESRD. Table 9-5 outlines the steps for evaluating the renal status of patients with diabetes.

Diabetic Renal Disease

To reduce complications and progression of disease, patients with diabetic nephropathy should control their blood pressure to levels <125/75 mm Hg, using β-blockers if necessary; strictly control their blood glucose level (the Hb A_{1c} goal should be <7%); and restrict their dietary sodium and protein intake. Therapy with an angiotensin-converting enzyme (ACE) inhibitor or angiotensin receptor blocker should be initiated if tolerated. Target cholesterol goals are LDL-C <100 mg/dL and non-HDL-C <130

Table 9-3: Guide to Primary Prevention of Cardiovascular Disease in Diabetic Patients

Risk Intervention	Recommendations
Smoking Goal: complete cessation	• Ask about smoking status as part of routine evaluation. Reinforce nonsmoking status. • Strongly encourage patient and family to stop smoking. • Provide counseling, nicotine replacement, and formal cessation programs as appropriate.
Blood pressure control Goal: <130/80 mm Hg	• Measure blood pressure at each visit. Consider home blood pressure monitoring. • Promote lifestyle modification: weight control, physical activity, moderation in alcohol, moderate sodium restriction. • Consider blood pressure medication. If initial blood pressure ≥130/80 mm Hg, add blood pressure medication. Individualize therapy to patient's other requirements and characteristics.

Risk Intervention	Recommendations
Cholesterol management Primary goal: LDL-C <100 mg/dL (some authorities recommend LDL-C ≤70 mg/dL for diabetic patients with multiple risk factors). Rule out secondary causes of high LDL (liver function tests, thyroid function tests, urinalysis).	• Ask about dietary habits as part of routine evaluation. • Measure total and HDL-C and TG; estimate LDL-C. • Start AHA diet (≤30% fat, <7% saturated fat, <200 mg cholesterol) and weight control. • Consider adding drug therapy to diet therapy for LDL-C levels >100 mg/dL. • Suggested drug therapy for LDL-C levels >130 mg/dL (drug selection priority modified according to TG level): TG <150 mg/dL—statin or cholesterol absorption inhibitor TG 150-400 mg/dL—statin ± fibrate TG >400 mg/dL—consider combination therapy (statin + fibrate or statin + niacin) • If LDL-C goal not achieved, consider combination drug therapy. • Risk factors to consider for more aggressive LDL-lowering therapy (ie, LDL-C goal ≤70 mg/dL): age (men ≥45 y, women ≥55 y or postmenopause), hypertension, diabetes, smoking, HDL-C <40 mg/dL, family history of CHD in first-degree relatives (male relatives <55 y, female relatives <65 y).

(continued on next page)

Table 9-3: Guide to Primary Prevention of Cardiovascular Disease in Diabetic Patients *(continued)*

Risk Intervention	Recommendations
Cholesterol management *(continued)* Secondary goals: HDL-C >40 mg/dL TG <150 mg/dL	• HDL-C <40 mg/dL: emphasize weight management and physical activity, avoidance of cigarette smoking.
Glucose control Goal: near-normal fasting glucose Hb A_{1c} ≤1% above normal	• First-step therapy: weight reduction and exercise. • Second-step therapy: oral hypoglycemic agents (sulfonylureas, metformin, acarbose, TZD). • Third-step therapy: insulin therapy.
Antiplatelet agents	• Some authorities recommend aspirin 80 to 325 mg/d if not contraindicated for primary prevention in high-risk diabetic patients.
Physical activity Goal: increase amount; exercise regularly 3-4 times/week for 30 min	• Ask about physical activity status and exercise habits as part of routine examination. • Encourage 30 min of moderate-intensity exercise 3-4 times/week as well as increased physical activity in daily life habits for patients who are inactive. • Encourage regular exercise to improve conditioning and optimize fitness level.

Risk Intervention	Recommendations
Physical activity *(continued)*	• Advise medically supervised programs for those with low functional capacity and/or comorbidities. • Promote environmental factors conducive to health (eg, golf courses that permit walking).
Weight management Goal: achieve and maintain desirable BMI and waist circumference	• Measure patient's height, weight, BMI, and waist circumference at each visit as part of routine evaluation. • Desirable BMI range: 21 to 25 kg/m^2. Desirable waist circumference for men, <102 cm (<40 inches); for women, <88 cm (<36 inches). • Start weight management and physical activity as appropriate.

AHA = American Heart Association, BMI = body mass index, CHD = coronary heart disease, Hb A_{1c} = hemoglobin A_{1c}, HDL-C = high-density lipoprotein cholesterol, LDL-C = low-density lipoprotein cholesterol, TG = triglycerides, TZD = thiazolidinedione.

Table 9-4: Detecting Clinical and Subclinical Cardiovascular Disease in the Diabetic Patient

Clinical Approach	Guidelines
Stress testing for coronary heart disease (CHD)	• Consult American Heart Association guidelines for exercise treadmill testing. *Special considerations for diabetic patients:* • Blood pressure and heart rate responses are often blunted because of elevated resting heart rate. • Painless ST-segment depression is common. • Diagnostic specificity of ST-segment depression is often reduced because of previous silent myocardial infarction (MI), conduction abnormalities, and increased left ventricular (LV) mass. • Exercise or pharmacologic stress thallium (or technetium) perfusion scintigraphy is a favorable alternative for exercise. • Ambulatory electrocardiographic (ECG) monitoring for silent ischemia may be helpful in some patients but is not routinely recommended.

Clinical Approach	Guidelines
Noninvasive evaluation of cardiac function	• Perform echocardiography (with Doppler) and radionuclide ventriculography. *Special considerations for diabetic patients:* • Diastolic dysfunction is common in asymptomatic diabetic patients. • Diastolic dysfunction often precedes systolic dysfunction. • LV wall motion abnormalities suggest diabetic cardiomyopathy.
Evaluation of autonomic dysfunction	• Perform bedside evaluation of autonomic dysfunction. • Autonomic dysfunction is present if two or more of the following tests are abnormal: – Resting heart rate (supine) >100 bpm – Excess diastolic blood pressure response to hand-grip exercise – Abnormal expiratory/inspiratory RR-interval ratio – Postural hypotension • Significance of autonomic dysfunction in diabetic patients: – Carries poor prognosis (50% mortality in 5 years) – Sudden death is common; consider electrophysiologic study for syncope workup

(continued on next page)

Table 9-4: Detecting Clinical and Subclinical Cardiovascular Disease in the Diabetic Patient *(continued)*

Clinical Approach	Guidelines
Evaluation of autonomic dysfunction *(continued)*	– Aggravated complications after elective surgical procedures – Increased danger with general anesthesia
Detection of subclinical CVD	• *History:* Carefully assess for claudication, angina, and dyspnea on exertion, cerebrovascular disease. • *Physical examination:* Conduct routine cardiovascular examination. Assess for carotid and femoral artery bruits; evaluate peripheral artery pulses, and ratio of ankle-to-brachial artery systolic blood pressure (marker of subclinical peripheral vascular disease). • *Laboratory:* Check for microalbuminuria (see Table 9-1). • *ECG*: LV hypertrophy is a strong predictor of CHD morbidity and mortality. • *Electron beam computed tomography*: coronary calcium score is highly correlated with total coronary atherosclerosis burden (role in risk assessment is under investigation). • *Carotid ultrasound*: detects subclinical carotid atherosclerosis (role in risk assessment is under investigation).

Table 9-5: Evaluating Renal Status

Clinical Approach	Guidelines
Urine albumin and protein	• Screen yearly for microalbuminuria for 7 years after onset of diabetes in all hypertensive patients with type 1 or 2 diabetes; thereafter, test urine yearly for albumin. • Microalbuminuria: urine albumin 30 to 300 mg/d or 30 to 300 mg/g creatinine in the first morning urine specimen.* • Rule out other kidney diseases that cause proteinuria (macroalbuminuria, nephrotic syndrome). • Detect increases in urine albumin and protein. – Macroalbuminuria: urine protein >300 mg/d (or >300 mg/g creatinine) in the first morning urine specimen. – Nephrotic syndrome: urine protein >3 g/d. – If either is present, further renal evaluation is needed. • Patients with microalbuminuria, proteinuria, high serum creatinine level, or the nephrotic syndrome should be evaluated by a nephrologist.

(continued on next page)

Table 9-5: Evaluating Renal Status *(continued)*

Clinical Approach	Guidelines
Urinalysis	• The presence of hematuria, pyuria, and a large number of casts (eg, red blood cell casts, white blood cell casts, >2 granular casts per high-power field) is often an indication that a nondiabetic disease is also affecting the kidney. Such patients should be evaluated by a nephrologist to develop a treatment strategy if needed.
Blood pressure evaluation	• If hypertension is present, exclude secondary causes, including advancing renal insufficiency. • Treatment with ACE inhibitor may be preferred unless hyperkalemia or other complications are present.

Clinical Approach	Guidelines
Blood urea nitrogen, serum creatinine, and glomerular filtration rate (GFR)	• The blood urea nitrogen is affected by the degree of renal insufficiency and level of dietary protein and, therefore, is not a satisfactory estimate of renal function. • The serum creatinine becomes high only after >50% of kidney function is lost and, therefore, is not useful for detecting early renal insufficiency. A rising serum creatinine level indicates progressive renal failure, and a plot of the reciprocal of serum creatinine vs time is useful for tracking the progressive decline in renal function. • The GFR is the most accurate estimate of the degree of renal dysfunction, but it generally requires administration of a radioisotope and ≥4 hours of the patient's time. The loss of GFR also provides the most accurate estimate of the rate of loss of kidney function.

* Urine collections must be done when there is no complicating condition that can elevate protein excretion (eg, fever, heavy exercise, poor glucose control, heart failure, urinary tract infection). Certain drugs, including nonsteroidal anti-inflammatory drugs and angiotensin-converting enzyme (ACE) inhibitors, can depress albumin excretion.

mg/dL. If the renal disease is progressive, the patient should be referred to a nephrologist.

Managing Risk Factors

Modifying the major risk factors for CVD in patients with diabetes should begin at the time of diabetes diagnosis because more than 80% of the medical complications in diabetes are vascular. Evidence that controlling CVD risk factors will reduce onset of CVD and its complications in patients with diabetes is increasing. Because these patients have a high CVD risk, risk factor treatment, beginning with lifestyle interventions and introducing pharmacologic interventions when warranted, should be undertaken at the same time as glycemic control. Comprehensive medical intervention in patients with established atherosclerotic CVD extends overall survival; improves quality of life; decreases the need for intervention procedures, such as angioplasty and coronary artery bypass graft surgery; and reduces the incidence of subsequent MI.[12] Table 9-6 outlines the goals for risk factor management in patients with diabetes.

Lifestyle Interventions

The best time to intervene is before diabetes develops. Two impressive studies have demonstrated that lifestyle changes are highly effective in preventing diabetes in patients with glucose intolerance. The US Diabetes Prevention Program assessed the effectiveness of a case-management approach to lifestyle interventions (goal loss of 7% body weight) vs the use of metformin (Glucophage®, Glucophage XR®).[13] The lifestyle program resulted in a 58% reduction in the incidence of diabetes compared with usual care, while the rate of diabetes prevention with metformin was only 31%. In the Finnish Diabetes Prevention study, the lifestyle program also had a 58% reduction in diabetes incidence, replicating the results of the US study.[14] The best way to achieve the success of these programs is to get patients with newly diagnosed glucose intolerance or type 2 diabetes into a structured weight-loss lifestyle program that includes dietary education, exercise, individual counseling, and group support.

Most patients with type 2 diabetes need to lose weight, but there is no universal agreement on a single diet for patients with diabetes, other than an emphasis on reduced caloric intake. According to the ADA, there is no 'diabetic diet' or 'ADA diet.' Dietary counseling should be individualized based on body mass index, body fat, underlying diseases, taste preferences, and other differences between patients. Medical nutrition therapy for diabetes is best performed by a registered dietitian or other qualified nutrition specialist. Sustained efforts that result in significant weight loss (7% to 10% of total body weight) using appropriate dietary change (nutritional variety and adequate intake for health) cause sustained decreases in Hb A_{1c}. Saturated fat and cholesterol intake should be reduced to levels consistent with the national cholesterol guidelines (less than 7% saturated fat calories and less than 250 mg of dietary cholesterol per day). Total fat intake should range between 25% and 30% of calories but should be consistent with a weight loss pattern if the patient is overweight. A reduction in protein intake to less than 10% of calories may reduce the progression of renal disease in those with diabetic nephropathy. A high intake of fruits and vegetables is recommended.[15]

Exercise is the most underused therapy for diabetes and can result in substantial improvement in glucose control by increasing insulin sensitivity in patients with type 2 diabetes. When exercise results in weight loss, the cholesterol profile and blood pressure are also improved.

Cigarette smoking is a major risk factor for CVD. When a patient who smokes also has diabetes, his or her risk for CVD is increased 200% to 400%. Clinicians should make a major effort to help diabetic patients who smoke overcome their smoking habit. Chapter 7 presents some practical guidelines for smoking cessation.

Table 9-6: Goals for Risk Factor Management in Patients With Diabetes

Risk Factor	Goal of Therapy	Recommending Body
Cigarette smoking	Complete cessation	ADA
Blood pressure	<130/80 mm Hg	JNC 7 (NHLBI), ADA
LDL cholesterol	<100 mg/dL, <70 mg/dL (optional)	ATP III (NHLBI), ADA
Triglycerides (TG) 200-499 mg/dL	Non-HDL cholesterol <130 mg/dL, TG <150 mg/dL	ATP III (NHLBI)
HDL cholesterol <40 mg/dL	Raise HDL (no set goal)	ATP III (NHLBI)
Prothrombotic state	Low-dose aspirin therapy (patients with coronary heart disease and other high-risk patients)	ADA
Glucose	Hemoglobin A_{1c} <7%	ADA
Overweight and obesity (body mass index ≥25 kg/m²)	Lose 10% of body weight in 1 year	OEI (NHLBI)
Physical inactivity	Exercise prescription dependent on patient status	ADA

Risk Factor	Goal of Therapy	Recommending Body
Adverse nutrition	• For type 2 diabetes, the main goals are to achieve and maintain goals for plasma glucose, lipids, and blood pressure. • For patients with evidence of diabetic nephropathy, reducing protein intake to <10% of calories may slow progression of kidney disease. • Saturated fat should be reduced to ≤7% of total calories. Total fat can range between 25% and 35% of total calories. • High intake of fruits and vegetables is recommended.	ADA, AHA, and NHLBI ATP III, OEI, and JNC 7

ADA = American Diabetes Association; AHA = American Heart Association; ATP III = Adult Treatment Panel III; JNC = Joint National Committee on the Prevention, Detection, Evaluation, and Treatment of High Blood Pressure; NHLBI = National Heart, Lung, and Blood Institute; OEI = Obesity Education Initiative Expert Panel on Identification, Evaluation, and Treatment of Overweight and Obesity in Adults.

Diabetes Care

Routine follow-up care for diabetes is critical to prevent complications. Routine patient self-care and comprehensive medical care can enhance the reduction of infections, ophthalmic complications, renal disease, peripheral vascular disease, and CVD. Guidelines for comprehensive care are available from many sources, including the ADA. Comprehensive risk-reduction guidelines are presented in Table 9-7. Other resources can be found at the state level, such as the Essential Diabetes Mellitus Care Guidelines developed by the State of Wisconsin (http://www.dhfs.state.wi.us/health/diabetes/DBMCGuidelns.htm).

Pharmacologic Intervention

Control of hyperglycemia is essential in preventing microvascular disease. Patients with type 1 diabetes require insulin therapy to achieve good glycemic control. Type 1 diabetes mellitus care is complex and beyond the scope of this chapter. General care for type 2 diabetes is covered here because approximately 95% of diabetic patients have type 2 diabetes, and appropriate patient care can reduce macrovascular complications.

The goal Hb A_{1c} level is less than 7%.[16] The UK Prospective Diabetes Study (UKPDS) trial and the European Prospective Investigation of Cancer and Nutrition (EPIC) Norfolk cohort demonstrated that the lower the Hb A_{1c}, the lower the rate of cardiac events, cardiac mortality, and total mortality.[17]

There are now four classes of oral agents for treating type 2 diabetes: sulfonylureas, biguanides, α-glucosidase inhibitors, and thiazolidinediones (TZDs).

The medications fit into three different functional classes based on their effects: (1) increasing insulin function (insulin sensitizers); (2) increasing insulin release (insulin secretagogues), and (3) decreasing glucose absorption.

Insulin Sensitizers

There are two types of insulin sensitizers: metformin and the TZDs (pioglitazone [Actos®] and rosiglitazone [Avandia®]). One combination agent is available (rosiglitazone/metformin [Avandamet®]). Metformin's primary effect is to decrease hepatic glucose production. There is also some effect on insulin action in peripheral muscle, perhaps mediated through the reduction in free fatty acid. Because of these two effects, a small amount of weight loss, and other favorable effects, metformin is usually the first-line therapy. It is relatively inexpensive and has the best outcome data. However, metformin may have a limited duration of effectiveness, losing potency after approximately 4 to 5 years.

Metformin is the only oral agent with randomized clinical trial evidence of reducing macrovascular events when used to treat type 2 diabetes.[18] The use of metformin was associated with a reduction of total mortality and every type of CVD outcome in the UKPDS study.[18] In the UKPDS study, metformin had significantly better outcomes, including reduced CVD outcomes and all-cause mortality, than a combination of a sulfonylurea and insulin therapy.[18,19]

The major side effects of metformin are dose-related mild gastrointestinal effects (nausea, abdominal pain, diarrhea) in about one third of patients. These effects can be reduced by taking metformin with food and titrating the dose slowly. Rarely, metformin causes fatal lactic acidosis in patients with renal failure or insufficiency. A creatinine level higher than 1.4 mg/dL in women or 1.5 mg/dL in men or a creatinine clearance less than 60 mL/min is considered a contraindication to metformin. Metformin should also be avoided in patients older than 80 years and patients with liver disease, alcoholism, cardiomyopathy, congestive heart failure, or other conditions that predispose them to renal acidosis. Metformin should be withheld from patients undergoing surgery or administration of intravenous contrast medium.[20]

TZDs are an important development in diabetes care. They decrease free fatty acid production by 20% to 40%, which results in an improvement in muscle tissue insulin sensitivity. In addition, reduced free fatty acid improves β-cell function, which appears to be a significant benefit of the TZDs. The TZDs also have beneficial effects on a number of metabolic parameters, including raising HDL-C, improving lipoprotein densities, and reducing inflammation. TZDs may raise LDL-C, but this usually involves shifting the smaller, more dense atherogenic particles to less atherogenic particles. TZDs can cause significant weight gain, but much of this seems to be from peripheral edema.

Glucose Absorption Inhibitors

There are two medications that fit this category: acarbose (Prandase®, Precose®) and miglitol (Glyset®). These medications reduce postprandial glucose levels by inhibiting carbohydrate absorption in the intestine. They do not cause hypoglycemia or weight changes. However, these agents are not widely used because they affect postprandial glucose levels and have significant gastrointestinal side effects (bloating, abdominal pain, diarrhea).

Insulin Secretagogues

Sulfonylureas (glimepiride [Amaryl®], glyburide [Diaβeta®, Glynase Pres Tab®, Micronase®], chlorpropamide [Diabinese®], glipizide [Glucotrol®]) were the only oral agents available from 1954 to 1994. Their primary action is to increase insulin secretion. Because hyperinsulinemia is a problem for most patients with type 2 diabetes, sulfonylureas are not a preferred initial treatment. Sulfonylureas have no proven benefit related to cardiovascular outcomes in patients with diabetes, and there is some evidence of harm.[1] The potential adverse effects associated with sulfonylureas include weight gain, increased insulin levels, diminished endothelial function, and increased vasoconstriction. In addition, patients with

Table 9-7: Guide to Comprehensive Risk Reduction for Diabetic Patients With Coronary and Other Vascular Disease

Risk Intervention	Recommendations
Smoking Goal: complete cessation	• Strongly encourage patient and family to stop smoking. • Provide counseling, nicotine replacement, and formal cessation programs as appropriate.
Blood pressure control Goal: <130/80 mm Hg	• Initiate lifestyle modification—weight control, physical activity, alcohol moderation, moderate sodium restriction—in all patients with blood pressure ≥130 mm Hg systolic or ≥80 mm Hg diastolic. • Add blood pressure medication individualized to patient requirements and characteristics (eg, age, race, need for drugs with specific benefits) if blood pressure is not <130 mm Hg systolic or <80 mm Hg diastolic.

(continued on next page)

Table 9-7: Guide to Comprehensive Risk Reduction for Diabetic Patients With Coronary and Other Vascular Disease *(continued)*

Risk Intervention	Recommendations
Lipid management Primary goal: LDL-C <70 mg/dL	• Start AHA diet (≤30% fat, <7% saturated fat, <200 mg/d cholesterol) in all patients. • Assess fasting lipid profile. • Immediately start cholesterol-lowering drugs when baseline LDL-C >130 mg/dL.
Secondary goals: HDL-C >35 mg/dL TG <150 mg/dL	• LDL-C 100-129 mg/dL: *consider* adding following drug therapy for TG to diet; LDL-C ≥130 mg/dL: *add* following drug therapy for TG to diet: – TG <150 mg/dL—statin or cholesterol absorption inhibitor – TG 150-400 mg/dL—statin, statin + fibrate, or statin + niacin – TG >400 mg/dL—consider combined therapy (statin + fibrate or statin + niacin) – HDL-C <40 mg/dL: emphasize weight management and physical activity; advise smoking cessation.
Glucose control Goal: near-normal fasting glucose Goal: Hb A_{1c} ≤1% above normal	• First-step therapy: weight reduction and exercise. • Second-step therapy: oral hypoglycemic agents (sulfonylureas, metformin, acarbose, TZD). • Third-step therapy: insulin therapy.

Risk Intervention	Recommendations
Physical activity Goal: minimum goal 30 min 3-4 times/week	• Assess risk, preferably with exercise test, to guide prescription. • Encourage minimum of 30 to 60 min of moderate-intensity activity (walking, jogging, cycling, or other aerobic activity) 3-4 times/week, supplemented by an increase in daily lifestyle activities (eg, walking breaks at work, using stairs, gardening, household work). • Maximum benefit 5 to 6 hours a week. • Advise medically supervised programs for moderate- to high-risk patients.
Weight management	• Start intensive dietary therapy and appropriate physical activity, as outlined above, in patients whose BMI is ≥ 25 kg/m^2. • Particularly emphasize need for weight loss in patients with hypertension, elevated TG, or elevated glucose levels.
Antiplatelet agents/ anticoagulants	• Start aspirin 80 to 325 mg/d if not contraindicated. • Manage warfarin to international normalized ratio 2.0-3.5 for post-MI patients not able to take aspirin.

(continued on next page)

Table 9-7: Guide to Comprehensive Risk Reduction for Diabetic Patients With Coronary and Other Vascular Disease *(continued)*

Risk Intervention	Recommendations
ACE inhibitors in post-MI patients	• Start early in stable, high-risk post-MI patients (anterior MI, previous MI, Killip class II [S3 gallop, rales, radiographic congestive heart failure). • Continue indefinitely for all with left ventricular dysfunction (ejection fraction ≤40%) or symptoms of failure. • Use as needed to manage blood pressure or symptoms in all other patients.
β-Blockers	• Start in high-risk post-MI patients (arrhythmia, left ventricular dysfunction, inducible ischemia) at 5 to 28 days. • Continue 6 months minimum. • Observe usual contraindications. Appropriate use of β-blockers not contraindicated in patients with diabetes. • Use as needed to manage angina, rhythm, or blood pressure in all other patients.

AHA = American Heart Association, ACE = angiotensin-converting enzyme, BMI = body mass index, Hb A_{1c} = hemoglobin A_{1c}, HDL-C = high-density lipoprotein cholesterol, LDL-C = low-density lipoprotein cholesterol, MI = myocardial infarction, TG = triglycerides, TZD = thiazolidinedione.

diabetes who take sulfonylureas have a predisposition to arrhythmias and are more likely to have unfavorable outcomes after CVD events.[1] Sulfonylureas are excreted significantly by the kidneys, so caution is recommended in patients with renal insufficiency.

The primary side effect associated with sulfonylureas that causes the greatest concern is hypoglycemia. Glyburide seems to have a higher rate of hypoglycemia than other oral agents. Weight gain is relatively common but variable.

The nonsulfonylurea secretagogues, repaglinide (Prandin®) and nateglinide (Starlix®), also increase insulin secretion. These agents are taken at each meal and carry less risk of hypoglycemia. They are primarily metabolized in the liver, so they can be more safely used in patients with renal insufficiency. In one study, repaglinide was associated with less progression of carotid atherosclerosis than glyburide.[21] They are significantly more expensive than sulfonylureas.

Insulin

Insulin is the oldest of the hypoglycemic agents. Higher doses nearly always result in lower glucose levels. The risks associated with insulin use include weight gain, hypoglycemia, and the need for increased insulin dosages. This is obviously the treatment of choice for type 1 diabetes. It is also used as a late-stage treatment for type 2 diabetes. Once-daily injections of intermediate- to long-acting insulin at breakfast and/or at bedtime are usually the initial treatment. Twice-daily combinations of intermediate- and rapid-acting insulin are frequently used to reduce glucose variability.

Oral Diabetes Agents and CVD Risk

Sulfonylureas were associated with an increased risk of CVD in the University Group Diabetes Program results, published in the 1970s.[22,23] This concern was abated by one of the UKPDS studies, which showed a decreased event rate with sulfonylureas when used with insulin. However, the CVD rate increased when sulfonylureas were used in conjunction with metformin.[17,18] Therefore, because of their initial action of increasing insulin secretion in hyperinsulinemic patients, their interference with myocardial ischemic preconditioning, and their lack of proven benefit in reducing CVD events, sulfonylureas are not recommended as first-line therapy for patients with type 2 diabetes and insulin resistance.

Because of the evidence supporting metformin, it is usually first-line therapy, especially in overweight, insulin-resistant patients. Occasionally, a patient presenting with type 2 diabetes will be lean and insulinopenic, but this is usually after the patient has had the disease for many years. Sulfonylureas, which promote insulin secretion, may be indicated in such patients. Patients with renal impairment who are not good candidates for metformin or who do not respond to metformin therapy because of insulin resistance should be considered for a TZD. Patients with extreme elevations of fasting glucose (higher than 300 mg/dL) and symptoms of hyperglycemia may need to be considered for insulin therapy. Ultimately, many patients with type 2 diabetes will need to be treated with a combination of oral agents to delay complications, and they may eventually require insulin therapy to achieve adequate hypoglycemic control.

Algorithms

A treatment algorithm for patients with type 2 diabetes is presented in Figure 9-1. Some of the oral hypoglycemic medications can have significant benefits in the overall metabolic profile for patients with type 2 diabetes. Metformin and the TZDs usually reduce triglycerides and LDL-C, and TZDs have a modest HDL-C-raising effect.

Medical Risk Reduction for CVD and Diabetes

Other medications that are routinely used for risk management in patients with CVD should be used to reduce the risk of coronary and other vascular diseases in patients who have diabetes.

Antiplatelet agents are routinely used in patients with atherosclerotic CVD and can be used in patients with diabetes who have established CVD. Caution is advised if the patient is at risk for hemorrhagic complications, such as hemorrhagic retinopathy or hemorrhagic stroke.

β-Blockers, which reduce cardiovascular mortality after MI, may be especially effective in patients with diabetes who are at risk for symptomatic ischemic episodes secondary to increased sympathetic activity.[24] However, β-blockers are often relatively contraindicated for patients with diabetes because they may raise glucose levels and may block tachycardia during hypoglycemia. However, these are not usually clinically significant issues in the well-controlled diabetic patient.

ACE inhibitors are widely prescribed following a heart attack to favorably influence myocardial remodeling and fibrosis. They should be continued indefinitely in all patients with symptoms of heart failure and in those with reduced left ventricular ejection fraction. They are recommended in patients with diabetes to reduce renal dysfunction (if renal function is not acutely worsened with this treatment). See Chapter 11 for information on β-blockers and ACE inhibitors.

Cholesterol medications (particularly statins) should also be considered as a preventive measure in patients with diabetes. In trials of these medications, diabetic patients have received considerable benefit in both primary and secondary prevention. Diabetes mellitus is considered a CHD risk equivalent in the National Cholesterol Education Program Adult Treatment Panel III guidelines, which set the LDL-C goal at less than 100 mg/dL for diabetic patients. Treatment of the specific cholesterol disorder with the appropriate cholesterol medication(s) is indicated (see Chapter 10 for information on cholesterol-lowering agents).

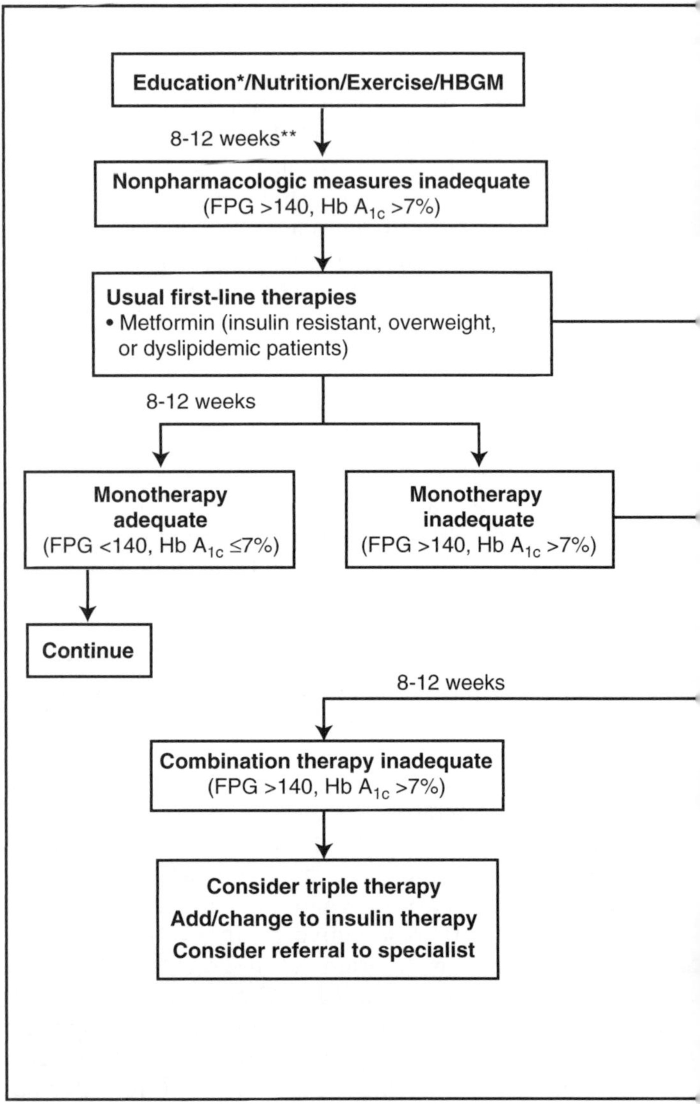

Figure 9-1: Treatment algorithm for type 2 diabetes.

Alternative first-line therapies

- AGIs (postprandial hyperglycemic patients)
- TZDs (insulin resistant or renally impaired patients)
- Meglitinides (patients with sulfa allergy or erratic meals)
- Insulin (if blood sugar >300 and patient symptomatic)
- Sulfonylurea (insulinopenic or lean patients)

Initiate oral combination therapy
(metformin + sulfonylurea)

Alternative combination therapy:

- TZD + sulfonylurea
- Metformin + TZD
- Metformin + meglitinide
- AGIs + any other agents

AGI = α-glucosidase inhibitor,

FPG = fasting plasma glucose,

Hb A_{1c} = hemoglobin A_{1c},

HBGM = home blood glucose monitoring,

TZD = thiazolidinedione.

* Refer to local diabetes education programs or diabetes educators.

** If glucose is consistently >250 and patient is symptomatic, may initiate therapy earlier.

References

1. O'Keefe JH Jr, Miles JM, Harris WH, et al: Improving the adverse cardiovascular prognosis of type 2 diabetes. *Mayo Clin Proc* 1999;74:171-180.

2. Haffner SM, Lehto S, Ronnemaa T, et al: Mortality from coronary heart disease in subjects with type 2 diabetes and in nondiabetic subjects with and without prior myocardial infarction. *N Engl J Med* 1998;339:229-234.

3. Howard BV, Rodriguez BL, Bennett PH, et al: Prevention Conference VI: diabetes and cardiovascular disease: Writing Group I: epidemiology. *Circulation* 2002;105:e132-e137.

4. Harris MI, Flegal KM, Cowie CC, et al: Prevalence of diabetes, impaired fasting glucose, and impaired glucose tolerance in U.S. adults. The Third National Health and Nutrition Examination Survey, 1988-1994. *Diabetes Care* 1998;21:518-524.

5. Harris MJ, Cowie CC, Stern MP, et al: *Diabetes in America.* 2nd ed. Bethesda, MD, National Institutes of Health, National Institute of Diabetes and Digestive and Kidney Diseases, 1995. NIH Publication No. 95-1468.

6. Centers for Disease Control and Prevention: Prevalence of diabetes. Number and percent of U.S. population with diagnosed diabetes. Available at: http://www.cdc.gov/diabetes/statistics/prev/national/index.htm. Accessed May 13, 2005.

7. Carter JS, Pugh JA, Monterrosa A: Non-insulin-dependent diabetes mellitus in minorities in the United States. *Ann Intern Med* 1996;125:221-232.

8. Whelton PK, Appel LJ, Espeland MA, et al: Sodium reduction and weight loss in the treatment of hypertension in older persons: a randomized controlled trial of nonpharmacologic interventions in the elderly (TONE). TONE Collaborative Research Group. *JAMA* 1998;279:839-846. Erratum in: *JAMA* 1998; 279:1954.

9. Genuth S, Alberti KG, Bennett P, et al: Follow-up report on the diagnosis of diabetes mellitus. *Diabetes Care* 2003;26: 3160-3167.

10. Nesto RW, Phillips RT: Asymptomatic myocardial ischemia in diabetic patients. *Am J Med* 1986;80:40-47.

11. Redberg RF, Greenland P, Foster V, et al: Prevention Conference VI: Diabetes and Cardiovascular Disease. Writing Group III:

risk assessment in persons with diabetes. *Circulation* 2002;105: e144-e152.

12. Smith SC Jr, Blair SN, Criqui MH, et al: Preventing heart attack and death in patients with coronary disease. *Circulation* 1995; 92:2-4.

13. Knowler WC, Barrett-Connor E, Fowler SE, et al: Reduction in the incidence of type 2 diabetes with lifestyle intervention or metformin. *N Engl J Med* 2002;346:393-403.

14. Tuomilehto J, Lindstrom J, Eriksson JG, et al: Prevention of type 2 diabetes mellitus by changes in lifestyle among subjects with impaired glucose tolerance. *N Engl J Med* 2001;344:1343-1350.

15. Grundy SM, Benjamin IJ, Burke GL, et al: Diabetes and cardiovascular disease: a statement for healthcare professionals from the American Heart Association. *Circulation* 1999;100:1134-1146. Erratum in: *Circulation* 2000;101:1629-1631.

16. Standards of medical care for patients with diabetes mellitus. *Diabetes Care* 2002;25(suppl):S33-S49.

17. Khaw KT, Wareham N, Luben R, et al: Glycated haemoglobin, diabetes, and mortality in men in Norfolk cohort of European Prospective Investigation of Cancer and Nutrition (EPIC-Norfolk). *BMJ* 2001;322:15-18.

18. Intensive blood-glucose control with sulfonylureas or insulin compared with conventional treatment and risk of complications in patients with type 2 diabetes (UKPDS 33). UK Prospective Diabetes Study (UKPDS) Group. *Lancet* 1998;352:837-853.

19. Effect of intensive blood-glucose control with metformin on complications in overweight patients with type 2 diabetes (UKPDS 34). UK Prospective Diabetes Study (UKPDS) Group. *Lancet* 1998; 352:854-865.

20. Zangeneh F, Kudva YC, Basu A: Insulin sensitizers. *Mayo Clin Proc* 2003;78:471-479.

21. Esposito K, Giiugliano D, Nappo F, et al: Regression of carotid atherosclerosis by control of postprandial hyperglycemia in type 2 diabetes mellitus. *Circulation* 2004;110:214-219.

22. Meinert CL, Knatterud GL, Prout TE, et al: A study of the effects of hypoglycemic agents on vascular complications in patients with adult-onset diabetes. II. Mortality results. *Diabetes* 1970; 19(suppl):789-830.

23. U.K. Prospective Diabetes Study 16. Overview of 6 years' therapy of type II diabetes: a progressive disease. U.K. Prospective Diabetes Study Group. *Diabetes* 1995;44:1249-1258.

24. Beckman JA, Creager MA, Libby P: Diabetes and atherosclerosis: epidemiology, pathophysiology, and management. *JAMA* 2002;287:2570-2581.

CHAPTER 10

Dyslipidemias

Cholesterol treatment is critical to atherosclerosis prevention and treatment.[1] Numerous primary and secondary prevention trials have demonstrated that treatment of lipoprotein disorders stabilizes plaques, improves endothelial function, prevents atherosclerotic lesion formation, and regresses existing plaques (Table 10-1). These processes reduce coronary heart disease (CHD) symptoms, adverse clinical events, and CHD mortality. For example, data from the Air Force/Texas Coronary Atherosclerosis Prevention Study (AFCAPS/TexCAPS),[2] published in 1998, demonstrated a 40% reduction in fatal and nonfatal coronary events and a 25% reduction in myocardial infarctions (MIs) and cardiac deaths in 6,605 persons with low-density lipoprotein cholesterol (LDL-C) levels greater than 130 mg/dL. Study participants, including 997 women and patients as old as 78 years, were randomized to receive either lovastatin (Mevacor®, Altocor™) or placebo therapy and were followed for an average of 5.2 years. Many other studies also support the effectiveness of lipid management in preventing CHD.

Dyslipidemias, including lipoprotein deficiencies or overproduction, are common clinical problems in family practice. An estimated 25% to 30% of adults in the United States have total cholesterol (TC) levels of 240 mg/dL or higher, and more than half of all Americans have a TC level that exceeds 200 mg/dL.[1] During the next several decades, the prevalence of CHD and the number of pa-

Table 10-1: Representative Clinical Trials for Cholesterol Treatment

Study	N	Years
Primary Prevention		
AFCAPS/ TexCAPS[2]	6,605	4.8
Helsinki Heart Study[3]	4,081	5
LRC-CPPT[4]	3,806	7.4
WOSCOPS[5]	6,595	4.9
ASCOT[6]	19,000	3.5
Secondary Prevention		
Lyon Diet Heart Study[7]	605	2.2
Indo-Mediterranean[8]	1,000	2
DART[9]	2,033	2
4S[10]	4,444	5.4
HPS[11]	20,536 (CHD, DM, or HTN)	5.5
CDP[12]	1,119	15
FATS[13]	146	2.5

Medication	Results
lovastatin	26%-36% event reduction (NNT=58)
gemfibrozil	34% event reduction (71% if TG >200)
cholestyramine	19% event reduction
pravastatin	31%-32% event reduction; 22% reduction in all-cause mortality (NNT=48)
atorvastatin	36% event reduction
Mediterranean diet	Decreased CVD events and mortality (NNT=58)
Mediterranean diet	Decreased CVD events and mortality (NNT=58)
Fish oil	29% reduction in all-cause mortality
simvastatin	42% event reduction, 30% all-cause mortality reduction (NNT=10)
simvastatin	Reduction in all-cause and CHD mortality and all vascular morbidity
niacin	Decreased all-cause mortality
niacin, colestipol, lovastatin	73% event reduction (NNT=7)

Table 10-2: Expert Panel III Classification of Total, LDL, and HDL Cholesterol and Triglycerides Levels

Total Cholesterol	
<200	Desirable
200-239	Borderline high
>240	High
LDL Cholesterol—Primary Target of Therapy	
<100	Optimal
100-129	Near optimal/above optimal
130-159	Borderline high
160-189	High
>190	Very high
HDL Cholesterol	
<40	Low
>60	High
Triglycerides	
<150	Normal
150-199	Borderline high
200-500	High
>500	Very high

LDL = low-density lipoprotein
HDL = high-density lipoprotein

tients eligible for cholesterol therapy are expected to increase dramatically because of the aging population, the increased prevalence of diabetes, and the increasing incidence of obesity in adults.

Despite what we know about the relationship between high cholesterol and heart disease, a recent study revealed that only 1 in 12 adults is screened annually for cholesterol levels[14] and only 32% of patients with known CHD are being treated for high cholesterol after MI.[15] In addition, based on the changes in the National Cholesterol Education Program (NCEP)-Expert Panel (ATP III) guidelines, it is now estimated that more than 50 million individuals are eligible for pharmacologic lipid-lowering therapy.[16,17] Primary care providers play an essential role in detecting, evaluating, and treating high blood cholesterol levels.

According to the NCEP ATP III, the patients who benefit most from lipid treatment are those with CHD or noncoronary atherosclerosis, genetic dyslipidemias, diabetes mellitus, and multiple risk factors, including lipoprotein abnormalities[1] (Tables 10-2 and 10-3).

The NCEP-ATP III guidelines recommend evaluation for underlying atherosclerosis and comprehensive risk assessment for all patients before determining lipoprotein goals. Low-density lipoprotein cholesterol treatment goals are risk-stratified using 10-year risk estimates derived from Framingham Heart Study data. A clinician can estimate CHD risk using downloadable risk calculators for the desktop or handheld computer. These risk calculators are available at the National Heart, Lung, and Blood Institute Web site: http://www.nhlbi.nih.gov/guidelines/cholesterol/index.htm. Another practical office version of a risk assessment tool is available for free download at: http://www.medicine.wisc.edu/mainweb/DOMPages.php?section=DOM&page=main. Table 10-2 outlines the ATP III classification of LDL-C, TC, HDL-C, and triglycerides (TG).

Table 10-3: LDL-C Goals Plus Cut-off Points for Initiating Lifestyle Changes or Medical Therapy (NCEP ATP III Guidelines)[1,17]

Patient Risk Group	LDL-C Goal (mg/dL)
CHD or CHD risk equivalent* (10-year risk >20%)	<100† (<70 optional)‡
2+ risk factors	<130
0-1 risk factors**	<160

*A coronary heart disease (CHD) risk equivalent is a condition that carries an absolute risk for developing new CHD equal to the risk for having recurrent CHD events in persons with established CHD.

**Almost all people with 0-1 risk factor have a 10-year risk less than 10%; thus, 10-year risk assessment in people with 0-1 risk factor is not necessary.

† LDL-C goal of <70 mg/dL is a treatment option in very high-risk patients.

Implications of Recent Trials for the NCEP ATP III Guidelines

The results of several recent studies have led many cardiologists to treat lipids to more aggressive targets than those suggested by the NCEP ATP III guidelines, especially in patients who have CHD or are at intermediate to high risk for CHD.[6,11,17-19] Readers are encouraged to review these

LDL-C Level (mg/dL) at Which to Start Lifestyle Changes	LDL-C Level (mg/dL) at Which to Consider Starting Medical Therapy
>100	>130 (100-129; medical therapy optional)[††]
>130	>130 (10-yr-risk= 10%-20%) (10-yr risk 10%-20%) >160 (10-yr risk = <10%)
>160	>160 (160-189: medical therapy optional)

‡ For patients with CHD, acute coronary syndrome, chronic kidney disease, or multiple risk factors.[17]

[††]Evidence now supports the use of low-density lipoprotein cholesterol (LDL-C)-lowering medications in this category even if LDL-C levels are less than 100 mg/dL because of recent statin clinical trials demonstrating risk reduction at any LDL-C level for CHD patients.[11,17] Consideration should be given to medications that modify TGs and HDL (eg, nicotinic acid, fibrate) in addition to LDL-C therapy.[17]

studies and the updates to the NCEP ATP III guidelines, published in July 2004. The results of these studies suggest that an LDL-C target of 70 mg/dL may be appropriate in very high risk patients, such as those with a recent acute coronary syndrome, established cardiovascular disease, and multiple or suboptimally treated risk factors (eg, diabetes mellitus, continued cigarette smoking, the metabolic syndrome), even when baseline LDL-C level is <100 mg/dL.[17] This more aggressive target may also be appropriate for patients with chronic kidney disease.

Certain intermediate-risk patients (those with two or more risk factors and a 10-year risk of 10% to 20%) may benefit from a target of 100 mg/dL. These patients include those with suboptimally treated risk factors (eg, continued smoking), the metabolic syndrome, or subclinical coronary artery disease.[17]

Appropriate non-HDL-C targets are 30 mg/dL higher than corresponding LDL-C targets.[17] An additional consideration is that for patients at high or very high risk, pharmacologic therapy (LDL-C lowering or HDL-C raising) should be started in conjunction with lifestyle changes when LDL-C (or non-HDL-C) is above target. For patients with LDL-C >160 mg/dL, LDL-C lowering should be considered, regardless of risk factor burden. Using the lipid targets for the next higher level of risk may be considered as a more aggressive option in any patient.

Screening

The NCEP ATP III guidelines recommend that all adults 20 years of age and older, and children from high-risk families (those with premature atherosclerosis or genetic dyslipidemias), have a fasting lipoprotein profile at baseline and approximately every 5 years. Because dyslipidemias may affect multiple members of high-risk families, a dyslipidemia or a family history of premature atherosclerosis (before 55 to 65 years of age) mandates a thorough screening evaluation of the patient and first-degree relatives. Routine screening of all children remains controversial, but children or adolescents who have parents, grandparents, or siblings with premature atherosclerosis or dyslipidemias should be screened for lipid disorders and other risk factors.[20,21]

Evidence indicates that HDL cholesterol (HDL-C) and LDL-C remain important risk factors in adults after age

65.[1,22] Older adults should be evaluated individually for dyslipidemia treatment, based on each patient's motivation, prognosis, comorbidities, and potential improvement in quality of life. See Chapter 13 for more information on dyslipidemias in children, adolescents, elderly people, and other special populations.

Because of the availability of advanced testing equipment and national standardization programs, office cholesterol testing is now practical and reliable. Nonfasting TC and HDL-C tests can also provide important information for an initial risk assessment. A fasting lipoprotein profile should be obtained at baseline if the patient has had previous cholesterol level records with a TC averaging greater than 200 mg/dL on two occasions; an HDL-C level of less than 40 mg/dL; or a family history of premature CHD or dyslipidemia. Because many people who develop atherosclerosis have TC levels less than 200 mg/dL, a lipoprotein profile, which includes LDL-C and TG as well as TC levels, is necessary for a thorough risk evaluation for patients with atherosclerosis, a family history of premature atherosclerosis, or multiple CHD risk factors. In these patients, the low TC level may be caused by low HDL-C, abnormalities of other lipoproteins, or multiple risk factors. Although lipoprotein evaluation is especially important for the high-risk individuals mentioned previously, approximately 50% of CHD events occur in individuals with no family history of CHD.[23] Therefore, treatment of lipid disorders is indicated independent of a patient's family history.

Measuring Cholesterol and Lipoprotein Levels

Note that TC and HDL-C levels are not affected by fasting and can be measured at any time of the day. Lipoprotein profiles must be assessed after a 12- to 14-hour fast, because TG measurements are variable in the nonfasting state. When TC, TG, and HDL-C levels are measured, and

Table 10-4: Factors That Can Affect Cholesterol Measurements[2]

- Acute or chronic illness (including MI, viral illness, or bacterial infection)
- Recent general surgery
- Pregnancy or lactation
- Poor nutritional status
- Nonfasting state (affects TG levels, not HDL-C or TC levels)
- Improper phlebotomy technique ('milking the finger' for fingerstick test)
- Day-to-day, or seasonal, variation

serum TG levels are less than 400 mg/dL, LDL-C can be estimated by this formula:

$$LDL\text{-}C = TC - (HDL\text{-}C - TG/5)$$

Dividing the clinical TG levels by 5 provides an estimate of very low-density lipoprotein cholesterol (VLDL-C). However, TC levels, HDL-C levels, and LDL-C calculations are not accurate if the TG level exceeds 400 mg/dL.[1]

A lipoprotein profile is usually sufficient to develop a clinical classification and treatment approach for dyslipidemias. However, when the TG level is more than 400 mg/dL, the TC, HDL-C, and LDL-C measurements are much less accurate in most clinical laboratories and should not be relied on for clinical decisions. When the TG level is more than 400 mg/dL, lipoprotein phenotyping to determine the specific biochemical abnormality may be useful to direct treatment (Table 10-4). Many factors can influence cholesterol measurements.[1]

Understanding 'Lipids,' Lipoproteins, and Atherosclerosis: Advanced Lipoprotein Testing

The total cholesterol in the plasma is carried by VLDL, LDL, and HDL. VLDL and LDL are considered atherogenic. HDL is considered protective. This designation, however, does not account for the complexity of the lipoproteins that underlie the clinical relationships between cholesterol concentrations and CHD risk. 'Lipids' are only surrogate markers for lipoproteins. To understand how lipids and lipoproteins relate to atherosclerosis, it is important to understand that atherogenicity is determined by lipoproteins, described quantitatively in terms of their concentration and qualitatively in terms of their size (see Table 10-5).

For example, not all LDL particles are of the same size and composition. Each lipoprotein concentration reflects a heterogeneous group of particles within that lipoprotein class of varying size and composition.[24] While all VLDL particles are atherogenic, larger VLDL particles are more associated with CHD, in part because they include chylomicron remnants and are common in patients with central obesity and type 2 diabetes mellitus.

While HDL particles in general are protective, an increased number of small HDL particles are a marker of increased atherogenic risk. This is not because small HDL particles are directly atherogenic, but instead because of impaired reverse cholesterol transport. Similarly, small LDL particles are more associated with CHD, whereas larger LDL particles are less atherogenic. At the upper end of LDL size, but included in clinical measurement of LDL-C, are IDL (intermediate density lipoprotein) particles, which also are atherogenic (see Figure 10-1).

Small, dense LDL particles have been called 'stealth LDL,' because they oxidize easily and are more atherogenic. When they are present, standard clinical laboratory determinations of LDL-C concentrations do not reflect adequately the number of LDL particles in the plasma,

Table 10-5: Measurements of Lipoproteins

- Total cholesterol refers to the concentration of cholesterol carried in all plasma lipoproteins. This is measured accurately in the clinical laboratory.
- The plasma HDL cholesterol (HDL-C) represents the concentration of cholesterol carried by plasma HDL and is a surrogate for the number of HDL particles.
- The plasma TG concentration represents the concentration of TGs carried by all plasma lipoproteins, but in general serves as a surrogate for the number of VLDL particles.
- LDL cholesterol (LDL-C) is the concentration of total cholesterol carried by plasma LDL particles. It is a surrogate for the number of LDL particles and is not usually measured directly in the laboratory. It is usually calculated for routine use by the Friedwald equation:

  $$LDL\text{-}C = TC - HDL\text{-}C - TG/5$$

  This equation takes advantage of the observation that total cholesterol is the sum of the major cholesterol-carrying lipoproteins, including LDL, HDL, and VLDL. In usual circumstances, VLDL is the major TG-carrying lipoprotein. The TG concentration divided by 5 is used to represent VLDL cholesterol, because on a mass basis about 20% of VLDL is cholesterol.

and this atherogenic state can be missed by simplistically interpreting a standard lipid profile. This is why the distinction between LDL (low-density lipoprotein) and LDL-C (the cholesterol concentration carried by LDL) is important. When TG levels are above normal, LDL levels may be high even though the LDL-C may be normal.

- The Friedwald equation is less accurate as TG levels increase, because the assumption that TG/5 equals the VLDL cholesterol concentration may no longer hold. There are several reasons for this, including the facts that lipoproteins other than VLDL may be carrying TG (such as chylomicrons and their remnants) and that compositional changes in VLDL make the relationship between VLDL cholesterol and the TG concentration nonlinear. Other sources of inaccuracy in the LDL-C calculation using the Friedewald equation include (1) cholesterol carried by IDL (intermediate-density lipoprotein) and lipoprotein(a) are included as 'LDL-C,' and (2) the LDL-C may be misleadingly low when small LDL particles are present.

When small particles are present, there are more opportunities to injure the endothelial wall; small particles traverse the endothelium more easily, have a longer circulatory time (because of impaired interaction with the LDL receptor), and are more easily oxidized ('stealth LDL'). Small LDL particles should be suspected when HDL-C is <40 mg/dL

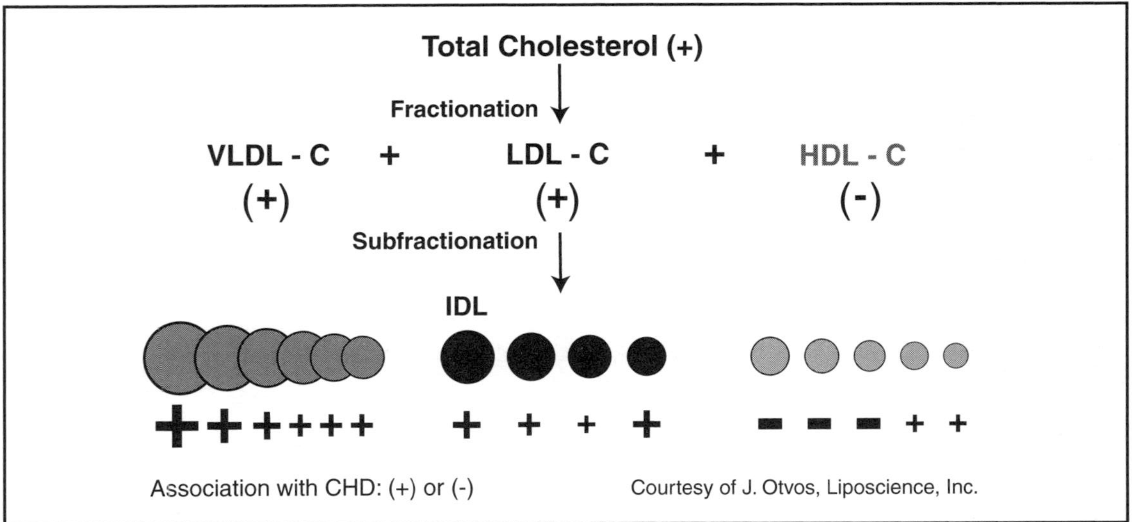

Figure 10-1: Lipoproteins (VLDL, LDL, and HDL) actually exist in varying particle size and density in humans. Atherogenicity varies according to density, with small dense LDL (and large VLDL and IDL) being highly atherogenic. Small, dense HDL is not as effective in reverse cholesterol transport as is normal density HDL, and is therefore associated with a higher risk of atherogenicity.

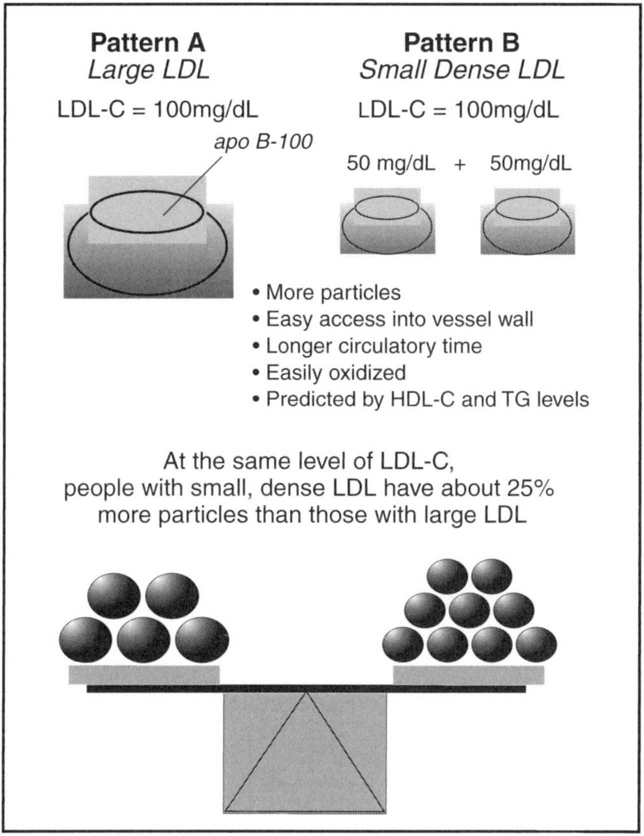

Figure 10-2: Differences in particle density for LDL-C: Pattern A and Pattern B. Large LDL, or "pattern A," has more cholesterol content, and is less atherogenic. Small, dense LDL, or "pattern B," has less cholesterol, is more easily oxidized, is associated with the presence of high triglyceride and low HDL-C states, and is more atherogenic. Because small, dense LDL contains less cholesterol, it is possible that one patient may have many more LDL particles but have less LDL-C on a lipid profile, or less cholesterol associated with LDL.

Table 10-6: Predictive Power of Lipoproteins

Study	Design	CVD Status
CHS 2002	Prospective	Primary Prevention
WHS 2002	Prospective	Primary Prevention
VA-HIT 2002	Prospective	Secondary Prevention
PLAC-I 2002	Prospective	Secondary Prevention
Framingham 2004	Prospective	Primary Prevention

*Significant and independent in multivariate models adjusting for lipids

in a male (or <50 mg/dL in a female) and TG levels are >120-200 mg/dL. In general, at the same level of LDL-C, people with small, dense LDL have approximately 25% more particles than those with large LDL (see Figure 10-2).

The number of LDL particles interacting with the arterial wall drives the disease, not the cholesterol within them. It is primarily the size of the particles that modulates the risk.[25]

In the clinical laboratory, when we want to know the number of LDL particles, for example, we should sim-

Recent Trials	
NMR Particle Atherosclerosis Endpoint	**Concentration Associations***
MI or Angina	↑ Total LDL Particles ↑ Small LDL Particles
MI, CHD death, Stroke	↑ Total LDL Particles ↑ Small LDL Particles
Nonfatal MI or CHD Death	↑ Total LDL Particles ↑ Small LDL Particles ↓ Total HDL Particles ↓ Small HDL Particles
Angiographic MLD	↑ Total LDL Particles ↑ Small LDL Particles ↓ Large HDL Particles
MI, Angina, Stroke, Claudication	↑ Total LDL Particles

ply be able to add up the number of LDL particles. The problem is that standard laboratory techniques do not allow direct measurement of the number of LDL particles, so instead we count the amount of cholesterol they carry. A limitation of this approach is that particle sizes differ within and between individuals, so the number of particles can be inaccurately estimated by standard techniques.

Advanced lipoprotein testing, specifically nuclear magnetic resonance (NMR),[26,27] which includes measurement of chylomicrons, VLDL, IDL, LDL, HDL and their subfractions, is necessary to measure particle number, size, and density. The rationale for this testing is based on limitations in standard enzymatic techniques for determining lipid levels in patients with hypertriglyceridemia and on data that lipoproteins are more directly correlated with atherosclerosis, and more predictive of CHD events, than standard lipid parameters.

The Usefulness of Advanced Lipoprotein Testing

The limitations of standard enzymatic determinations of lipid levels are well known. When serum triglycerides are >200 mg/dL, the estimated LDL-C using the Friedwald formula is less accurate, and is not valid if the triglycerides are >400 mg/dL. Accordingly, the 20% relationship between serum triglycerides and VLDL cholesterol becomes less accurate. Because of neutral lipid exchange, catalyzed by cholesterol ester transfer protein, cholesterol-depleted LDL and HDL particles predominate. Use of standard laboratory techniques results in falsely low impressions of the amount of LDL and HDL particles that actually are present. Although direct measurement of LDL cholesterol partially mitigates this problem, it does not address the lipid changes in other atherogenic lipoproteins such as VLDL, IDL, and HDL, or the issue of neutral lipid exchange.

Multiple cohort studies and clinical trials have found that LDL particle number (LDL-P) is more predictive than LDL-C [28] (see Table 10-6). Thus, the test is especially useful in higher-risk patients, especially those with TG levels >120 to 150 mg/dL, where LDL-P is likely to be elevated, and monitoring LDL-P to get to goal could be useful. For patients with atherosclerosis and diabetes, or those whose Framingham 10-year risk calculates to greater than 20% (a 'CHD equivalent' according to the NCEP ATP III), the LDL-P recommended goal is less than 1,000 mg/dL (see www.liposcience.com).

Table 10-7: Secondary Causes of Hyperlipidemias

Before conducting extensive testing or making treatment decisions, the clinician must rule out the following potential secondary causes of dyslipidemias:

- Poorly controlled diabetes mellitus
- Obesity and the metabolic syndrome
- Medications (steroids, including estrogen, progesterone, prednisone, anabolic steroids, and others; β-blockers; or cis-retinoic acid)
- Obstructive liver disease
- Nephrotic syndrome
- Multiple myeloma
- Hypothyroidism
- Excessive dietary alcohol, fat, or caloric intake.

Types of Dyslipidemias

A directed medical history, nutrition history, thyroid-stimulating hormone assay, and fasting blood chemistry survey (including glucose, liver enzymes, and creatinine) can rule out most of the common secondary causes of dyslipidemias (Table 10-7). Hypothyroidism should be considered, especially in an older patient or a patient with previously normal lipid levels who develops a sudden elevation of LDL-C or TG. Treating the secondary cause usually results in a marked improvement, or normalization, of abnormal lipoprotein levels.

Table 10-8 presents a practical system for classifying dyslipidemias into four categories based on clinical, genetic, and biochemical parameters. This approach uses screening lipoprotein results and is compatible with the more complex Fredrickson-Levy system.

Table 10-8: Classifications of Dyslipidemias

Lipoprotein Levels (mg/dL)	Fredrickson-Levy Class
LDL-C elevated	
LDL-C >130	IIA
TG <150	
HDL-C >40	
Triglycerides elevated	
TG >500*	I, V
LDL-C NA	
HDL-C NA	
HDL-C decreased	
HDL-C <40	—
TG <150	
LDL-C <130	
Combined dyslipidemia	
LDL-C >130	IIB, III, IV
TG >150	
HDL-C <40	

NA = not applicable

Elevated Low-density Lipoprotein Cholesterol

As the table indicates, elevated LDL-C levels, without an elevation of TG, are considered either primary or familial hypercholesterolemia (FH), a relatively common disorder caused by defects in the LDL receptor gene. FH is expressed during childhood and is autosomal dominant, with selective elevation of LDL-C, usually more than 220 mg/dL in adults or more than 170-200 mg/dL in children, and often with xanthomas or extensor tendon thickening, primar-

Genetic Disorder

Familial hypercholesterolemia (LDL-C >200)
Primary hypercholesterolemia (LDL-C = 130-199)

Lipoprotein lipase deficiency

Apo C-III deficiency
Familial hypertriglyceridemia

Hypoalphalipoproteinemia
Tangier disease
Fish eye disease

Familial combined hyperlipidemia
Familial dysbetalipoproteinemia

Low-density lipoprotein cholesterol (LDL-C), high-density lipoprotein cholesterol (HDL-C), and total cholesterol (TC) levels are not accurate when triglycerides (TG) are more than 400 mg/dL.

ily Achilles tenderness. Most patients with isolated LDL-C level elevations less than 200 mg/dL do not have FH and are considered to have primary hypercholesterolemia, which is probably attributable to multiple causes, including nutrition, obesity, and behavioral and genetic factors.

Hypertriglyceridemias

Hypertriglyceridemias are elevations of chylomicrons, intermediate-density lipoproteins (IDL), or VLDL. Because all of these forms of dyslipidemia result in elevated TG, lipoprotein phenotyping may help the clinician distinguish among them. Fasting TG levels of more than 1,000 mg/dL in patients with an underlying moderated hypertriglyceridemia can be caused by either genetic influences or a combination of genetic predisposition and secondary causes, such as alcohol abuse, poorly controlled diabetes, obesity, renal disease, or corticosteroid use.[29,30] Most commonly, estrogen in women (in any form) can dramatically raise TG levels and is contraindicated for women with elevated TG levels, especially when baseline levels exceed 400 mg/dL.

Patients with TG levels of more than 1,000 mg/dL have a relatively low risk of CHD but a high risk of pancreatitis, so the priority of medical therapy in these patients is preventing pancreatitis. VLDL particles in these patients are small and less atherogenic. Clinicians should note that TG levels drop precipitously during acute attacks, and may mask the cause of this life-threatening condition. To determine if a patient's pancreatitis was caused by hypertriglyceridemia, wait until after recovery and remeasure TG levels, take a careful family history, and conduct family lipid screening.

Combined Dyslipidemias

Combined dyslipidemias are common and important disorders found in a large percentage of patients who survive MI or who have coronary revascularization.[31] Combined dyslipidemias include abnormalities of several lipoproteins, usually elevated LDL-C and TG levels with low HDL-C. Family history will often reveal multiple first-degree family members with CHD. Affected patients and family members often present with many dyslipidemias, including elevated TG levels, elevated LDL-C levels, and combined dyslipidemias.[23] This disorder is not usually expressed until adulthood, but it is now being identified in children because of the recent increase in childhood obesity in the United States.

Although TG is not metabolically independent from other lipoproteins, research documenting increased atherosclerosis risk, while accounting for the interaction of TG, LDL-C, HDL-C, and other risk factors, has led to designating TG an independent CHD risk factor.[1] Moderate hypertriglyceridemia (TG level 200 to 499 mg/dL) is usually associated with alteration of LDL-C and VLDL-C into highly atherogenic forms; with low HDL-C caused by reduced HDL-C production; and with altered HDL-C effectiveness in reverse cholesterol transport.[1]

Non-HDL Cholesterol

Non-HDL-C (TC minus HDL cholesterol) can be used to monitor treatment of patients who have had an initial TG measurement of 200 to 499 mg/dL. It does not require a fasting blood test, and its value more accurately assesses risk in patients with TG 200-499 mg/dL. Non-HDL-C includes all of the atherogenic lipoproteins (LDL, VLDL, IDL) and should be less than 30 points higher than the LDL-C goal. For example, the non-HDL-C goal for a patient with CHD or diabetes, or with a 10-year risk greater than 20%, should be less than 130 mg/dL, and the goal for a patient with a 10-year CHD risk of 10% to 20% is less than 160 mg/dL.[1]

The Metabolic Syndrome

The metabolic syndrome is a common, high-risk syndrome that resembles familial combined hyperlipidemia and frequently results in premature clinical manifestations. Previously known as syndrome X or the insulin-resistance syndrome, it has multiple risk factors caused by abnormal metabolism that is caused by the central deposition of body fat, and to secondary insulin resistance that causes hyperinsulinemia. These conditions cause a combined dyslipidemia, glucose intolerance or type II diabetes, and hypertension, all of which are considered important CHD risk factors. The metabolic syndrome can be effectively detected in the office by measuring the patient's waist circumference, at the iliac crest, on exhalation. Table 10-9 outlines specific measures that identify this syndrome.

Table 10-9: Clinical Identification of the Metabolic Syndrome (Any Three of the Following Levels)

Risk Factor	Defining Level
Abdominal obesity*	Waist circumference
Men	>102 cm (>40 in)
Women	>88 cm (>35 in)
Triglycerides	>150 mg/dL
HDL cholesterol	
Men	<40 mg/dL
Women	<50 mg/dL
Blood pressure	>130/ >85 mm Hg
Fasting glucose	>110 mg/dL

*waist circumference measured at iliac crest

Overweight and obesity are associated with insulin resistance and the metabolic syndrome. However, abdominal obesity is more highly correlated with the metabolic risk factors than is an elevated body mass index. Therefore, waist circumference (measured at the iliac crest during exhalation) is recommended to identify the body weight component of the metabolic syndrome.

In addition to the metabolic syndrome, other causes of combined dyslipidemias include a lack of physical activity, hypothyroidism, diabetes mellitus, alcohol abuse, nephrotic syndrome, and use of glucocorticoids.

Familial dysbetalipoproteinemia (type III), a rare subtype of the combined dyslipidemias, is associated with premature CHD and peripheral arterial disease. This disorder is characterized by elevations of fasting TC, TG levels exceeding 300 mg/dL, and the presence of xanthomas. When levels of both LDL-C and TG are high, lipoprotein electrophoresis is recommended, because treatment recommendations differ from those for other combined dyslipidemias.

Low HDL Cholesterol

HDL cholesterol is an independent risk factor and the most powerful predictor of premature CHD.[1,29] Low HDL-C (HDL-C <40 mg/dL, TG <150 mg/dL) is associated with genetic factors, male sex, hypertriglyceridemias, smoking, obesity, and a sedentary lifestyle. Familial hypoalphalipoproteinemia (low HDL-C), a syndrome found in 7% to 10% of CHD patients younger than 60 years of age, is characterized by an HDL-C level of less than 40 mg/dL, a TG level of less than 200 mg/dL, and an autosomal dominant inheritance.[31] Many other genetic forms of HDL-C exist, but they are far less common. Medications, including β-blockers (nonsympathomimetic), retinoids, progestins, and anabolic steroids, can significantly lower HDL-C levels. Weight loss, lowering TG levels, exercise (if HDL-C >30 mg/dL), smoking cessation, and some medications (niacin, fibrates) can raise HDL-C levels.

Lifestyle Interventions

Lifestyle changes, including improved nutrition, weight management, exercise, and smoking cessation, are the cornerstones of any treatment program to modify serum lipid levels. Weight reduction and increased physical activity are critical for managing all dyslipidemias and improving cardiovascular fitness.

Nutrition and Weight Management

Because dietary improvements have been shown to reduce LDL-C levels and the risk of CHD, they are recommended as the first step in therapeutic lifestyle changes. Table 10-10 summarizes nutritional recommendations demonstrated to reduce CHD events.

Patients with dyslipidemias or a diagnosis of CHD should use the NCEP ATP III guidelines,[1] but should also consider the specific proven recommendations in Table 10-11.

Table 10-10: Nutritional Recommendations

	AHA/NCEP* General Population
Total fat (% of calories)	<30%
Saturated fat	<10%
Monounsaturated fat	10%-15%
Polyunsaturated fat	≤10%
Carbohydrate	50%-60%
Protein	10%-20%
Cholesterol	<300 mg

*American Heart Association/National Cholesterol Education Program guidelines for the general healthy American population.[1]

Debate continues about how much fat should be included in the diet for treating dyslipidemia. A diet in which less than 10% of calories comes from fat can reduce LDL-C, but may also reduce HDL-C and increase TG because of a higher carbohydrate content.[32] In the Mediterranean diet, 30% to 40% of calories come from fat; monounsaturated fat is emphasized, and saturated fat is limited to less than 7% of calories. This diet can reduce LDL-C without decreasing HDL-C and increasing TG, but the higher fat intake may make calorie control and weight loss more difficult. This well-balanced eating plan has proven to dramatically lower CHD events and total mortality in patients with known CHD.[7,8]

Serum cholesterol reduction from diet modification varies significantly among individuals, but averages 10% to

AHA/NCEP** Dyslipidemia or CHD	Very Low Fat Diet	Mediterranean Dietary Pattern[7,8]
<30%	10%	30%-40%
<7%	—	7%-10%
10%-15%	—	15%-30%
≤10%	—	<10%
50%-60%	70%-75%	40%-55%
10%-20%	15%-20%	15%-20%
<200 mg	5 mg	<200 mg

**AHA/NCEP guidelines for anyone with coronary heart disease (CHD), CHD risk equivalent, or dyslipidemia.[1]

15%.[1] The TG level is responsive to diet change, weight loss, and exercise. The main dietary influences on HDL-C are weight loss and the balance of fat and carbohydrate in the diet. For these reasons, diet recommendations for dyslipidemia should be individualized based on the patient's lipid pattern, body weight, food preferences, and level of motivation. For medical nutrition therapy, it is a good idea to have your patient consult with a registered dietitian who can tailor guidelines and maximize the lipid response to diet.

Special Considerations

Although patients with familial hypercholesterolemia (LDL-C >200-220 mg/dL) are less responsive to diet changes than those with other forms of hypercholester-

Table 10-11: Proven Lifestyle Recommendations

- Reduce intake of saturated fat to less than 7% of daily caloric intake.
- Reduce intake of cholesterol to less than 200 mg per day.
- Use plant stanols and sterols.
- Use soluble fiber.
- Limit trans-fat by considering it part of the daily saturated fat intake.
- Consume two to three fish meals per week.
- Include soy protein in the diet.

olemia, all patients with elevated TC levels should reduce their intake of saturated fat, trans-fat, and cholesterol. For some patients with elevated LDL-C levels, increased consumption of foods high in soluble fiber—oats, barley, dried beans and peas, nuts, fruits, and some vegetables—may be beneficial. It is preferable to obtain fiber from food, because of the additional nutrients provided by high-fiber foods; however, fiber supplements (psyllium) may be recommended for patients who are not able to consume adequate fiber through diet. Stanols and sterols, which are marketed as margarines, other food products, and soy protein, can also reduce LDL-C levels in some people.

For patients with very high TG levels (500 to 1,000 mg/dL), emphasis should be on weight reduction. TG levels are influenced by the total amount of fat and carbohydrate consumed, but not by the type of fat (Table 10-12).

Patients with combined dyslipidemia and the metabolic syndrome should make weight control and regular exercise priorities. These changes will favorably affect all se-

Table 10-12: Additional Considerations for Patients With Hypertriglyceridemia

- Very low-fat diets, which are higher in carbohydrates, can lead to significant increases in serum triglycerides (TG) in some people, particularly those with the metabolic syndrome.
- Patients with high TG levels should limit or avoid alcohol.
- Patients with glucose intolerance and high TG levels should limit their consumption of simple carbohydrates and total calories and increase regular, sustained, physical activity.
- To avoid pancreatitis, severely hypertriglyceridemic patients (TG ≥1,000 mg/dL) should strictly control total fat to 10%-15% of calories.

rum lipoproteins, abdominal obesity, insulin resistance, glucose intolerance, and hypertension that are associated with this type of dyslipidemia. These patients should attempt to reduce body weight by limiting fat intake to 25% to 30% of calories and saturated fat to <7% of calories. In addition, they should limit their total carbohydrate intake to 60%, or less, of calories, emphasizing complex carbohydrates, such as whole grains and vegetables, rather than simple carbohydrates, such as sweetened drinks and desserts.

Normalization of body weight through caloric restriction and increased exercise is the primary goal for patients with low HDL-C levels. Alcohol and monounsaturated fatty acids may raise HDL-C levels. However, alcohol should not be recommended as a specific treatment for low HDL-C, because it is addictive, myotonic, and caloric, and it raises blood pressure and TG levels. Consumption of alcohol in

Table 10-13: Percentage of Calories as Fat Translated to Fat in Grams

Calorie Intake	30% of Calories (g)
1,500	50
1,800	60
2,000	67
2,400	80

moderation is reasonable; moderation is the equivalent of one alcoholic drink per day (1.5 oz alcohol, 6 oz of wine, 12 oz of beer). HDL-C levels may also increase in response to a diet higher in monounsaturated fats, such as nuts, avocado, and canola or olive oil, or the ω-3 unsaturated fats found in fish, but these fat calories must displace other calories in the diet to limit weight gain.

Applying the Guidelines

The specific identity, function, and safe doses of protective nutrients (such as antioxidants, flavonoids, fish oils, and folic acid) are not understood, so it is not possible to establish appropriate guidelines for using these supplements. Until more information is available, the best advice a clinician can give patients is that reasonable amounts of these and other potentially beneficial nutrients can be obtained by consuming at least five servings of fruits and vegetables per day; at least six servings of grain products (at least half of which should be whole grain), soy, or legumes several times per week; fish two to three times per week, and a handful of nuts several times per week.

Because elevated LDL-C levels in combination with elevated HDL-C levels in older women are associated with only a modestly increased risk, nutritional assess-

10% of Calories (g)	7% of Calories (g)
17	12
20	14
22	16
27	19

ment and counseling may be adequate for this group. Refer to Table 10-2 to help determine the best approach for these patients.

The clinician can help patients apply nutritional guidelines in a practical way by counseling them to make changes in their behavior and by translating recommended fat allowances into calories. Table 10-13 lists the daily total fat and saturated fat gram allowances at different calorie levels and fat recommendations.

The five food categories listed in Table 10-14 account for more than 90% of the fat, saturated fat, and cholesterol consumed in the typical American diet.[33] Counseling for low-fat and low-cholesterol eating should focus on substitution in these five food categories—because of their significant contributions to dietary fat—and on recommendations to increase consumption of plant-based foods.

Exercise

Physical activity is associated with improvement in the lipoprotein profile, but results depend on baseline life-style habits, presence of obesity or diabetes, type of dyslipidemia, and the specific exercise program. Both endurance and resistance exercises are helpful in achieving weight reduction, reducing TG, and raising HDL-C levels, but have little influence on LDL-C levels unless weight loss is signifi-

Table 10-14: Major Food Group Sources of Saturated Fat and Cholesterol

Food Group	Suggestions
Meat	Eat smaller portions (6 to 8 oz per day). Use lean meats, and trim fat. Broil, bake, or grill. Include fish several times per week. Plan some meatless meals using soy, dried beans, or peas.
Dairy products	Use skim or low-fat products. Use part-skim or low-fat cheeses as meat substitutes. Substitute low-fat frozen desserts for ice cream.
Eggs	Limit yolks to four per week. Use egg whites or egg substitutes when baking.
Fish/oils	Use smaller amounts of all fats. Substitute unsaturated fats, such as olive oil, canola oil, or soft margarine, for butter, stick margarine, or shortening. Use reduced-fat mayonnaise and salad dressings.
Snacks/desserts	Substitute low-fat snack foods (pretzels, popcorn, fruit) for fried snacks. Eat smaller servings of desserts. Substitute fruit for other desserts. Eat small amounts of nuts or seeds several times per week.

cant.[1,34] Daily physical activity increases the clearance of TG-rich lipoproteins and glucose, and is often effective in treating hypertriglyceridemia and combined dyslipidemia.

A clear physician message about the importance of physical activity can have a significant impact on increasing a patient's physical activity. Exercise of moderate intensity, longer duration, and increased frequency appears to have more benefit for dyslipidemia and weight loss than higher-intensity, less-frequent exercise.[1,29,34] However, both resistance and endurance exercise will improve dyslipidemias. Encourage any regular activity that a patient enjoys.

Smoking Cessation

Cigarette smoking is associated with metabolic processes that affect lipoproteins, including increasing plasma free fatty acids, glucose, and VLDL-C, and lowering HDL-C. Smoking also oxidizes LDL-C and is associated with metabolic and physiologic changes that significantly increase CHD events.[35] Smoking cessation is associated with an average increase in HDL-C level of 6 to 8 mg/dL.[35]

Pharmacologic Management

Medications for cholesterol treatment should be used only after careful consideration and implementation of the therapeutic lifestyle changes. The guidelines in this section are general recommendations and are not meant to replace your clinical judgment in dealing with an individual patient. Treatment should be individualized based on overall risk, pattern of dyslipidemia, associated medical conditions, cost, prognosis, and patient motivation.

Indications

Medication use is recommended for those patients at highest risk who fail to reach goal cholesterol levels after an adequate trial of lifestyle change, usually 3 to 6 months. Early pharmacologic treatment, combined with lifestyle changes, may be advisable for the highest-risk patients, including those with prior CHD events or CHD equivalents, and those with genetic lipid disorders.

Table 10-15: Cholesterol-lowering Medications

Medication	Dose Range
Statins*	
Atorvastatin (Lipitor®)	10 mg q.d., min 80 mg q.d., max
Rosuvastatin (Crestor®)	5 mg q.d. min 40 mg q.d. max
Fluvastatin (Lescol®)	20 mg q.h.s., min 40 mg b.i.d. or 80
Lovastatin (Mevacor®, Altocor™)	10 mg q.h.s., min 80 mg q.h.s. or 40 mg b.i.d. or 80 mg XL, max
Pravastatin (Pravachol®)	10 mg q.h.s., min 40 mg q.h.s., max
Simvastatin (Zocor®)	10 mg q.h.s., min

*All statins have moderate triglyceride (TG)-lowering (15% to 40+%) and high-density-lipoprotein (HDL)-raising (5% to 12%) effects.

**Increased myositis in combination with fibrates and niacin (approximately 1% to 3%).

LDL-C Reduction (%)	Side Effects and Special Considerations
35-38 50-60	For all statins*,**: • Most of LDL-C level reduction with statins occurs with the initial dose. • Increased hepatic, transaminases, and other minor GI effects (2%-3%). • May continue if liver function test results are elevated, but <2-3 times normal—remonitor. • Myalgias/arthralgias (2%-3%).**,†
20-25	
20-25 34-40	Lovastatin is now available as a generic medication.**,†
25-32 30-35	
35-40	

†Cytochrome CYP450 metabolism. Interaction with other medications that are metabolized by CYP450; may result in higher statin levels and possible myositis and/or rhabdomyolysis.

(continued on next page)

Table 10-15: Cholesterol-lowering Medications *(continued)*

Medication	Dose Range
Cholesterol Absorption Inhibitors	
Colestipol (Colestid®)	4-8 g b.i.d.-t.i.d
Cholestyramine (Questran®)	5-10 g b.i.d.-t.i.d. (start at low dose)
Colesevelam (WelChol®)	6 capsules (3 capsules b.i.d. or 6 q.d. with meal)
Ezetimibe (Zetia®)	10 mg daily
Psyllium	5-15 g b.i.d.-t.i.d.
Plant stanols or sterols (dietary supplement)	3 tablespoons of margarine (Benecol®, Take Control®) t.i.d., or orange juice (Heartwise®) or other future food products
Fish oils (EPA + DHA) supplements	Dose range 1-18 g (total of EPA + DHA)

LDL-C Reduction (%)	Side Effects and Special Considerations
10-25	May increase TG level; bloating, constipation
TG may increase moderately	Interferes with some medications and fat-soluble vitamin absorption
	Colesevelam has less GI toxicity and may interfere less with absorption of other medications
18% monotherapy, 22%-25% combination	Minimal—occasional GI upset, mild liver enzyme elevation; for LDL-C disorders; potent combination with statins
0%-10%	Bloating/diarrhea/constipation—titrate slowly
8%-15%	Minimal to no side effects; weight gain may occur because of increased calorie intake from oils in the food portion of the product
TG reduction of 30%-50% No LDL-C effect, minimal HDL-C effect	Fishy taste, belching, loose stools, greasy/foul smelling stools, nausea

(continued on next page)

Table 10-15: Cholesterol-lowering Medications *(continued)*

Medication	Dose Range
Niacin	
Niacin plain** (crystalline) (Niacor®)	500-1,500 mg b.i.d.-t.i.d.
Extended release (Niaspan®, Slo-Niacin®)	Niaspan®: Starting dose 500 mg, maximum dose 2,000 mg q.h.s. Slo-Niacin®: Starting dose 250 mg b.i.d. maximum dose 1,000 mg b.i.d.
Fibrates	
Gemfibrozil** (Lopid®)	600 mg b.i.d.
Fenofibrate** (Tricor®, Lofibra®, Antara™)	48-200 mg q.i.d.

** Increased myositis with gemfibrozil, and possibly fenofibrate and niacin, in combination with statins (approximately 1% to 3%)

To guide your treatment decisions, the new NCEP-ATP III guidelines use 10-year CHD risk estimates to stratify risk for primary prevention patients with two or more CHD risk factors into LDL-C treatment goal categories. The risk estimate tools mentioned previously are simple and can be used to calculate risk in a minimal amount of time. Table 10-3 shows LDL cholesterol goals

LDL-C Reduction (%)	Side Effects and Special Considerations
20%-25% (at high dose) 50% TG reduction	Flushing, dry skin, rash, glucose intolerance, hepatitis, elevated uric acid
Also: 50% TG decrease and 25% HDL-C increase	Dyspepsia or ulcer; Caution with diabetes, gout, history of gastritis or peptic ulcer
TG 50% decrease HDL-C 5%-20% increase; LDL-C 10% increase 20% decrease	Nausea Rare hepatitis Myositis (2%-6%) with statins and cyclosporine; Cautious use in renal failure

(continued on next page)

and the cut points for initiating lifestyle changes or medical therapy.

Medications

The number of available cholesterol-lowering medications is limited, and each medication has specific uses. There are now four classes of medications used to treat dyslipidemias: statins (HMG-CoA reductase inhibitors),

Table 10-15: Cholesterol-lowering Medications *(continued)*

Combination Medication	Doses Available
Advicor® (lovastatin/Niaspan®)	20/500, 20/1,000 mg
Vytorin® (ezetimibe/simvastatin)	10/10, 10/20, 10/40, 10/80 mg
Caduet® (amlodipine/atorvastatin)	2.5/10, 2.5/20, 2.5/40, 5/10, 5/20, 5/40, 5/80, 10/10, 10/20, 10/40, 10/80 mg

fibrates, niacin, and cholesterol absorption inhibitors. Psyllium and plant stanols or sterols are less frequently used because of only modest LDL-C reductions and less clinical evidence. Table 10-15 lists available medications in each class and gives important information about their use. To effectively treat dyslipidemias, it is important that primary care physicians become familiar with all the medication classes. Although some of the medications are expensive, cost-effective therapy is possible with good knowledge and appropriate use of the medications.[30]

Medications within each class have similar effects and side effects. However, because pharmacokinetics vary, medications may be cautiously substituted within a class if side effects occur.

Combination therapy

In January 2004, the US Food and Drug Administration (FDA) approved the first medicine to treat two different conditions with one pill. The drug, which is marketed by Pfizer under the trade name Caduet®, combines amlodipine (Norvasc®, Lotrel®) and atorvastatin (Lipitor®). Caduet® is indicated for the treatment of hypertension,

LDL-C Reduction	Side Effects
29%, 30%	Same as for niacin and/or lovastatin
45%, 52%, 55%, 60%	Same as for ezetimibe and/or simvastatin
Based on atorvastatin dose: 10 mg, 39%; 20 mg, 43%; 40 mg, 50%; 80 mg, 60%	Same as for amlodipine and atorvastatin

chronic stable angina, vasospastic angina, dysbetalipoproteinemia, elevated serum TG levels, hypercholesterolemia, and mixed dyslipidemia. The dosage should be individualized based on the effectiveness and tolerance for each drug in the combination. The usual beginning dose of the antihypertensive amlodipine is 5 mg once a day, with a maximum dose of 10 mg once a day.

Choosing the right medication for specific dyslipidemias

The pattern of dyslipidemia will dictate the choice of medication for each patient. Figure 10-3, a dyslipidemia treatment summary, can help you tailor your treatment to a patient's specific needs, as can the information in Table 10-16 and Table 10-17.

Treating Hypertriglyceridemias

After secondary causes are evaluated and treated, niacin (Niaspan®) and gemfibrozil (Lopid®) are the best and most cost-effective treatments for patients with hypertriglyceridemias (TG >400 to 500 mg/dL). When the TG level is >400 mg/dL, TG must be controlled before TC and LDL-C levels can be successfully lowered. Table 10-18 gives specific guidelines.

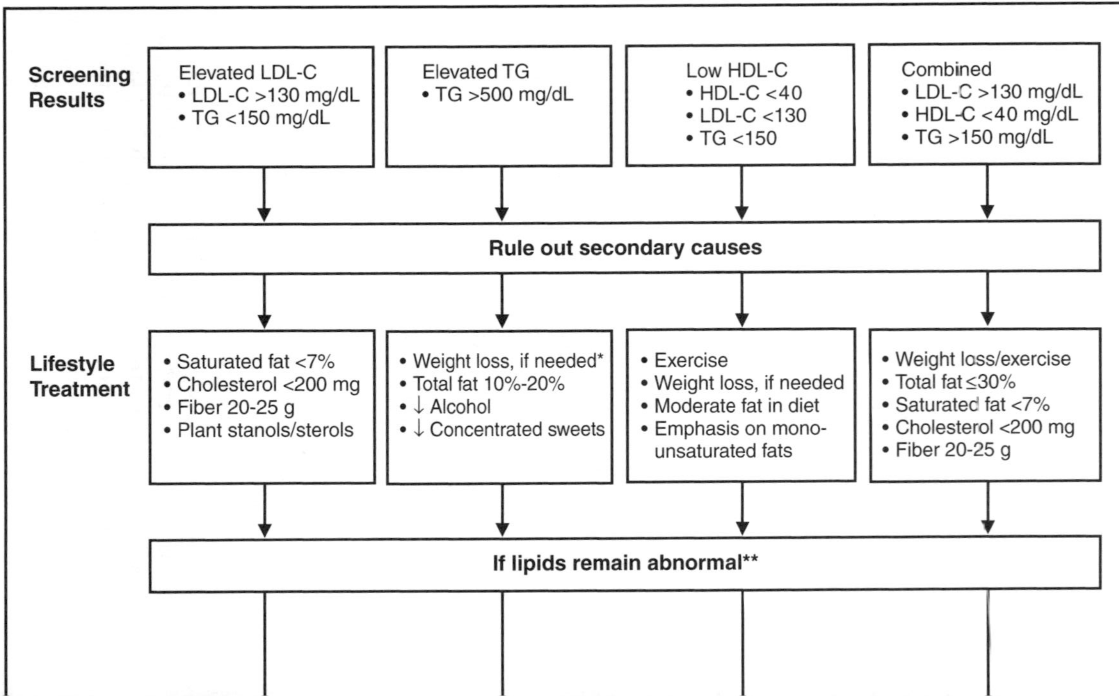

Screening Results
Elevated LDL-C
• LDL-C >130 mg/dL
• TG <150 mg/dL
Elevated TG
• TG >500 mg/dL
Low HDL-C
• HDL-C <40
• LDL-C <130
• TG <150
Combined
• LDL-C >130 mg/dL
• HDL-C <40 mg/dL
• TG >150 mg/dL
Rule out secondary causes
Lifestyle Treatment
• Saturated fat <7%
• Cholesterol <200 mg
• Fiber 20-25 g
• Plant stanols/sterols
• Weight loss, if needed*
• Total fat 10%-20%
• ↓ Alcohol
• ↓ Concentrated sweets
• Exercise
• Weight loss, if needed
• Moderate fat in diet
• Emphasis on mono-unsaturated fats
• Weight loss/exercise
• Total fat ≤30%
• Saturated fat <7%
• Cholesterol <200 mg
• Fiber 20-25 g
If lipids remain abnormal**

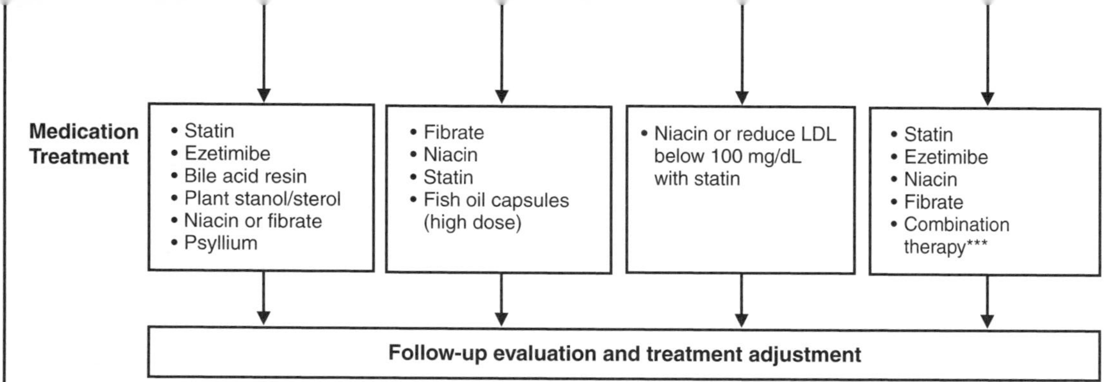

*Exception: immediate medication (fibrate or niacin) for patients with TG >1,000 mg/dL because of high risk of pancreatitis, or LDL-C >220 mg/dL because of genetic disorders and resistance to non-pharmacologic treatment after ruling out secondary causes.

**(1) Goal LDL-C <100 mg/dL with CHD/noncoronary atherosclerosis; diabetes mellitus, or 10-yr CHD-risk >20%; (2) Goal LDL-C <130 mg/dL if no known CHD but high risk (LDL-C >160 mg/dL with two or more risk factors or LDL-C >190 mg/dL in isolation).

***See text: statins and fibrates and/or niacin may be used in combination with monitoring for risk of myositis (risk of interaction 1%-3%).

Figure 10-3: Dyslipidemia treatment algorithm.

Table 10-16: Special Considerations for Medications

- Statins primarily reduce LDL-C, but also moderately reduce TG and raise HDL-C.
- Ezetimibe is more effective in combination with statins (25% LDL-C and 14% Tg decrease) and is only used in 10-mg doses.
- Bile acid resins primarily lower LDL-C, but may exacerbate TG elevations.
- Plant sterols and psyllium are food derivatives that lower LDL-C levels modestly, but this effect can be enhanced in combination with other medications.
- Niacin is effective for elevated TG and low HDL levels, but lowers LDL only at higher doses. Its use is somewhat limited by side effects.
- The fibrates, including gemfibrozil and fenofibrate, primarily reduce TG and subsequently raise HDL-C. However, as the TG is lowered, it may also elevate LDL-C.

LDL-C = low-density lipoprotein cholesterol
TG = triglycerides
HDL-C = high-density lipoprotein cholesterol

The treatments of choice for combined dyslipidemia, which is commonly associated with the metabolic syndrome and premature CHD, are statins, niacin, gemfibrozil (Lopid®), and fenofibrate (Tricor®, Lofibra®, Antara™). Additional guidelines for treating combined dyslipidemia appear in Table 10-19.

Table 10-17: Treating Elevated Low-density Lipoprotein Cholesterol

- Statins are the most effective treatment for isolated LDL-C level elevations, or elevated LDL-C with combined dyslipidemias, after TG is controlled.
- Ezetimibe is effective as monotherapy (18% LDL-C reduction) but is more effective in combination with statins (25% LDL-C reduction). A combination of ezetimibe and simvastatin is scheduled for release in 2004.
- The side effects of bile acid resins, plant sterols, and psyllium are limited to the gastrointestinal tract, but the LDL-C efficacy is only 5% to 24%.
- Niacin is a potent and inexpensive agent, especially in low-dose combination with bile acid resins, but high doses are usually required to lower LDL-C levels significantly (niacin 2,000 mg daily total reduces LDL-C by 20% to 25%).

LDL-C = low-density lipoprotein cholesterol
TG = triglycerides
HDL-C = high-density lipoprotein cholesterol

Low HDL-cholesterol

Niacin is the only medication that effectively raises isolated low HDL-C levels (<40 mg/dL). Isolated low HDL-C deficiencies are slow to respond to treatment, if they respond at all.[36]

Patients with documented atherosclerosis or a high-risk family profile with low HDL-C levels must lower LDL-C to <100 mg/dL and may be candidates for prolonged trial of low-to-moderate-dose niacin (250 mg to 500 mg b.i.d.) to determine whether HDL-C levels can be

Table 10-18: Specific Guidelines for Treating Hypertriglyceridemia

- Before considering medication, identify and treat any secondary cause for triglyceride (TG) level elevation.
- Estrogens, progestins, and other steroids are contraindicated for patients with hypertriglyceridemia, because they significantly elevate TG levels, which may lead to pancreatitis.
- Fibrates are the treatment of choice for hypertriglyceridemia associated with diabetes, gout, gastritis, or ulcer disease, because niacin may exacerbate these conditions.
- Patients with well-controlled diabetes may tolerate niacin without significant worsening of hyperglycemia, but caution and careful monitoring are advised.
- If TG levels are reduced with fibrates, the LDL-C level often rises and may require additional treatment.
- Fenofibrate is safe and effective for TG reduction, but it is more expensive than gemfibrozil.
- Omega-3 fish oil capsules can lower TG levels safely and effectively, but may cause abdominal bloating, belching, flatulence, or loose stools.
- Bile acid resins or estrogens may exacerbate TG elevations.

LDL-C = low-density lipoprotein cholesterol

Table 10-19: Additional Guidelines for Treating Dyslipidemia

- Combined dyslipidemias are frequently associated with glucose intolerance and gout, which are relative contraindications for using niacin.
- Treatment with fibrates may be effective, but to reduce LDL-C levels effectively they may need to be combined with a low-dose statin, ezetimibe, or bile acid resin.
- Statins may be useful if TG levels are moderately elevated, but may not be as effective if the TG level is more than 300 to 400 mg/dL. In that case, treat with a TG-lowering medication such as niacin, fibrates, or fish oil capsules.
- Patients taking contraceptives or hormone replacement therapy should have baseline lipoprotein screening and follow-up testing to ensure that TG levels are not significantly elevated.

LDL-C = low-density lipoprotein cholesterol
TG = triglycerides

increased without significant side effects. Some studies have demonstrated that using statins to lower LDL-C levels below target levels can reduce CHD events when HDL-C levels cannot be raised.[1,2,37]

Combination therapy

Combining medications to treat dyslipidemia may be effective when a single agent is insufficient, or when the goal is to reduce the dosage and side effects of a single medication. Combining a statin or other medication that reduces lipoprotein production with a medication that reduces bile acid reabsorption is effective in reducing LDL-

Table 10-20: Guidelines for Monitoring Medications

- Results of liver function tests (such as ALT or AST) that are less than 2 to 3 times normal and are not progressive are acceptable with the use of cholesterol medications, especially the statins.
- More frequent monitoring is recommended for patients with severe underlying clinical disease or liver enzyme elevations or underlying liver disease, and patients who are on combination cholesterol therapy or are taking other medications that could interact to cause drug-induced hepatitis.
- Because physical activity often causes benign elevations of CK, measuring CK levels is only recommended if patients complain of generalized myalgias.
- When lipoprotein levels reach treatment goals, monitoring every 4 to 6 months to assess the side effects, check laboratory studies, and verify diet and medication adherence is appropriate.

CK = creatinine kinase, ALT = alanine transaminase, AST = aspartate transaminase

C levels. Although statins can be combined with niacin or fibrates, the patient should be taught to identify and report any myalgia symptoms, and blood chemistry should be monitored every 3 to 4 months.

Monitoring medications

Until lipid goals are reached, patients taking medications should be monitored for elevations of liver function levels and should have a lipoprotein profile every 4 to 6 weeks to adjust medications and evaluate side effects. *Because dyslipidemias are asymptomatic conditions, an initial visit 4 to 6 weeks after therapy is started provides an opportunity for valuable physician feedback on medication effectiveness. If patients do not get feedback within that time frame, there is a significant drop in medication adherence.*[1] Some additional guidelines for monitoring medications appear in Table 10-20.

Patient Education

Patient education and counseling are important parts of the family practice professional's role in preventing and treating dyslipidemias. According to the US Preventive Services Task Force, there is good evidence from high-quality studies that primary care clinicians can change patient behavior through simple counseling interventions. Although patients bear the primary responsibility for following through with preventive behaviors, the keys to their effective participation are education, motivation, and counseling. A busy clinician certainly cannot fill all his patients' educational needs but can play a pivotal role in starting and guiding the process.

Because dyslipidemia, like hypertension, is largely a 'silent' condition, patient education and counseling are important prevention strategies, especially for patients who are at high risk for CHD. Providing them with printed information about cholesterol—its relationship to CHD and the factors affecting cholesterol levels, such as good nutrition, weight control, and exercise—and presenting evidence that they can actually do something to improve their health are important first steps in prevention. However, effective patient education takes much more than an instructional pamphlet and a few words of encouragement. Chapter 14 offers detailed information on prevention strategies to incorporate into an existing practice setting. Many of them can be implemented during routine patient visits.

References

1. National Cholesterol Education Program (NCEP) Expert Panel (ATP III): Executive summary of the third report of the National Cholesterol Education Program (NCEP) expert panel on detection, evaluation and treatment of high blood cholesterol in adults (Adult Treatment Panel III). *JAMA* 2001;285:2486-2497.

2. Downs JR, Clearfield M, Weis S, et al: Primary prevention of acute coronary events with lovastatin in men and women with average cholesterol levels: results of AFCAPS/TexCAPS. Air Force/ Texas Coronary Atherosclerosis Prevention Study. *JAMA* 1998;279:1615-1622.

3. Manninen V, Tenkanen L, Koskinen P, et al: Joint effects of serum triglyceride and LDL cholesterol and HDL cholesterol concentrations on coronary heart disease risk in the Helsinki Heart Study: Implications for treatment. *Circulation* 1992;85:37-45.

4. The Lipid Research Clinics Coronary Primary Prevention Trial results: I. Reduction in incidence of coronary heart disease. *JAMA* 1984;344:351-364.

5. Shepherd J, Cobbe SM, Ford I, et al: Prevention of coronary heart disease with pravastatin in men with hypercholesterolemia. West of Scotland Coronary Prevention Study Group. *N Engl J Med* 1995;333:1301-1307.

6. Sever PS, Dahlof B, Poulter N, et al, for the ASCOT Investigators: Prevention of coronary and stroke events with atorvastatin in hypertensive patients who have average or lower-than-average cholesterol concentrations, in the Anglo-Scandinavian Cardiac Outcomes Trial—Lipid Lowering Arm (ASCOT-LLA): a multicentre randomised controlled trial. *Lancet* 2003;361:1149-1158.

7. de Lorgeril M, Salen P, Martin JL, et al: Mediterranean diet, traditional risk factors, and the rate of cardiovascular complications after myocardial infarction: final report of the Lyon Diet Heart Study. *Circulation* 1999;99:779-785.

8. Singh RB, Dubnov G, Niaz MA, et al: Effect of an Indo-Mediterranean diet on progression of coronary artery disease in high risk patients (Indo-Mediterranean Diet Study): a randomised, single-blind trial. *Lancet* 2002;360:1455-1461.

9. Burr ML, Fehily AM, Gilbert JF, et al: Effects of changes in fat, fish, and fibre intakes on myocardial reinfarction: Diet and Reinfarction Trial (DART). *Lancet* 1989;2:757-761.

10. Scandinavian Simvastatin Survival Study Group: Randomised trial of cholesterol lowering in 4,444 patients with coronary heart disease: the Scandinavian Simvastatin Survival Study (4S). *Lancet* 1994;344:1383-1389.

11. Heart Protection Study Collaborative Group: MRC/BHF Heart Protection Study of cholesterol lowering with simvastatin in 20,536 high-risk individuals: a randomised placebo-controlled trial. *Lancet* 2002;360:7-22.

12. Canner PL, Berge KG, Wenger NK, et al: Fifteen year mortality in Coronary Drug Project patients: long-term benefit with niacin. *J Am Coll Cardiol* 1986;8:1245-1255.

13. Brown G, Albers JJ, Fisher LD, et al: Regression of coronary artery disease as a result of intensive lipid-lowering therapy in men with high levels of apolipoprotein B. *N Engl J Med* 1990;323:1289-1298.

14. Amsterdam EA: Cholesterol and coronary artery disease. *Med Economics* 2001;(suppl):3.

15. Fonarow GC, French WJ, Parsons LS, et al: Use of lipid-lowering medications at discharge in patients with acute myocardial infarction: data From the National Registry of Myocardial Infarction 3. *Circulation* 2001;103:38-44.

16. Fedder D, Koro CT, L'Italien GJ: New National Cholesterol Education Program III guidelines for primary prevention lipid-lowering drug therapy: projected impact on the size, sex, and age distribution of the treatment-eligible population. *Circulation* 2002;105:152-156.

17. Grundy SM, Cleeman JI, Merz CN, et al: Implications of recent clinical trials for the National Cholesterol Education Program Adult Treatment Panel III guidelines. *Circulation* 2004;110:227-239.

18. Cannon CP, Braunwald E, McCabe CH, et al: Intensive versus moderate lipid lowering with statins after acute coronary syndromes. *N Engl J Med* 2004;350:1495-1504.

19. Nissen SE, Tuzcu EM, Schoenhagen P, et al: Effect of intensive compared with moderate lipid-lowering therapy on progression of coronary atherosclerosis: a randomized controlled trial. *JAMA* 2004;291:1071-1080.

20. National Cholesterol Education Program: Highlights of the report of the expert panel on blood cholesterol levels in children and adolescents. *Am Family Physician* 1992;45:2127-2182 and PHS-NIH Publication No. 91-2731, Sept 1991.

21. Williams CL, Hayman LL, Daniels SR, et al: Cardiovascular health in childhood: a statement for health professionals from the Committee on Atherosclerosis, Hypertension, and Obesity in the Young (AHOY) of the Council on Cardiovascular Disease in the Young, American Heart Association. *Circulation* 2002;106:143-160.

22. Carlsson CM, Carnes M, McBride PE, et al: Managing dyslipidemia in older adults. *J Am Geriatrics Soc* 1999;47:1458-1465.

23. Williams RR, Hunt SC, Heiss G, et al: Usefulness of cardiovascular family history data for population-based preventive medicine and medical research (the Health Family Tree Study and the NHLBI Family Study). *Am J Cardiol* 2001;87:129-35.

24. Blanke GJ, Otvos JD, Rifai N, et al: LDL particle concentration and size as determined by NMR spectroscopy as predictors of cardiovascular disease in women. *Circulation* 2002;106:1930-1937.

25. Otvos JD, Freedman DS, Pegus C, et al: LDL and HDL particle subclasses are independent predictors of cardiovascular events in the Veterans Affairs HDL Intervention Trial (VA-HIT). Paper presented at American Heart Association Scientific Sessions, Chicago, IL, 2002.

26. Kuller L, Arnold A, Tracy R, et al: Nuclear magnetic resonance spectroscopy of lipoproteins and risk of coronary heart disease in the cardiovascular health study. *Arterioscler Thromb Vasc Biol* 2002;22:1175-1180.

27. Rosenson RS, Otvos JD, Freedman DS: Relations of lipoprotein subclass levels and low-density lipoprotein size to progression of coronary artery disease in the Pravastatin Limitation of Atherosclerosis in the Coronary Arteries (PLAC-1) trial. *Am J Cardiol* 2002;90:89-94.

28. Cromwell WC, Otvos JD: Low-density lipoprotein particle number and risk for cardiovascular disease. *Curr Atheroscler Rep* 2004;6:381-387.

29. Oberman A, Kreisberg RA, Henkin Y: *Principles and Management of Lipid Disorders: A Primary Care Approach*. Baltimore, Williams & Wilkins, 1992.

30. Knopp RH: Drug treatment of lipid disorders. *N Engl J Med* 1999;341:498-511.

31. Genest J, Martin-Munley S, McNamara JR, et al: Frequency of genetic dyslipidemias in patients with premature-coronary artery disease. *Arteriosclerosis* 1989;9:701A.

32. Grundy SM: The optimal ratio of fat-to-carbohydrate in the diet. *Annu Rev Nutr* 1999;19:325-341.

33. Subar AF, Krebs-Smith SM, Cook A, et al: Dietary sources of nutrients among US adults, 1989 to 1991. *J Am Diet Assoc* 1998; 98:537-547.

34. Thompson PD, Cullinane EM, Sady SP, et al: Modest changes in high-density lipoprotein concentration and metabolism with prolonged exercise training. *Circulation* 1988;78:25-34.

35. McBride PE: The health consequences of smoking. Cardiovascular diseases. *Med Clin North Am* 1992;76:333-353.

36. Martin-Jadraque R, Tato F, Mostaza JM, et al: Effectiveness of low-dose crystalline nicotinic acid in men with low high-density lipoprotein cholesterol levels. *Arch Intern Med* 1996;156:1081-1088.

37. Sacks FM, Pfeffer MA, Moye LA, et al: The effect of pravastatin on coronary events after myocardial infarction in patients with average cholesterol levels. Cholesterol and Recurrent Events (CARE) Trial investigators. *N Engl J Med* 1996;335:1001-1009.

CHAPTER 11

Hypertension

Blood pressure control is critical for preventing cardiovascular disease (CVD), especially congestive heart failure and stroke. The Seventh Report of the Joint National Committee on Prevention, Detection, Evaluation, and Treatment of High Blood Pressure (JNC 7)[1,2] states that the relationship between blood pressure and the risk of CVD events is 'continuous, consistent, and independent of other risk factors.' The higher the systolic and/or diastolic pressure, the greater the chance of myocardial infarction (MI), stroke, and kidney disease.[1,2]

Hypertension is the most common primary diagnosis in the United States.[3] Approximately 50 million people in the United States, and 1 billion people worldwide, are affected by hypertension, and as the population ages, this prevalence will increase unless effective preventive measures are taken. Despite progress made in improving blood pressure control rates in recent years, 30% of individuals with hypertension are still unaware that they have it. Even more alarming, a study conducted in 2002 showed that although all physicians polled were familiar with the guidelines for treating hypertension presented in the sixth JNC report (JNC 6), and 76% agreed with them, only 14% followed them.[4]

Benefits of Lowering Blood Pressure

Clinical trials have demonstrated that antihypertensive therapy is associated with a 35% to 40% reduction in the incidence of stroke, a 20% to 25% reduction in MI, and more than a 50% reduction in heart failure.[5] For example, achieving a sustained 12 mm Hg decrease in systolic blood pressure for 10 years in patients with stage 1 hypertension (systolic blood pressure of 140 to 149 mm Hg and/or diastolic blood pressure of 90 to 99 mm Hg) and additional cardiovascular risk factors will prevent 1 death for every 11 patients treated.[6] Table 11-1 lists recent clinical trials that tested a variety of medications and resulted in specific indications for specific medications.

The New Joint National Committee Guideline

The JNC 7 report, released in May 2003,[1] simplified the classification of blood pressure by establishing a new guideline for hypertension prevention and management based on the results of numerous large-scale clinical trials published after the release of JNC 6. Key messages of the new guideline are outlined in Table 11-2.

Table 11-3 outlines the revised blood pressure classification categories for adults 18 years of age or older that were proposed by JNC 7.

Obtaining Accurate Blood Pressure Readings

To obtain an accurate blood pressure measurement, the patient should be seated in a chair quietly for 5 minutes with feet on the floor and an arm supported at heart level; fitted with an appropriately sized cuff; measured with a properly calibrated and validated instrument; and evaluated with two readings taken about 5 minutes apart. If the reading is high, it should be confirmed by checking the other arm.

Because older patients are more likely to experience an orthostatic drop in blood pressure, their blood pressure should be checked while they are standing up and while they are lying down. Patients should be given their specific blood pressure numbers and blood pressure goals verbally and in writing.

Home blood pressure measurements or ambulatory blood pressure monitoring should be considered if a patient's hy-

Table 11-1: Clinical Trial and Guideline Basis for Compelling Indications for Individual Drug Classes

Compelling Indication*
Heart failure
Post-myocardial infarction
High coronary disease risk
Diabetes
Chronic kidney disease
Recurrent stroke prevention

* Compelling indications for antihypertensive drugs are based on benefits from outcome studies or existing clinical guidelines; the compelling indication is managed in parallel with the blood pressure.

** Conditions for which clinical trials demonstrate benefit of specific classes of antihypertensive drugs

BB = β-blocker; ACEI = angiotensin-converting enzyme inhibitor; ARB = angiotensin II receptor blocker;

Recommended Drugs

Diuretic	BB	ACEI	ARB	CCB	Aldo ANT	Clinical Trial Basis**
•	•	•	•		•	ACC/AHA Heart Failure Guideline, MERIT-HF, COPERNICUS, CIBIS, SOLVD, AIRE, TRACE, ValHEFT, RALES
	•	•			•	ACC/AHA Post-MI Guideline, BHAT, SAVE, CAPRICORN, EPHESUS
•	•	•		•		ALLHAT, HOPE, ANBP2, LIFE, CONVINCE
•	•	•	•	•		NKF-ADA Guideline, UKPDS, ALLHAT
		•	•			NKF Guideline, Captopril Trial, RENAAL, IDNT, REIN, AASK
•		•				PROGRESS

CCB = calcium channel blocker; Aldo ANT = aldosterone antagonist

National Heart, Lung, and Blood Institute: *JNC 7 Express: The Seventh Report of the Joint National Committee on Prevention, Detection, Evaluation, and Treatment of High Blood Pressure.* Rockville, MD, US Department of Health and Human Services; May 2003. NIH Publication no. 03-5233.

Table 11-2: Key Messages of JNC 7 Guideline

- For individuals older than 50 years, systolic blood pressure is more important as a risk factor for CVD than diastolic blood pressure.
- Beginning at 115/75 mm Hg, CVD risk doubles with each increment of 20/10 mm Hg.
- Individuals with normal blood pressure at age 55 have a 90% lifetime risk for developing hypertension.
- Persons with systolic blood pressure ranging from 120 to 139 mm Hg or diastolic blood pressure ranging from 80 to 89 mm Hg should be considered prehypertensive and should make lifestyle modifications to prevent CVD.
- Thiazide diuretics, either alone or combined with other medication classes, should be the initial medication therapy for most individuals with hypertension.
- Diuretics are synergistic with every other class of hypertension medications, because other hypertension medications increase plasma volume.

pertension could be caused by 'white-coat' syndrome. Home and ambulatory blood pressures predict target organ changes (Table 11-4) caused by hypertension as well as office blood pressure does. Ambulatory blood pressure monitoring is conducted with an instrument worn for at least 24 hours and measures blood pressure at predetermined intervals during sleep and waking hours. Ambulatory blood pressure values are usually lower than readings taken in a clinician's office. Patients with hypertension have an aver-

- Certain high-risk conditions (eg, diabetes mellitus, chronic kidney disease) provide compelling evidence for using other medication classes.
- Many patients require two or more antihypertensive medications to achieve their blood pressure goals.
- Therapy with two agents should be considered if blood pressure is more than 20/10 mm Hg greater than the goal, with one agent being a thiazide diuretic.
- The most effective therapy prescribed by the careful physician will control hypertension only if patients are motivated.
- Clinician empathy builds trust and is a potent motivator.
- The responsible clinician's judgment remains paramount.

CVD = cardiovascular disease

age blood pressure of >135/85 mm Hg when they are awake and a reading of >120/75 mm Hg when they are sleeping. Blood pressure should drop by 10% to 20% during the night. If it does not, the patient may be at increased risk for cardiovascular events. Self-measurement of blood pressure can improve adherence to therapy, evaluate white-coat or anxiety-related hypertension, and provide information on the causes of elevated blood pressure and the response to antihypertensive therapy.

Table 11-3: Classification of Blood Pressure for Adults 18 Years of Age or Older

BP Classification	SBP mm Hg		DBP mm Hg
Normal	<120	and	<80
Prehypertension	120-129	or	80-90
Stage 1 hypertension	140-159	or	90-99
Stage 2 hypertension	≥160	or	≥100

BP = blood pressure; SBP = systolic blood pressure; DBP = diastolic blood pressure

A home reading of more than 135/85 mm Hg is considered to be hypertensive. Home measurement devices should be checked regularly for accuracy.

History and Physical Examination

A complete history and physical examination establishes the diagnosis of hypertension and assesses for target organ changes. Eye and cardiovascular examinations are helpful in assessing the patient with a history of 'borderline high blood pressure' who claims to have white-coat hypertension. A patient has hypertension with confirmed target organ damage if arteriovenous nicking is present on the retina, S4 gallop is present in the cardiac examination, and arterial bruits are present on the physical examination.

Assessing Hypertensive Patients

Evaluation of patients with documented hypertension has three major objectives: (1) to assess the presence or absence of target organ damage and CVD (Table 11-4);

Table 11-4: Target Organ Damage

- Heart
  - Left ventricular hypertrophy
  - Angina or prior myocardial infarction
  - Prior coronary revascularization
  - Heart failure
- Brain
  - Stroke or transient ischemic attack (including cerebral hemorrhage and/or atherosclerosis)
- Chronic kidney disease
- Peripheral arterial disease
- Retinopathy

(2) to assess the patient's lifestyle and identify other cardiovascular risk factors or concomitant disorders that may affect prognosis and guide treatment (Table 11-5); and (3) to reveal identifiable causes of high blood pressure (Table 11-6).

Laboratory tests and other diagnostic procedures should be performed to rule out the more common, reversible causes of hypertension before treatment is prescribed. These routine tests are listed in Table 11-7. A fasting lipid profile, which includes high- and low-density lipoprotein cholesterol and triglycerides, is also recommended to assess overall cardiovascular risk and to guide risk reduction plans.

Optional tests include measurement of urinary albumin excretion or albumin/creatinine ratio. More extensive testing for identifiable causes of hypertension is not indicated unless the history or examination suggests a secondary cause or a prescribed treatment does not result in blood pressure control.

Table 11-5: Major Cardiovascular Risk Factors

- Hypertension*
- Cigarette smoking
- Obesity* (BMI ≥30 kg/m^2)
- Physical inactivity
- Dyslipidemia*
- Diabetes mellitus*
- Microalbuminuria or estimated GFR less than 60 mL/min
- Age (older than 55 years for men and 65 years for women)
- Family history of premature cardiovascular disease (men younger than 55 years and women younger than 65 years)

*Components of metabolic syndrome or insulin resistance.
BMI = body mass index; GFR = glomerular filtration rate

Treating the Hypertensive Patient

The primary goal of antihypertensive therapy is to reduce cardiovascular and renal morbidity and mortality. The main focus of treatment should be on achieving the systolic blood pressure goal. Once this goal has been reached, most patients, especially those older than 50 years, will also reach the diastolic blood pressure goal. Achieving treatment goals of less than 140/90 mm Hg for most patients, and less than 130/80 mm Hg for patients with diabetes or chronic kidney disease, is associated with a decrease in cardiovascular complications.[7,8] Figure 11-1 outlines the JNC 7 blood pressure management recommendations for adults.

Table 11-6: Identifiable Causes of Hypertension

- Sleep apnea
- Drug-induced or drug-related causes
- Chronic kidney disease
- Primary aldosteronism
- Renovascular disease
- Chronic steroid therapy and Cushing's syndrome
- Pheochromocytoma
- Coarctation of the aorta
- Thyroid or parathyroid disease

Table 11-7: Routine Laboratory Tests for Hypertension

- Electrocardiogram (evaluate for left ventricular hypertrophy, prior myocardial infarction, other heart disease)
- Urinalysis (test for glucose, protein, microalbuminuria)
- Blood glucose
- Hematocrit
- Serum potassium and calcium
- Creatinine or the corresponding estimated glomerular filtration rate

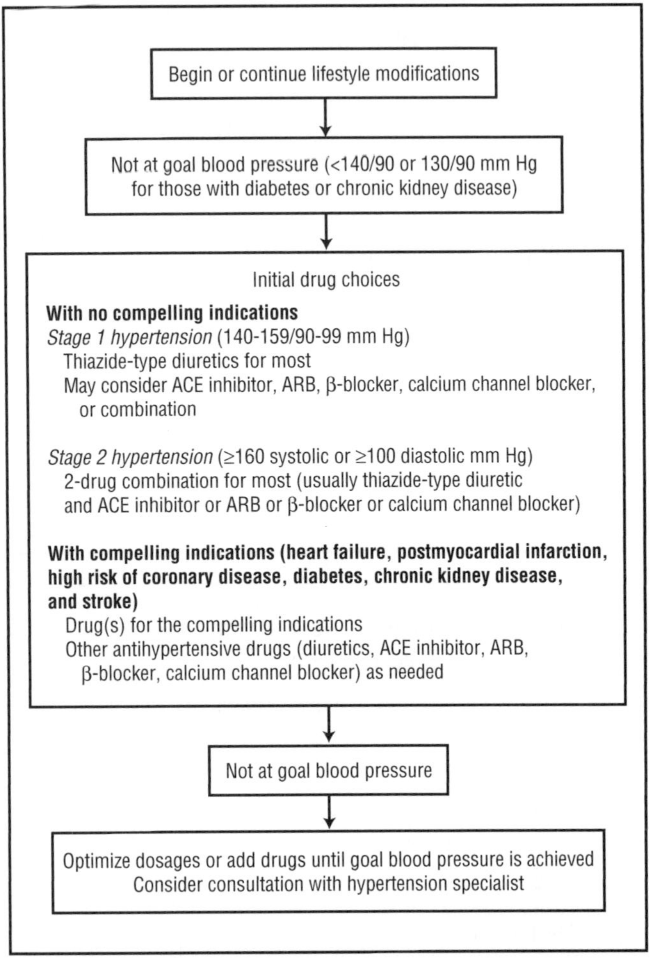

Figure 11-1: Algorithm for the treatment of hypertension. *JNC 7 Express: The Seventh Report of the Joint National Committee on Prevention, Detection, Evaluation, and Treatment of High Blood Pressure.* Bethesda, MD, National Heart, Lung, and Blood Institute, 2003. NIH publication no. 03-5233.

Table 11-8: Beneficial Lifestyle Changes

- Lose weight, if overweight
- Stop smoking
- Increase physical activity
- Moderate alcohol consumption
- Moderate dietary sodium intake
- Maintain adequate intake of dietary potassium, calcium, and magnesium

Lifestyle Interventions

Adopting a healthy lifestyle is the most important step patients can take to prevent hypertension. It is also an indispensable part of any treatment plan for managing patients with hypertension. Table 11-8 lists beneficial lifestyle changes for individuals with hypertension.

Lifestyle changes have been shown to be effective in lowering blood pressure and reducing other cardiovascular risk factors.[1,2,9-11] They can also enhance the efficacy of antihypertensive medications. Table 11-9 shows the effect some lifestyle changes can have on reducing systolic blood pressure. Combining two or more of the recommended lifestyle changes can achieve even more favorable results.

Pharmacologic Interventions

Several classes of medications have been proven effective in lowering blood pressure and reducing the complications of hypertension, including angiotensin-converting enzyme (ACE) inhibitors, angiotensin-receptor blockers (ARBs), β-blockers, calcium channel blockers, and thiazide diuretics. Thiazide diuretics have been the basis of antihypertensive therapy in many outcome trials[1,17] and should be considered the initial treatment for most patients with hypertension unless there is a compelling indication to use

Table 11-9: Lifestyle Modifications to Manage Hypertension*

Modifications	Recommendation	Approximate SBP Reduction, Range
Weight reduction	Maintain normal body weight (BMI, 18.5-24.9 kg/m^2)	5-20 mm Hg/10 kg weight loss[8,9,12]
Adopt DASH eating plan	Consume a diet rich in fruits, vegetables, and low-fat dairy products (reduced content of saturated and total fat).	8-14 mm Hg[13,14]
Dietary sodium reduction	Reduce dietary sodium intake to no more than 100 mEq/L (2.4 g sodium or 6 g sodium chloride).	2-8 mm Hg[13,15]

*For overall cardiovascular risk reduction, stop smoking. The effects of implementing these modifications are dose and time dependent and could be higher for some individuals.

Modifications	Recommendation	Approximate SBP Reduction, Range
Physical activity	Engage in regular aerobic physical activity, such as brisk walking (at least 30 minutes per day, most days of the week).	4-9 mm Hg[11,16]
Moderation of alcohol consumption	Limit consumption to no more than two drinks per day (1 oz or 30 mL ethanol [eg, 24 oz beer, 10 oz wine, or 3 oz 80-proof whiskey]) in most men and no more than one drink per day in women and lighter-weight people.	2-4 mm Hg[10]

BMI=body mass index, calculated as weight in kilograms, divided by the square of height in meters; BP=blood pressure; DASH=Dietary Approaches to Stop Hypertension, SBP=systolic blood pressure

Table 11-10: Oral Antihypertensive Drugs*

Drug	Usual Dose Range, mg/d (daily frequency)
Thiazide diuretics	
Chlorothiazide (Diuril®)	125-500 (1)
Chlorthalidone	12.5-25 (1)
Hydrochlorothiazide (Microzide™, HydroDIURIL®)	12.5-50 (1)
Polythiazide (Renese®)	2-4 (1)
Indapamide (Lozol®)	1.25-2.5 (1)
Metolazone	
Mykrox®	0.5-1.0 (1)
Zaroxolyn®	2.5-5 (1)
Loop diuretics	
Bumetanide (Bumex®)	0.5-2 (2)
Furosemide (Lasix®)	20-80 (2)
Torsemide (Demadex®)	2.5-10 (1)
Potassium-sparing diuretics	
Amiloride (Midamor®)	5-10 (1-2)
Triamterene (Dyrenium®)	50-100 (1-2)
Aldosterone receptor blockers	
Eplerenone (Inspra®)	50-100 (1-2)
Spironolactone (Aldactone®)	25-50 (1-2)
β-Blockers	
Atenolol (Tenormin®)	25-100 (1)
Betaxolol (Kerlone®)	5-20 (1)
Bisoprolol (Zebeta®)	2.5-10 (1)
Metoprolol	
Lopressor®	50-100 (1-2)
Toprol XL® (extended release)	50-100 (1)
Nadolol (Corgard®)	40-120 (1)

Drug	Usual Dose Range, mg/d (daily frequency)
***β-Blockers** (continued)*	
Propranolol	
Inderal®	40-160 (1)
Inderal® LA (long acting)	60-180 (1)
Timolol (Blocadren®)	20-40 (2)
β-Blockers with intrinsic sympathomimetic activity	
Acebutolol (Sectral®)	200-800 (2)
Penbutolol (Levatol®)	10-40 (1)
Pindolol (Visken®)	10-40 (2)
Combined α- and β-blockers	
Carvedilol (Coreg®)	12.5-50 (2)
Labetalol (Normodyne®, Trandate®)	200-800 (2)
Angiotensin-converting enzyme inhibitors	
Benazepril (Lotensin®)	10-40 (1-2)
Captopril (Capoten®)	25-100 (2)
Enalapril (Vasotec®)	2.5-40 (1-2)
Fosinopril (Monopril®)	10-40 (1)
Lisinopril (Prinivil®, Zestril®)	10-40 (1)
Moexipril (Univasc®)	7.5-30 (1)
Perindopril (Aceon®)	4-8 (1-2)
Quinapril (Accupril®)	10-40 (1)
Ramipril (Altace®)	2.5-20 (1)
Trandolapril (Mavik®)	1-4 (1)

(continued on next page)

Table 11-10: Oral Antihypertensive Drugs* (continued)

Drug	Usual Dose Range, mg/d (daily frequency)
Angiotensin II antagonists	
Candesartan (Atacand®)	8-32 (1)
Eprosartan (Teveten®)	400-800 (1-2)
Irbesartan (Avapro®)	150-300 (1)
Losartan (Cozaar®)	25-100 (1-2)
Olmesartan (Benicar®)	20-40 (1)
Telmisartan (Micardis®)	20-80 (1)
Valsartan (Diovan®)	80-320 (1)
Calcium channel blockers	
Nondihydropyridines	
Diltiazem (extended release)	
Cardizem® CD, Dilacor XR®, Tiazac®	180-420 (1)
Cardizem® LA	120-540 (1)
Verapamil	
Calan®, Isoptin® (immediate release)	80-320 (2)
Calan® SR, Isoptin® SR (extended release)	120-360 (1-2)
Covera HS®, Verelan® PM (extended release)	120-360 (1)

National Heart, Lung, and Blood Institute: *JNC 7 Express: The Seventh Report of the Joint National Committee on Prevention, Detection, Evaluation, and Treatment of High Blood Pressure*. Rockville, MD, US Department of Health and Human Services, 2003. NIH publication no. 03-5233.

Drug	Usual Dose Range, mg/d (daily frequency)
Dihydropyridines	
Amlodipine (Norvasc®)	2.5-10 (1)
Felodipine (Plendil®)	2.5-20 (1)
Isradipine (DynaCirc® CR)	2.5-10 (2)
Nicardipine, sustained release (Cardene® SR)	60-120 (2)
Nifedipine, long acting (Adalat® CC, Procardia XL®)	30-60 (1)
Nisoldipine (Sular®)	10-40 (1)
α_1-Blockers	
Doxazosin (Cardura®)	1-16 (1)
Prazosin (Minipress®)	2-20 (2-3)
Terazosin (Hytrin®)	1-20 (1-2)
Centrally acting drugs	
Clonidine	
Catapres®	0.1-0.8 (2)
Catapres-TTS® (patch)	0.1-0.3 (1/wk)
Methyldopa (Aldomet®)	250-1,000 (2)
Reserpine	0.05**-0.25 (1)
Guanfacine	0.5-2 (1)
Direct vasodilators	
Hydralazine (Apresoline®)	25-100 (2)
Minoxidil (Loniten®)	2.5-80 (1-2)

*Dosages may vary from those listed in the *Physician's Desk Reference.*

**A 0.1-mg dose may be given every other day to achieve this dosage.

Table 11-11: Fixed-dose Combination Drugs for Hypertension*

ACEI and CCB	Trade Name
Amlodipine/benazepril hydrochloride (2.5/10, 5/10, 5/20, 10/20)	Lotrel®
Enalapril maleate/felodipine (5/5)	Lexxel®
Trandolapril/verapamil (2/180, 1/240, 2/240, 4/240)	Tarka®
ACEI and Diuretic	**Trade Name**
Benazepril/hydrochlorothiazide (5/6.25, 10/12.5, 20/12.5, 20/25)	Lotensin HCT®
Captopril/hydrochlorothiazide (25/15, 25/25, 50/15, 50/25)	Capozide®
Enalapril maleate/hydrochloro-thiazide (5/12.5, 10/25)	Vaseretic®
Lisinopril/hydrochlorothiazide (10/12.5, 20/12.5, 20/25)	Prinzide®
Moexipril/hydrochlorothiazide (7.5/12.5, 15/25)	Uniretic®
Quinapril/hydrochlorothiazide (10/12.5, 20/12.5, 20/25)	Accuretic®

ARB and Diuretic	Trade Name
Candesartan cilexetil/hydro-chlorothiazide (16/12.5, 32/12.5)	Atacand HCT®
Eprosartan mesylate/hydro-chlorothiazide (600/12.5, 600/25)	Teveten® HCT
Irbesartan/hydrochlorothiazide (150/12.5, 300/12.5)	Avalide®
Losartan potassium/hydro-chlorothiazide (50/12.5, 100/25)	Hyzaar®
Telmisartan/hydrochlorothiazide (40/12.5, 80/12.5)	Micardis® HCT
Valsartan/hydrochlorothiazide (80/12.5, 160/12.5)	Diovan-HCT®

BB and Diuretic	Trade Name
Atenolol/chlorthalidone (50/25, 100/25)	Tenoretic®
Bisoprolol fumarate/ hydrochlorothiazide (2.5/6.25, 5/6.25, 10/6.25)	Ziac®
Propranolol LA/hydrochloro-thiazide (40/25, 80/25)	Inderide®
Metoprolol tartrate/hydro-chlorothiazide (50/25, 100/25)	Lopressor HCT®
Nadolol/bendroflumethiazide (40/5, 80/5)	Corzide®
Timolol maleate/hydro-chlorothiazide (10/25)	Timolide®

(continued on next page)

Table 11-11: Fixed-dose Combination Drugs for Hypertension* *(continued)*

CCB and Statin	Trade Name
Amlodipine/atorvastatin (2.5/10, 2.5/20, 2.5/40, 5/10, 5/20, 5/40, 5/80, 10/10, 10/20, 10/40, 10/80)	Caduet®

Centrally Acting Drug and Diuretic	Trade Name
Methyldopa/hydrochlorothiazide (250/15, 250/25, 500/30, 500/50)	Aldoril®
Reserpine/chlorothiazide (0.125/250, 0.25/500)	Diupres®
Reserpine/hydrochlorothiazide (0.125/25, 0.125/50)	Hydropres®

ACEI = angiotensin converting enzyme inhibitor, ARB = angiotensin receptor blocker, BB = β-blocker, CCB = calcium channel blocker

*Some drug combinations are available in multiple fixed doses. Each drug dose is listed in milligrams.

another class of medication. Diuretics, which are more affordable than other antihypertensive medications, can be used either alone to achieve blood pressure control or in combination therapy to enhance the antihypertensive efficacy of multidrug regimens. Thiazide diuretics are especially effective in combination with other antihypertensive medications because all nondiuretic antihypertensives increase plasma volume, and the effects of thiazide diuretics on blood pressure generally last for 24 hours. Despite their proven efficacy, diuretics continue to be underused.[18]

Diuretic	Trade Name
Amiloride HCl/hydrochlorothiazide (5/50)	Moduretic®
Spironolactone/hydrochlorothiazide (25/25, 50/50)	Aldactazide®
Triamterene/hydrochlorothiazide (37.5/25, 50/25, 75/50)	Dyazide®, Maxzide®

National Heart, Lung, and Blood Institute: *JNC 7 Express: the Seventh Report of the Joint National Committee on Prevention, Detection, Evaluation, and Treatment of High Blood Pressure.* Bethesda, MD, US Department of Health and Human Services, 2003. NIH publication no. 03-5233.

If the medication selected is not well tolerated or is contraindicated for a particular patient, a medication from one of the other classes proven to reduce cardiovascular events should be used. Table 11-10 lists commonly used antihypertensive agents.

Most patients with hypertension need two or more antihypertensive medications to achieve their blood pressure goals. When a single medication in adequate doses fails to achieve the goal (eg, when blood pressure is more than 20/10 mm Hg higher than goal), a second medica-

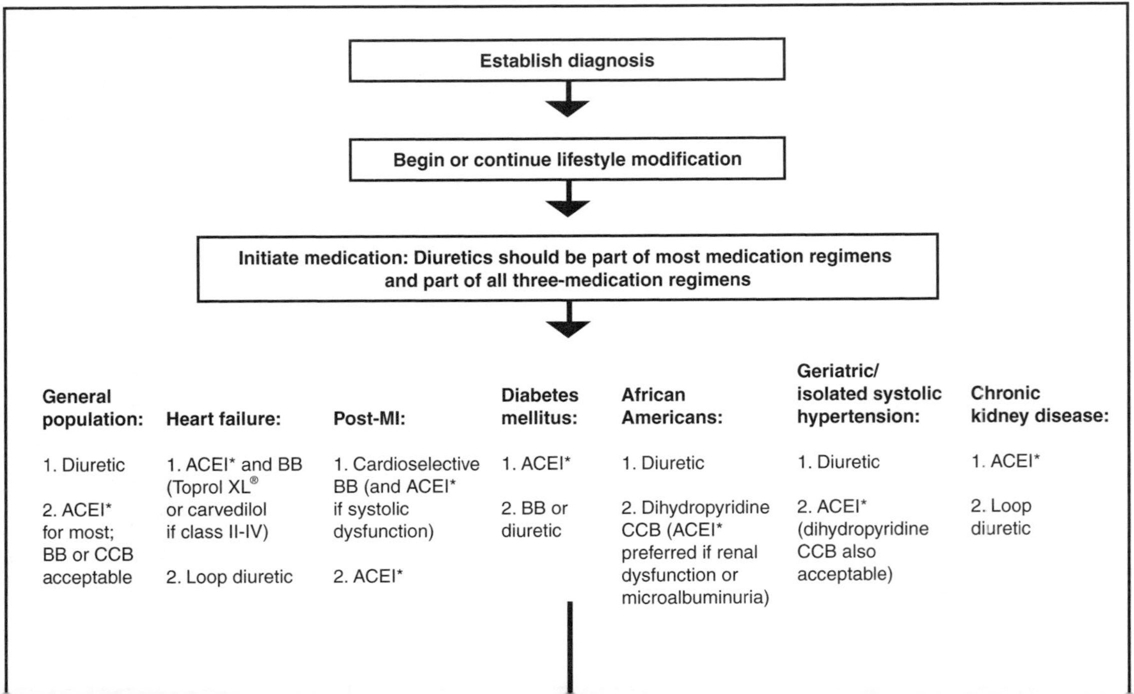
Establish diagnosis
Begin or continue lifestyle modification
Initiate medication: Diuretics should be part of most medication regimens and part of all three-medication regimens
General population:
1. Diuretic
2. ACEI* for most; BB or CCB acceptable
Heart failure:
1. ACEI* and BB (Toprol XL® or carvedilol if class II-IV)
2. Loop diuretic
Post-MI:
1. Cardioselective BB (and ACEI* if systolic dysfunction)
2. ACEI*
Diabetes mellitus:
1. ACEI*
2. BB or diuretic
African Americans:
1. Diuretic
2. Dihydropyridine CCB (ACEI* preferred if renal dysfunction or microalbuminuria)
Geriatric/ isolated systolic hypertension:
1. Diuretic
2. ACEI* (dihydropyridine CCB also acceptable)
Chronic kidney disease:
1. ACEI*
2. Loop diuretic

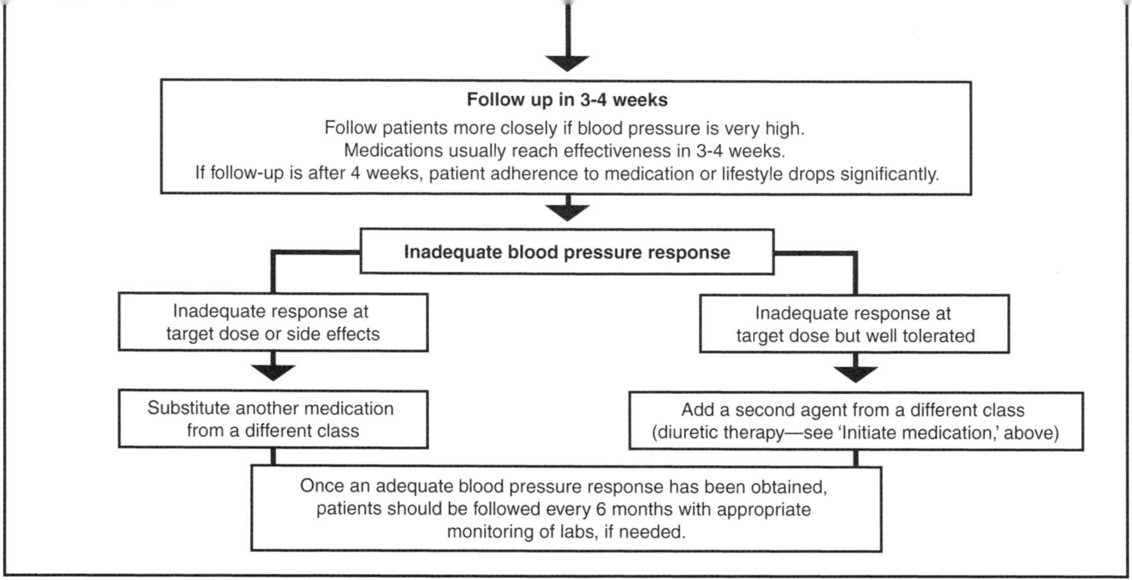

Figure 11-2: Treatment of hypertension. This is a simplified algorithm to cover most hypertensive patients. Selection of drug therapy should be based on the patient's clinical status and comorbidities. * Angiotensin receptor blocker if cough or angioedema with ACEI. ACEI = angiotensin converting enzyme inhibitor, BB = β-blocker, CCB = calcium channel blocker.

Table 11-12: Initial Hypertension Therapy in Patients With Comorbid Disease[1]

Diabetes Mellitus

- Combinations of two or more drugs are usually needed to achieve the target blood pressure goal of <130/80 mm Hg.
- ACE inhibitor provides maximum cardiovascular and renal benefits.
- In patients with microalbuminuria or clinical albuminuria, use ACE inhibitor or ARB.
- β-Blockers and diuretics are second-line agents.
- Benefit from myocardial infarction/stroke reduction from β-blockade outweighs the risk of masking hypoglycemia.
- β-Blockers and long-acting diltiazem are appropriate alternatives for patients who cannot tolerate, or whose hypertension is not controlled by, ACE inhibitor plus low-dose diuretic therapy.
- ACE inhibitors have been the primary agents studied for type 2 diabetes.

tion should be added to increase the likelihood of achieving the blood pressure goal more quickly. Thiazide diuretics are particularly synergistic with other classes of medications and should be considered with any other class of medication as the second choice. However, they should be used with caution in patients who are at risk for orthostatic hypotension, patients with diabetes, and some older patients. Table 11-11 lists combination medications for hypertension.

Heart Failure

- Mild symptoms—start with ACE inhibitor.
- ACE inhibitor should be titrated to the highest dose tolerated, even if blood pressure is low, as long as the patient does not become symptomatic or develop impaired renal function.
- ARB may be substituted for ACE inhibitor when ACE inhibitor is not tolerated.
- β-Blockers should be started if the patient has ischemic heart disease, is post myocardial infarction, has angina, or has reached ACE inhibitor target dose. Titrate to the highest dose tolerated.
- Spironolactone should be considered after the patient is placed on the maximum doses of ACE inhibitor and β-blocker.
- Diuretics (usually loop) are often used acutely for fluid management.

(continued on next page)

In January 2004, the US Food and Drug Administration (FDA) approved the first medicine to treat two different conditions with one pill. The drug, which is marketed by Pfizer under the trade name Caduet®, combines amlodipine (Norvasc®) and atorvastatin (Lipitor®). Caduet® is indicated for the treatment of hypertension, chronic stable angina, vasospastic angina, dysbetalipoproteinemia, elevated serum TG levels, hypercholesterolemia, and mixed dyslipidemia. The dosage should be individu-

Table 11-12: Initial Hypertension Therapy in Patients With Comorbid Disease[1] *(continued)*

Chronic Kidney Failure

- Goal is to slow deterioration of renal function and prevent cardiovascular disease.
- Chronic kidney failure is defined as reduced excretory function with an estimated glomerular filtration rate of <60 mL/min per 1.73 m^2 (approximate creatinine of >1.5 mg/dL [132.6 µmol/L] in men and >1.3 mg/dL [>114.9 µmol/l] in women) **or** the presence of albuminuria (>300 mg/d or 200 mg albumin per gram of creatinine).
- Use of ACE inhibitor or ARB has demonstrated favorable effect on renal disease.
- A limited increase in serum creatinine of as much as 35% above baseline with an ACE inhibitor or an ARB is acceptable and not a reason to withhold treatment unless hyperkalemia develops.
- In patients with advanced renal disease (estimated glomerular filtration rate <30 mL/min per 1.73 m^2), increasing doses of loop diuretics are usually needed in combination with other drug classes.

ACE = angiotensin-converting enzyme,
ARB = angiotensin receptor blocker

alized based on the effectiveness and tolerance for each drug in the combination. The usual beginning dose of the antihypertensive amlodipine is 5 mg once a day, with a maximum dose of 10 mg once a day.

Compelling evidence exists for initiating treatment with a medication other than a thiazide diuretic in some patients with hypertension and certain comorbidities including heart failure, high coronary heart disease risk, diabetes, chronic kidney disease, recurrent stroke, and previous MI.

Figure 11-2 presents an algorithm for initial therapy for patients with these comorbidities, and Tables 11-12 and 11-13 present the clinical basis for the guideline.

Special Considerations in Medication Choices

Antihypertensive medications can have favorable and unfavorable effects that clinicians should know about when making treatment decisions. Some favorable effects that specific antihypertensive medication classes may have on other conditions are listed below.

- Thiazide diuretics are useful in slowing demineralization in osteoporosis.
- β-Blockers are useful in treating atrial tachyarrhythmia/fibrillation, migraine headaches, essential tremor, or perioperative hypertension. They may also have short-term usefulness in treating thyrotoxicosis.
- Calcium channel blockers may be useful in treating Raynaud's syndrome and certain arrhythmias.
- α-Blockers may be useful in treating prostatism.

Contraindications and Common Side Effects of Antihypertensive Medications

Similar to most medications, antihypertensives also can adversely affect some patients. Some possible unfavorable effects of specific classes of antihypertensive medications are listed below.

Table 11-13: Medication Notes for Treatment of Hypertension

Diuretics

- Diuretics are recommended for initial therapy unless a compelling indication is met.
- Diuretics are synergistic with all other classes of antihypertensive medications and should be part of most medication regimens.
- Low doses (12.5-25 mg hydrochlorothiazide) should be used unless the patient has heart failure or chronic kidney disease, in which case a loop diuretic (furosemide) should be used.
- Diuretics should be considered part of all three-medication regimens.
- JNC 7 defines resistant hypertension as the failure to reach goal blood pressure in patients who are adhering to full doses of an appropriate three-drug regimen that includes a diuretic.
- Diuretics reduce reflex fluid retention associated with lowering blood pressure and must be added before diagnosing resistant hypertension.
- Check blood urea nitrogen, creatinine, and potassium 6 weeks after initiation and yearly thereafter, unless symptoms suggest renal or electrolyte disorders. More frequent monitoring is recommended if other drugs that affect renal function or potassium homeostasis are being used.

ACE Inhibitors and ARBs

- ACE inhibitors and ARBs have once-daily dosing.
- With the exception of captopril, based on kinetics and mechanism of action, twice-daily dosing is not more effective in treating hypertension. Twice-daily dosing may be better tolerated in older patients and those with congestive heart failure.
- ARBs are alternatives for patients with ACE inhibitor-associated cough or angioedema.
- Check blood urea nitrogen, creatinine, and potassium 6 weeks after initiation and yearly thereafter, unless symptoms suggest renal or electrolyte disorders. More frequent monitoring is recommended if other drugs that affect renal function or potassium homeostasis are being used.

ACE = angiotensin-converting enzyme,
ARB = angiotensin receptor blocker,
JNC 7 = *Seventh Report of the Joint National Committee on Prevention, Detection, Evaluation, and Treatment of High Blood Pressure.*

- Thiazide diuretics should be used cautiously in patients who have gout or a history of significant hyponatremia.
- β-Blockers should be avoided in patients with asthma, reactive airway disease, or second- or third-degree heart block.
- ACE inhibitors and ARBs are contraindicated in pregnant women and women who are likely to become pregnant. Caution should also be used for patients with significant renal failure.
- ACE inhibitors should not be prescribed for patients with a history of angioedema.
- Aldosterone antagonists and potassium-sparing diuretics cause hyperkalemia and should be avoided in patients with baseline serum potassium values of more than 5.0 mmol/L.

Follow-up and Monitoring

Once antihypertensive therapy has been initiated, patients should return approximately once a month for follow-up to adjust their treatment and medications until they have reached their blood pressure goals. These visits are essential, because high blood pressure is an asymptomatic condition, and patient adherence drops quickly after 1 month if there is no feedback on the effects of the treatment. Follow-up visits can be provided by a health professional other than a physician and can be brief, but they must provide enough time for blood pressure evaluation, interim history, and a treatment plan. For patients with stage 2 hypertension or with complicating comorbid conditions, physician visits may be needed.

Serum potassium and creatinine levels should be checked once or twice a year. In patients with renal insufficiency and patients whose medication needs adjustment, these levels should be checked more often. When patients have reached their blood pressure goals and remain stable, follow-up visits can be scheduled at 3- to 6-month intervals, depending on comorbidities and the need for laboratory testing.

Special Treatment Considerations

Treatment for hypertension is similar for all demographic groups. However, socioeconomic factors and lifestyle can present barriers to blood pressure control. The following are special considerations that may affect treatment decisions.

- African-Americans: Hypertension is more prevalent and tends to be more severe. These patients demonstrate somewhat reduced blood pressure responses to monotherapy with β-blockers, ACE inhibitors, or ARBs than with diuretics or calcium channel blockers. However, any of these medications combined with a diuretic provides a good response.
- Obesity and the metabolic syndrome: These risk factors for developing hypertension are becoming increasingly prevalent in the United States, including in children, young adults, and, especially, minorities.
- Left ventricular hypertrophy (LVH): LVH is an independent risk factor that increases the risk of adverse CVD outcomes. Effective therapy requires aggressive blood pressure management, weight loss, sodium restriction, and treatment with all classes of medications except the direct vasodilators, hydralazine, and minoxidil.
- Peripheral arterial disease (PAD): PAD is equivalent in risk to ischemic heart disease. Hypertension in most patients with PAD can be treated with any class of antihypertensive medications. Additionally, other risk factors should be managed aggressively and aspirin should be used.
- Elderly patients: More than two thirds of people older than 65 years have hypertension, but this population has the lowest rate of blood pressure control. Treatment should follow the general principles of hypertension care, but lower initial doses may be indicated to avoid adverse reactions. Ultimately, standard doses and multiple medications will be needed to reach blood pressure control.

- Postural hypotension: Caution should be used to avoid volume depletion and excessively rapid dose titration of antihypertensive medications.
- Dementia and cognitive impairment: These conditions occur more commonly in people with hypertension. Effective antihypertensive therapy can reduce the progression of cognitive impairment.
- Women: Oral contraceptives may cause an increase in blood pressure, so it should be checked regularly. In contrast, hormone replacement therapy does not raise blood pressure.[19] Women taking oral contraceptives who develop hypertension should consider other forms of contraception.
- Pregnant women: Pregnant women with hypertension should be followed carefully to reduce complications. For the safety of the fetus, methyldopa, β-blockers, and vasodilators are the preferred treatment. ACE inhibitors and ARBs are contraindicated in pregnancy.
- Children and adolescents: Secondary causes are more common in these patients. Lifestyle interventions are the preferred initial therapy. For children with higher levels of blood pressure or an insufficient response to lifestyle modifications, medication choices are similar to those in adults, but doses are usually lower. Children and adolescents with uncomplicated hypertension that is well controlled do not need to restrict physical activity.
- Patients with severe hypertension and acute target organ damage ('hypertensive emergency'): These patients require hospitalization and immediate parenteral medication therapy.[20]
- Patients with unusually high blood pressure but no acute target organ damage ('hypertensive urgency'): These patients do not need to be hospitalized, but they should receive immediate treatment with combination oral antihypertensive therapy.

Algorithms

Figure 11-2 outlines the strategy proposed by the JNC 7 report for treating hypertension.

Improving Hypertension Control

Even the most effective therapy prescribed by the most careful physician will not successfully control hypertension if the patient is not motivated to take the prescribed medication and make the recommended lifestyle changes. The clinician's ability to empathize with patients is a key factor in earning their trust and thereby in increasing their motivation to adhere to the therapy prescribed.

Before deciding on a treatment strategy, it is important that:

- The clinician understands the patient's cultural beliefs and attitudes toward the health care system that may affect his or her acceptance of the prescribed therapy and trust in physicians.
- The clinician and the patient agree on the blood pressure goal and the strategy to achieve it.
- The clinician helps the patient feel comfortable about sharing concerns and fears about treatment.

Patient Education

Because hypertension, like dyslipidemia, is largely a 'silent' condition, patient education and counseling are critical to prevention and treatment, especially for patients who are at risk for CVD. Patients resist modifying their lifestyle or taking medication when they are experiencing no symptoms. Blood pressure screenings for all patients should be conducted routinely. Physicians and patients should talk about the dangers of hypertension and about healthy lifestyle choices, such as exercising regularly, reducing intake of calories, sodium, and saturated fats, and stopping smoking.

Patients who require antihypertensive medications need to be informed about the dangers of uncontrolled hyperten-

Table 11-14: Critical Factors Affecting Patient Adherence to Hypertension Therapy

- Misunderstanding of the condition or the treatment
- Denial of illness, because of the absence of symptoms
- Belief that medications are a symbol of ill health
- Personal lack of involvement in the care plan
- Unexpected adverse effects of medications
- Concern about the cost of treatment
- Difficulty in scheduling appointments
- Competing demands on their time

sion and the importance of taking medications as prescribed. To encourage adherence, a daily routine for taking medications should be established. Patients should inform their physicians of any side effects they may experience so that medication dosage can be adjusted or the medication changed to a different class that can help them reach their blood pressure goals with a minimum of troublesome side effects. Chapter 14 offers detailed information on prevention and patient education strategies physicians can incorporate into their existing practice settings. Many of them can be implemented during routine patient visits. Table 11-14 lists critical factors affecting adherence to hypertension therapy.

Resistant Hypertension

When a patient fails to reach his or her goal blood pressure despite adhering to full doses of an appropriate three-medication regimen, the clinician should first rule out identifiable causes of resistant hypertension (Tables 11-6 and 11-15), paying particular attention to the type of diuretic

Table 11-15: Causes of Resistant Hypertension

Improper Blood Pressure Measurement

Volume Overload and Pseudotolerance

- Excessive sodium intake
- Volume retention from kidney disease
- Inadequate diuretic therapy

Medication-induced or Other Causes

- Lack of adherence to the prescribed therapy
- Inadequate doses
- Inappropriate combinations
- Nonsteroidal anti-inflammatory medications
- Cocaine, amphetamines, or other illicit drugs
- Sympathomimetics (decongestants, anorectics)
- Oral contraceptives
- Adrenal steroids
- Cyclosporine and tacrolimus
- Erythropoietin
- Consuming licorice or chewing tobacco
- Selected over-the-counter dietary supplements and medicines (eg, ephedra, ma huang, bitter orange)

Associated Conditions

- Obesity
- Excess alcohol intake

and the dose in relation to renal function. If the blood pressure goal still cannot be achieved, consultation with a hypertension specialist should be considered.

A Public Health Approach

Clinicians can reduce the risk for hypertension by promoting public health approaches. The epidemic of obesity will have such an enormous impact on the health of the population that medical care will not be able to respond adequately. According to JNC 7, advocating public health intervention strategies such as reducing daily dietary caloric and salt intake (especially in processed foods), reducing body weight, increasing community and school opportunities for physical activity, and eliminating smoking in public places will 'provide an attractive opportunity to interrupt and prevent the continuing costly cycle of managing hypertension and its complications.'[1] Physicians can help by promoting and supporting community health efforts. Community health efforts to prevent hypertension and obesity, especially in children, have the greatest potential effect on long-term health outcomes.[1]

References

1. Chobanian AV, Bakris GL, Black HR, et al: The Seventh Report of the Joint National Committee on Prevention, Detection, Evaluation, and Treatment of High Blood Pressure: the JNC 7 report. *JAMA* 2003;289:2560-2572.

2. National Heart, Lung, and Blood Institute: *JNC 7 Express: The Seventh Report of the Joint National Committee on Prevention, Detection, Evaluation and Treatment of High Blood Pressure*. Rockville, MD, US Department of Health and Human Services, 2003. NIH publication no. 03-5233.

3. Izzo JL Jr, Levy D, Black HR: Clinical advisory statement: importance of systolic blood pressure in older Americans. *Hypertension* 2000;35:1021-1024.

4. Oliveria SA, Lapuerta P, McCarthy BD, et al: Physician-related barriers to the effective management of uncontrolled hypertension. *Arch Intern Med* 2002;162:413-420.

5. Neal B, MacMahon S, Chapman N: Effects of ACE inhibitors, calcium antagonists, and other blood-pressure-lowering drugs: results of prospectively designed overviews of randomised trials. Blood Pressure Lowering Treatment Trialists' Collaboration. *Lancet* 2000;356:1955-1964.

6. Ogden LG, He J, Lydeck E, et al: Long-term absolute benefit of lowering blood pressure in hypertensive patients, according to JNC VI risk stratification. *Hypertension* 2000;35:539-543.

7. American Diabetes Association: Treatment of hypertension in adults with diabetes. *Diabetes Care* 2003;26(suppl 1):580-582.

8. National Kidney Foundation (NKF) Kidney Disease Outcome Quality Initiative (K/DOQI) Advisory Board: K/DOQI clinical practice guidelines for chronic kidney disease: evaluation, classification, and stratification. *Am J Kidney Dis* 2002;39(suppl 2): S1-S246.

9. The Trials of Hypertension Prevention Collaborative Research Group: Effects of weight loss and sodium reduction intervention on blood pressure and hypertension incidence in overweight people with high-normal blood pressure. The Trials of Hypertension Prevention, Phase II. *Arch Intern Med* 1997;157:657-667.

10. Xin X, He J, Frontini MG, et al: Effects of alcohol reduction on blood pressure: a meta-analysis of randomized controlled trials. *Hypertension* 2001;38:1112-1117.

11. Whelton SP, Chin A, Xin X, et al: Effect of aerobic exercise on blood pressure: a meta-analysis of randomized controlled trials. *Ann Intern Med* 2002;136:493-503.

12. He J, Whelton PK, Appel LJ, et al: Long-term effects of weight loss and dietary sodium reduction on incidence of hypertension. *Hypertension* 2000;35:544-549.

13. Sacks FM, Svetkey LP, Vollmer WM, et al: Effects on blood pressure of reduced dietary sodium and the Dietary Approaches to Stop Hypertension (DASH) diet. DASH-Sodium Collaborative Research Group. *N Engl J Med* 2001;344:3-10.

14. Vollmer WM, Sacks FM, Ard J, et al: Effects of diet and sodium intake on blood pressure: subgroup analysis of the DASH-Sodium trial. *Ann Intern Med* 2001;135:1019-1028.

15. Chobanian AV, Hill M: National Heart, Lung, and Blood Institute Workshop on Sodium and Blood Pressure: a critical review of current scientific evidence. *Hypertension* 2000;35:858-863.

16. Kelley GA, Kelley KS: Progressive resistance exercise and resting blood pressure: A meta-analysis of randomized controlled trials. *Hypertension* 2000;35:838-843.

17. Psaty BM, Smith NL, Siscoveck DS, et al: Health outcomes associated with antihypertensive therapies used as first-line agents. A systematic review and meta-analysis. *JAMA* 1997;277:739-745.

18. Psaty BM, Manolio TA, Smith NL, et al: Time trends in high blood pressure control and the use of antihypertensive medications in older adults: the Cardiovascular Health Study. *Arch Intern Med* 2002;162:2325-2332.

19. Risks and benefits of estrogen plus progestin in healthy postmenopausal women: principal results from the Women's Health Initiative randomized controlled trial. *JAMA* 2002;288:321-333.

20. The Sixth Report of the Joint National Committee on Prevention, Detection, Evaluation and Treatment of High Blood Pressure. *Arch Intern Med* 1997;157:2413-2446.

CHAPTER 12

Emerging Cardiovascular Risk Factors

The established cardiovascular disease (CVD) risk factors (examined in Chapter 1) account for most but not all of the defined CVD risk, including the risk within a specific population and between different populations.[1] Although new trials of treatment for elevated cholesterol levels, hypertension, diabetes, and smoking show marked reductions in risk for coronary heart disease (CHD), a significant proportion of CHD events occur in those with conventional risk factors treated to target. Less commonly, patients experience CVD events with major abnormalities of risk factors. Although cholesterol-lowering therapy has been shown to prevent adverse cardiac events in several large clinical trials, the incidence of myocardial infarction (MI) and cardiac-related deaths remains unacceptably high.[2] As a result, the medical community has intensified its search for new risk factors for CHD. Many additional factors are emerging as possible determinants of coronary disease or other atherosclerotic disease, including homocysteine, lipoprotein (a) [Lp(a)], and markers of inflammation such as C-reactive protein, fibrinogen, and interleukin (IL)-6.

Although these factors are not included in the typical risk evaluation system, convincing evidence suggests that some or all of them may play a role in determining CHD risk. Many other promising factors are under evaluation as well.

Homocysteine

Homocysteine (Hcy), an amino acid that intermediates in methionine metabolism, is normally found in small amounts in the blood. Vitamins B_6 and B_{12}, plus folate and several enzyme systems, promote the conversion of Hcy to cysteine. Deficiencies in these vitamins lead to elevated Hcy levels, which are associated with an increased risk of coronary disease.[3] Patients with homozygous homocystinuria (high serum Hcy levels) have a greater than 50% likelihood of CHD by age 30.[1] In fact, high plasma Hcy levels can be detected in 20% to 30% of patients with premature coronary artery disease (CAD).[3] A direct causal link has not been established, but evidence suggests that Hcy may contribute to atherosclerosis by damaging the arterial endothelium and promoting thrombosis. Several studies have demonstrated strong associations between hyperhomocysteinemia and CHD, cerebrovascular disease, and peripheral vascular disease (PVD).[3-15] Although more research is needed, elevated Hcy levels are an emerging CHD risk factor, and our broadening understanding of Hcy may be helpful in secondary CHD prevention and in warning patients with a strong family history of premature CHD.

Hyperhomocysteinemia may result from abnormalities in the function of any of the enzymes involved in Hcy metabolism or from deficiencies of enzyme cofactors or cosubstrates. Clinically, total Hcy levels increase as people age and with tobacco use.[16,17] Men have higher total Hcy levels than women, and total Hcy levels tend to be elevated in individuals with renal dysfunction, unexplained deep venous thrombosis, and other chronic medical disorders (Table 12-1).[18]

Because there are a limited number of clinical trials demonstrating that lowering Hcy levels reduces the risk of CVD, population-wide screening for elevated Hcy is not recommended. In one trial, patients given folic acid, vitamin B_6, and vitamin B_{12} after percutaneous transluminal coronary angioplasty had a 48% reduction in restenosis.[1]

A recent clinical trial testing whether treatment of Hcy could reduce recurrent stroke revealed that the use of a multivitamin vs high-dose folate and vitamins B_6 and B_{12} made no difference.[19] However, screening may be useful for patients with a personal or family history of CVD who do not have the well-established risk factors but might benefit from Hcy-lowering therapy. Other groups for whom screening may be useful include individuals with the following conditions: chronic renal failure; unexplained deep venous thrombosis; systemic lupus erythematosus; severe psoriasis; those who have undergone a solid organ transplant; and those who take medications known to raise Hcy levels (Table 12-1).

Homocysteine concentrations exceeding the target value of 10 mmol/L are a sensitive marker for folate deficiency, and levels greater than 20 mmol/L may indicate an inherited enzyme or nutritional vitamin B_6 or B_{12} deficiency. In the United States, some adults, especially pregnant women, consume inadequate levels of folate and have functional folate deficiency.[3] The recognition of this condition gave rise to a government mandate requiring that flour be fortified with folic acid to help people achieve a minimal daily intake of 200 mg. Clinicians should advise all patients at high risk for CHD to get enough folic acid and vitamins B_6 and B_{12} in their diets by eating foods such as green leafy vegetables and grain fortified with folic acid.

Treatment for patients with known hyperhomocysteinemia should include dietary counseling and folate supplementation with a daily multivitamin containing at least 400 mg of folic acid.[20] To assess the response to treatment, the clinician should recheck Hcy levels in 8 weeks. If levels are still elevated, the dose of the folic acid supplement may be safely increased to 5 mg (5,000 μg) daily. Another amino acid, trimethlyglycine (often called TMG or betaine), is effective at lowering Hcy levels and is being investigated for Hcy treatment. Figure 12-1 illustrates a recommended treatment plan for patients with hyperhomocysteinemia.

Table 12-1: Causes of Hyperhomocysteinemia

Enzyme Deficiencies

- cystathionine β-synthase
- methionine synthase
- 5-methyltetrahydrofolate reductase

Vitamin Deficiencies

- folate
- vitamin B_6
- vitamin B_{12}

Demographics

- increasing age
- male sex
- tobacco users
- solid organ transplant recipients

Lipoprotein(a)

Lp(a) is a cholesterol-like particle that binds to low-density lipoprotein (LDL). Levels are genetically determined and are unaffected by diet or lifestyle. Lp(a) is an acute-phase reactant that acts in both atherogenesis and atherothrombosis (because a portion of the molecule is similar to plasminogen). Lp(a) is a large glycoprotein, apolipoprotein-A that binds to LDL cholesterol (LDL-C) and then to the arterial endothelium, causing increased cholesterol accumulation. It further increases thrombotic risk by competing for plasminogen receptors, which increases free plasminogen.[21,22] High Lp(a) levels indicate a patient at high risk for premature atherosclerosis.[1] Several large, prospective studies have recently identified

Chronic Medical Disorders

- chronic renal dysfunction
- systemic lupus erythematosus
- malignant neoplasm
- psoriasis

Acute-phase Response to Systemic Illness

Medication use

- methotrexate
- nitrous oxide
- antiseizure agents (phenytoin and carbamazepine)
- nicotinic acid
- colestipol
- thiazide diuretics

excess Lp(a), which is commonly detected in both men and women with premature CHD, as a powerful predictor of premature CHD[23-32] (Table 12-2).

An important component of the increased CHD risk associated with increased levels of Lp(a) is elevated LDL-C. Lipoprotein(a) appears to interact with LDL-C to promote atherogenesis by increasing the oxidative susceptibility of LDL-C, which is a critical first step in the development of atherosclerosis.[33,34] Lipoprotein(a) also contributes to atherothrombotic risk by[35] impairing fibrinolysis, increasing cholesterol deposits in the arterial wall, and enhancing oxidation of LDL-C.

Clinicians should consider Lp(a) screening for patients with atherosclerosis (particularly premature atheroscler o-

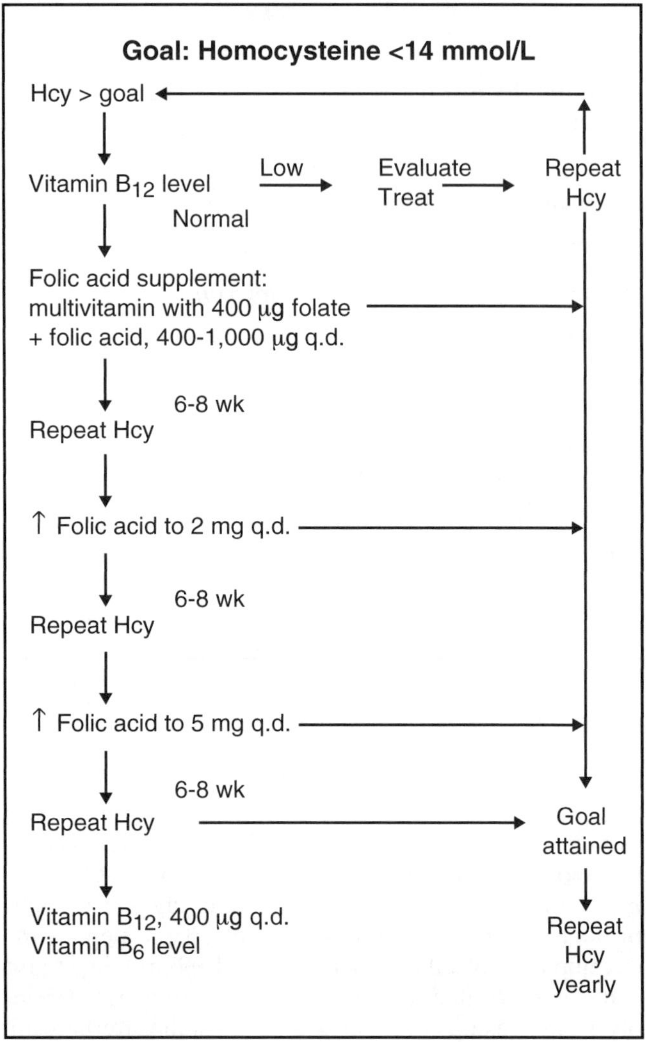

Figure 12-1: Treatment algorithm for patients with hyperhomocysteinemia. Hcy = total homocysteine level (fasting), q.d. = every day.

sis without obvious risk factors), and for those with a family history of premature CHD. Screening can identify high-risk individuals and high-risk families, and can promote early testing and treatment for family members. In addition, because of the high risk of Lp(a) in conjunction with LDL, LDL-C treatment targets of <110 mg/dL are suggested for primary prevention. Therapy aimed at lowering LDL-C has been proven to reduce cardiovascular events. Furthermore, according to the results of clinical trials that demonstrated decreased progression of atherosclerosis, lowering LDL-C in patients with high Lp(a) was sufficient to achieve the benefits.[32] Because there are still no clinical data to confirm that treating Lp(a) reduces cardiovascular events, LDL-C treatment is the primary intervention strategy for patients with high Lp(a).

Markers of Inflammation

Research indicates that atherosclerosis, in addition to being a disease of lipid accumulation, is a chronic inflammatory process.[36] Both basic science and epidemiologic studies have shown that atherogenesis is an inflammatory response that leads to the development of acute coronary and cerebrovascular syndromes.[36] As a result, atherosclerosis is now widely accepted as a chronic inflammatory disorder initiated by vascular injury induced by oxidized LDL, reactive oxygen species, diabetes mellitus, and other conditions.[37] Researchers have suggested that inflammatory markers such as high sensitivity C-reactive protein (hs-CRP), P-selectin, tumor necrosis factor-α, and IL-6 may provide additional methods for assessing cardiovascular risk in primary and secondary prevention.[36,38,39]

Although each of these emerging risk factors has been correlated with CHD, further investigation is needed before they can be firmly established as clinical markers for predicting CHD risk. In addition, evidence of benefits from treatment must be confirmed and treatment algorithms must be developed.

Table 12-2: Prospective Studies of Lp(a) Excess and CHD Risk

	Mean/Range of Follow-up Years	N Cases
Gothenburg	6	26
Helsinki	5	138
Guernsey	N/A	51
Reykjavik	8.6	104
Physician's Health	5.2	296
LRC-CPPT	7-10	233
BUPA	5-12	229

Lp(a) = lipoprotein(a), CHD = coronary heart disease, LRC-CPPT = Lipid Research Clinics Coronary Primary Prevention Trial, BUPA = British United Provident Association

N Controls	RR (95% CI)	*P* value	Comments
101	N/A	.01	Small
130	1.3 (0.8-2.0)	.37	Hypercholester-olemic cohort; no CHD
3,583	2.1 (1.0-4.7)	.07	Women; no CHD
1,228	1.2 (N/A)	.01	Similar to SBP, TG; weaker than TC and apo A-1
296	1.1 (0.7-1/8)	.80	No CHD
390	1.1 (1.0-1.2)	<.02	Hypercholester-olemic cohort Similar to LDL-C; weaker than HDL-C and tobacco use
1,145	2.3 (1.5-3.6)	<.05	All with CHD family history; weaker than apo B and apo A-1

SBP = systolic blood pressure, TG = triglyceride, TC = total cholesterol, LDL-C = low-density lipoprotein cholesterol, HDL-C = high-density lipoprotein cholesterol

(continued on next page)

Table 12-2: Prospective Studies of Lp(a) Excess and CHD Risk *(continued)*

	Mean/Range of Follow-up Years	N Cases
GRIPS	5	107
Framingham	15.4*	248
Framingham	12	174
Quebec	5	116

*Counteracted elevated high-density lipoprotein
GRIPS = Gottingham Risk Incidence and Prevalence Study

C-reactive Protein

High sensitivity C-reactive protein (CRP) measures inflammation at levels much lower than those previously used clinically—below 1 mg/L—and is a reliable predictor of CHD risk.[36,40-49] CRP is a signaling protein produced by the liver that has numerous effects on atherogenesis and metabolism, including increasing insulin resistance, LDL-oxidation, and endothelial damage. Clinical investigations have suggested a number of associations between hs-CRP and CHD. For example, recent

N Controls	RR (95% CI)	*P* value	Comments
5,728	2.4	<.01	No CHD
	(1.5-3.9)		Weaker than LDL-C, family history, fibrinogen, and HDL-C
1,943	1.9 (1.2-2.9)	<.05	Men <55 years Similar to LDL-C, diabetes mellitus; weaker than tobacco
1,165	1.6 (1.1-2.3)	<.05	Women; no CHD
2,040	1.2 (0.7-1.85)	NS	Increased risk of mildly elevated LDL-C

investigations suggest an association between elevated hs-CRP levels and sudden death,[50,51] and some studies have shown that increased hs-CRP levels are a predictor of second events in patients with known CHD.[36,52-60]

Other research suggests that hs-CRP may be a marker for risk of restenosis after angioplasty[61,62] and that CRP predicts risk of stroke, MI, PVD, and CVD death.[63] Finally, CRP and IL-6 both affect metabolism, resulting in inflammation and insulin resistance.[64]

Combining CRP with lipid testing may help target patients who will benefit from more aggressive cholesterol and aspirin therapy. Studies are in progress.

The American Heart Association has produced guidelines on the use of inflammatory markers for CVD risk prediction, and has classified CRP as a Class IIa/B indication (conflicting evidence, but the weight of the evidence in favor).[36] CRP has a testing advantage in that it has a long half-life, is stable over time, and does not require fasting.[63] CRP is independent of lipid levels, and, in combination with lipid levels, improves risk prediction compared with lipid levels alone.[46] CRP level of <1 mg/L is low risk, 1 to 3 mg/L is average risk, and >3 mg/L is considered high risk.[36]

Despite evidence of hs-CRP's predictive potential, there is no direct confirmation that lowering it results in reduced risk of CHD events. However, data from randomized clinical trials of aspirin[65] and statin therapy suggest that they achieve greater risk reductions when hs-CRP is elevated.[36,66,67] Many agents have been shown to lower hs-CRP, but studies attempting to show a decrease in events have not been completed. Because hs-CRP is an inflammatory marker (acute-phase reactant), levels will increase with infection, vigorous exercise, trauma, and acute or chronic illness.[36,67] Although the use of hs-CRP as a marker for risk prediction shows promise, more randomized, controlled trials with outcome measures are needed before conclusions can be drawn and clinical recommendations can be established.

Fibrinogen

Fibrinogen, a circulating glycoprotein made in the liver, plays a central role in thrombus formation and destruction, and binds to endothelial cells and platelets in the process.[36] A known positive association exists between fibrinogen and the risk of future CHD events. Fibrinogen is involved in endothelial cell changes, vasoconstriction, platelet aggregation, and increased blood viscosity.[1] Data from a study by Junker et al showed a positive correlation between fibrinogen level and many diseased vessels detected during angiography.[68] Many other studies demonstrate that fibrinogen levels increase with obesity, smoking, and aging, and decrease with regular exercise and moderate alcohol intake.[42,69-72] Fibrinogen is an acute-phase reactant and increases up to fourfold with inflammatory triggers. However, no studies to date show that decreasing the fibrinogen levels leads to a decrease in CHD events. Further research is needed before recommendations about fibrinogen screening and treatment can be made.

Interleukin-6

Interleukin-6 is an inflammatory cytokine that is secreted by macrophages, lymphocytes, and endothelial cells. It activates platelet production and endothelial and macrophage function, and stimulates the hypothalamic-pituitary-adrenal axis, which is associated with central obesity, hypertension, and insulin resistance.[72] Although IL-6 has been linked to CHD, it is not yet known whether it is a marker for, or a cause of, disease.[65,73,74] Large prospective studies of healthy populations have shown that elevated IL-6 levels independently predict risk of premature CHD and death. This relationship exists after controlling for CRP levels,[51,75] and it indicates a possible role for IL-6 in the progression of CHD.[76] Data from a recent study of 2,225 people 70 to 79 years of age suggest that IL-6 is a stronger predictor of heart attack or stroke in elderly people than is CRP.[77]

IL-6 and CRP levels are highly correlated in patients with CHD, but the nature of the relationship is still unclear.[78] Increased levels of systemic markers of inflammation such as IL-6 are common in patients with active CHD, and research continues into the mechanism of interaction of IL-6 and atherosclerosis.[79-83] Currently, testing for IL-6 levels is not recommended in primary or secondary prevention.

Other Inflammation Markers

Research to find additional inflammation markers linked to heart disease is ongoing. In a prospective study of 1,229 patients with documented CAD, serum IL-18 was identified as a strong independent predictor of death from cardiovascular events.[84] Results from the study also strongly support the possibility that inhibiting IL-18 might be a new treatment strategy for stabilizing plaque.[84] However, more studies are needed before treatment recommendations can be made.

Much interest also exists in the potential role of infections caused by specific microorganisms (such as *Chlamydia pneumoniae*, *Helicobacter pylori*, and cytomegalovirus) in the pathogenesis of atherosclerosis and the precipitation of clinical signs of CHD and other atherosclerotic disease. However, the results from clinical studies have been conflicting and difficult to interpret.[85] Research does not support infectious causes of CHD, but clinical investigations and trials continue.

References

1. Hackam DG, Anand SS: Emerging risk factors for atherosclerotic vascular disease: a critical review of the evidence. *JAMA* 2003;290:932-940.

2. Superko HR: Beyond LDL cholesterol reduction. *Circulation* 1996;94:2351-2354.

3. Boushey C, Beresford SA, Omen GS, et al: A quantitative assessment of plasma homocysteine as a risk factor for vascular disease. Probable benefits of increasing folic acid intakes. *JAMA* 1995;274:1049-1057.

4. Arnesen E, Refsum H, Bonaa KH, et al: Serum total homocysteine and coronary heart disease. *Int J Epidemiol* 1995;24:704-709.

5. Brattstrom L, Israelsson B, Norrving B, et al: Impaired homocysteine metabolism in early-onset cerebral and peripheral

occlusive arterial disease. Effects of pyridoxine and folic acid treatment. *Atherosclerosis* 1990;81:51-60.

6. Clarke R, Daly L, Robinson K, et al: Hyperhomocysteinemia: an independent risk factor for vascular disease. *N Engl J Med* 1991;324:1149-1155.

7. Dalery K, Lussier-Cacan S, Selhub J, et al: Homocysteine and coronary artery disease in French Canadian subjects: relation with vitamins B_{12}, B_6, pyridoxal phosphate, and folate. *Am J Cardiol* 1995;75:1107-1111.

8. Graham IM, Daly LE, Refsum HM, et al: Plasma homocysteine as a risk factor for vascular disease. The European Concerted Action Project. *JAMA* 1997;277:1775-1781.

9. Pancharuniti N, Lewis CA, Sauberlich HE, et al: Plasma homocyst(e)ine, folate, and vitamin B-12 concentrations and risk for early-onset coronary artery disease. *Am J Clin Nutr* 1994;59: 940-948.

10. Perry IJ, Refsum H, Morris RW, et al: Prospective study of serum total homocysteine concentration and risk of stroke in middle-aged British men. *Lancet* 1995;346:1395-1398.

11. Robinson K, Mayer EL, Miller DP, et al: Hyperhomocysteinemia and low pyridoxal phosphate. Common and independent reversible risk factors for coronary artery disease. *Circulation* 1995;92:2825-2830.

12. Selhub J, Jacques PF, Bostom AG, et al: Association between plasma homocysteine concentrations and extracranial carotid-artery stenosis. *N Engl J Med* 1995;332:286-291.

13. Stampfer MJ, Malinow MR, Willett WC, et al: A prospective study of plasma homocyst(e)ine and risk of myocardial infarction in US physicians. *JAMA* 1992;268:877-881.

14. Verhoef P, Stampfer MJ, Buring JE, et al: Homocysteine metabolism and risk of myocardial infarction: relation with vitamins B_6, B_{12}, and folate. *Am J Epidemiol* 1996;143:845-859.

15. Wu LL, Wu J, Hunt SC, et al: Plasma homocyst(e)ine as a risk factor for early familial coronary artery disease. *Clin Chem* 1994;40: 552-561.

16. Kang SS, Wong PW, Cook HY, et al: Protein-bound homocyst(e)ine. A possible risk factor for coronary artery disease. *J Clin Invest* 1986;77:1482-1486.

17. Glueck CJ, Shaw P, Lang JE, et al: Evidence that homocysteine is an independent risk factor for atherosclerosis in hyperlipidemic patients. *Am J Cardiol* 1995;75:132-136.

18. Stein JH, McBride PE: Hyperhomocysteinemia and atherosclerotic vascular disease: pathophysiology, screening, and treatment. *Arch Intern Med* 1998;158:1301-1306.

19. Toole JF, Malinow MR, Chambless LI, et al: Lowering homocysteine in patients with ischemic stroke to prevent recurrent stroke, myocardial infarction, and death: the Vitamin Intervention for Stroke Prevention (VISP) randomized controlled trial. *JAMA* 2004;291:565-575.

20. Keevil JG, Stein JH, McBride PE: Cardiovascular disease prevention. *Prim Care Clin Office Pract* 2002;29:667-696.

21. Brown MS, Goldstein JL: Plasma lipoproteins: teaching old dogmas new tricks. *Nature* 1987;330:113-114.

22. Scanu AM, Lawn RM, Berg K: Lipoprotein(a) and atherosclerosis. *Ann Intern Med* 1991;115:209-218.

23. Bostom AG, Gagnon DR, Cupples LA, et al: A prospective investigation of elevated lipoprotein (a) detected by electrophoresis and cardiovascular disease in women. The Framingham Heart Study. *Circulation* 1994;90:1688-1695.

24. Bostom AG, Cupples LA, Jenner JL, et al: Elevated plasma lipoprotein (a) and coronary heart disease in men aged 55 years and younger. A prospective study. *JAMA* 1996;276:544-548.

25. Cremer P, Nagel D, Labrot B, et al: Lipoprotein Lp(a) as predictor of myocardial infarction in comparison to fibrinogen, LDL cholesterol and other risk factors: results from the prospective Gottingen Risk Incidence and Prevalence Study (GRIPS). *Eur J Clin Invest* 1994;24:444-453.

26. Genest JJ Jr, Martin-Munley SS, McNamara JR, et al: Familial lipoprotein disorders in patients with premature coronary artery disease. *Circulation* 1992;85:2025-2033.

27. Rosengren A, Wilhelmsen L, Eriksson E, et al: Lipoprotein(a) and coronary heart disease: a prospective case-control study in a general population sample of middle aged men. *BMJ* 1990;301:1248-1251.

28. Rosenson RS: Beyond low-density lipoprotein cholesterol. A perspective on low high-density lipoprotein disorders and Lp(a) lipoprotein excess. *Arch Intern Med* 1996;156:1278-1284.

29. Schaefer EJ, Lamon-Fava S, Jenner JL, et al: Lipoprotein(a) levels and risk of coronary heart disease in men. The Lipid Research Clinics Coronary Primary Prevention Trial. *JAMA* 1994;271:999-1003.

30. Sigurdsson G, Baldursdottir A, Sigvaldason H, et al: Predictive value of apolipoproteins in a prospective survey of coronary artery disease in men. *Am J Cardiol* 1991;69:1251-1254.

31. Wald NJ, Law M, Watt HC, et al: Apolipoproteins and ischemic heart disease: implications for screening. *Lancet* 1994;343:75-79.

32. Stein JH, McBride PE: Screening and managing patients with lipoprotein(a) excess. *Internal Medicine* 1999;20:9-21.

33. Hajjar KA, Gavish D, Breslow JL, et al: Lipoprotein(a) modulation of endothelial cell surface fibrinolysis and its potential role in atherosclerosis. *Nature* 1989;339:303-305.

34. Cushing GL, Gaubatz JW, Nava ML, et al: Quantitation and localization of apolipoproteins (a) and B in coronary artery bypass vein grafts resected at re-operation. *Arteriosclerosis* 1989;9:593-603.

35. Stein JH, Rosenson RS: Lipoprotein Lp(a) excess and coronary heart disease. *Arch Intern Med* 1997;157:1170-1176.

36. Pearson TA, Mensah GA, Alexander RW, et al: Markers of inflammation and cardiovascular disease: application to clinical and public health practice: A statement for healthcare professionals from the Centers for Disease Control and Prevention and the American Heart Association. *Circulation* 2003;107:499-511.

37. Ross R: Atherosclerosis—an inflammatory disease. *N Engl J Med* 1999;340:115-126.

38. Lagrand WK, Visser CA, Hermens WT, et al: C-reactive protein as a cardiovascular risk factor: more than an epi-phenomenon? *Circulation* 1999;100:96-102.

39. Ridker PM: Evaluating novel cardiovascular risk factors: can we better predict heart attacks? *Ann Intern Med* 1999;130:933-937.

40. Danesh J, Collins R, Appleby P, et al: Association of fibrinogen, C-reactive protein, albumin, or leukocyte count with coronary heart disease: meta-analyses of prospective studies. *JAMA* 1998;279:1477-1482.

41. Danesh J, Whincup P, Walker M, et al: Low grade inflammation and coronary heart disease: prospective study and updated meta-analyses. *BMJ* 2000;321:199-204.

42. Folsom AR, Aleksic N, Catellier D, et al: C-reactive protein and incident coronary heart disease in the Atherosclerosis Risk In Communities (ARIC) study. *Am Heart J* 2002;144:233-238.

43. Kop WL, Gottdiener JS, Tangen CM, et al: Inflammation and coagulation factors in persons >65 years of age with symptoms of depression but without evidence of myocardial ischemia. *Am J Cardiol* 2002;89:419-424.

44. Kuller LH, Tracy RP, Shaten J, et al: Relation of C-reactive protein and coronary heart disease in the MRFIT nested case-control study. Multiple Risk Factor Intervention Trial. *Am J Epidemiol* 1996;144:537-547.

45. Ridker PM, Haughie P: Prospective studies of C-reactive protein as a risk factor for cardiovascular disease. *J Investig Med* 1998;46:391-395.

46. Ridker PM, Rifai N, Rose L, et al: Comparison of C-reactive protein and low-density lipoprotein cholesterol levels in the prediction of first cardiovascular events. *N Engl J Med* 2002;347:1557-1565.

47. Sakkinen P, Abbott RD, Curb JD, et al: C-reactive protein and myocardial infarction. *J Clin Epidemiol* 2002;55:445-451.

48. Tracy RP, Lemaitre RN, Psaty BM, et al: Relationship of C-reactive protein to risk of cardiovascular disease in the elderly. Results from the Cardiovascular Health Study and the Rural Health Promotion Project. *Arterioscler Thromb Vasc Biol* 1997;17:1121-1127.

49. Tracy RP: Hemostatic and inflammatory markers as risk factors for coronary disease in the elderly. *Am J Geriatr Cardiol* 2002;11:93-100.

50. Albert CM, Ma J, Rifai N, et al: Prospective study of C-reactive protein, homocysteine, and plasma lipid levels as predictors of sudden cardiac death. *Circulation* 2002;105:2595-2599.

51. Harris TB, Ferrucci L, Tracy RP, et al: Associations of elevated interleukin-6 and C-reactive protein levels with mortality in the elderly. *Am J Med* 1999;106:506-512.

52. Bazzino O, Ferreiros ER, Pizarro R, et al: C-reactive protein and the stress tests for the risk stratification of patients recovering from unstable angina pectoris. *Am J Cardiol* 2001;87:1235-1239.

53. Biasucci LM: C-reactive protein and secondary prevention of coronary events. *Clin Chim Acta* 2001;311:49-52.

54. Bickel C, Rupprecht HJ, Blankenberg S, et al: Relation of markers of inflammation (C-reactive protein, fibrinogen, von Willebrand factor, and leukocyte count) and statin therapy to long-term mortality in patients with angiographically proven coronary artery disease. *Am J Cardiol* 2002;89:901-908.

55. De Sutter J, De Buyzere M, Gheeraert P, et al: Fibrinogen and C-reactive protein on admission as markers of final infarct size after primary angioplasty for acute myocardial infarction. *Atherosclerosis* 2002;157:189-196.

56. Haverkate F, Thompson SG, Pyke SD, et al: Production of C-reactive protein and risk of coronary events in stable and unstable angina. European Concerted Action on Thrombosis and Disabilities Angina Pectoris Study Group. *Lancet* 1997;349:462-466.

57. Lindahl B, Toss H, Siegbahn A, et al: Markers of myocardial damage and inflammation in relation to long-term mortality in unstable coronary artery disease. FRISC Study Group. Fragmin during Instability in Coronary Artery Disease. *N Engl J Med* 2000;343:1139-1147.

58. Milazzo D, Biasucci LM, Luciani N, et al: Elevated levels of C-reactive protein before coronary artery bypass grafting predict recurrence of ischemic events. *Am J Cardiol* 1999;84:459-461, A9.

59. Zebrack JS, Muhlestein JB, Horne BD, et al: C-reactive protein and angiographic coronary artery disease: independent and additive predictors of risk in subjects with angina. *J Am Coll Cardiol* 2002;39:632-637.

60. Zebrack JS, Anderson JL, Maycock CA, et al: Usefulness of high-sensitivity C-reactive protein in predicting long-term risk of death or acute myocardial infarction in patients with unstable or stable angina pectoris or acute myocardial infarction. *Am J Cardiol* 2002;89:145-149.

61. Chew DP, Bhatt DL, Robbins MA, et al: Incremental prognostic value of elevated baseline C-reactive protein among established markers of risk in percutaneous coronary intervention. *Circulation* 2001;104:992-997.

62. Walter DH, Fichtlscherer S, Britten MB, et al: Statin therapy, inflammation and recurrent coronary events in patients following coronary stent implantation. *J Am Coll Cardiol* 2001;38:2006-2012.

63. Blake GJ: Inflammation and biomarkers. In: Topol E, ed, *Textbook of Cardiovascular Medicine*, Vol 6, 2003, Lippincott, Williams, and Wilkins, New York, NY.

64. Verma S, Li SH, Badiwala MV: Endothelin antagonism and interleukin-6 inhibition attenuate the proatherogenic effects of C-reactive protein. *Circulation* 2002;105:1890-1896.

65. Ridker PM, Cushman M, Stampfer MJ, et al: Inflammation, aspirin, and the risk of cardiovascular disease in apparently healthy men. *N Engl J Med* 1997;336:973-979.

66. Ridker PM: High-sensitivity C-reactive protein: potential adjunct for global risk assessment in the primary prevention of cardiovascular disease. *Circulation* 2001;103:1813-1818.

67. Ridker PM: Clinical application of C-reactive protein for cardiovascular disease detection and prevention. *Circulation* 2002;107: 363-369.

68. Junker R, Heinrich J, Ulbrich H, et al: Relationship between plasma viscosity and the severity of coronary heart disease. *Arterioscler Thromb Vasc Biol* 1998;18:870-875.

69. Yarnell JW, Sweetnam PM, Rumley A, et al: Lifestyle and hemostatic risk factors for ischemic heart disease: the Caerphilly Study. *Arterioscler Thromb Vasc Biol* 2000;20:271-279.

70. Tracy RP: Inflammation markers and coronary heart disease. *Curr Opin Lipidol* 1999;10:435-441.

71. Tracy RP: Epidemiological evidence for inflammation in cardiovascular disease. *Thromb Haemost* 1999;82:826-831.

72. Yudkin JS, Stehouwer CD, Emeis JJ, et al: C-reactive protein in healthy subjects: associations with obesity, insulin resistance, and endothelial dysfunction: a potential role for cytokines originating from adipose tissue? *Arterioscler Thromb Vasc Biol* 1999;19:972-978.

73. Ridker PM, Rifai N, Stampfer MJ, et al: Plasma concentration of interleukin-6 and the risk of future myocardial infarction among apparently healthy men. *Circulation* 2000;101:1767-1772.

74. Yudkin JS, Kumari M, Humphries SE, et al: Inflammation, obesity, stress, and coronary heart disease: is interleukin-6 the link? *Atherosclerosis* 2000;148:209-214.

75. Ridker PM, Rifai N, Clearfield M: Measurement of C-reactive protein for the targeting of statin therapy in the primary prevention of acute coronary events. *N Engl J Med* 2001;344:1959-1965.

76. Lindmark E, Diderholm E, Wallentin L, et al: Relationship between interleukin 6 and mortality in patients with unstable coro-

nary artery disease: effects of an early invasive or noninvasive strategy. *JAMA* 2001;286:2107-2113.

77. Cesari M, Pennix BW, Newman AB, et al: Inflammatory markers and onset of cardiovascular events. *Circulation* 2003;109:2317.

78. Teramoto S, Yamamoto H, Ouchi Y: Increased C-reactive protein and increased plasma interleukin-6 may synergistically affect the progression of coronary atherosclerosis in obstructive sleep apnea syndrome. *Circulation* 2003;107:E40.

79. Simon AD, Yazdani S, Wang W, et al: Circulating levels of IL-1β, a prothrombotic cytokine, are elevated in unstable angina versus stable angina. *J Thromb Thrombolysis* 2000;9:217-222.

80. Berk BC, Weintraub WS, Alexander RW: Elevation of C-reactive protein in 'active' coronary artery disease. *Am J Cardiol* 1990;65:168-172.

81. Biasucci LM, Vitelli A, Liuzzo G, et al: Elevated levels of interleukin 6 in unstable angina. *Circulation* 1995;94:874-877.

82. Biasucci LM, Liuzzo G, Fantuzzi G, et al: Increasing levels of interleukin(IL)-IRa and IL-6 during the first 2 days of hospitalization in unstable angina are associated with increased risk of in-hospital coronary events. *Circulation* 1999;99:2079-2084.

83. Toss H, Lindahl B, Siegbahn A, et al: Prognostic influence of increased fibrinogen and C-reactive protein levels in unstable coronary artery disease. FRISC Study Group. Fragmin during Instability in Coronary Artery Disease. *Circulation* 1997;96:204-4210.

84. Blankenberg S, Tiret L, Bickel C, et al: Interleukin-18 is a strong predictor of cardiovascular death in stable and unstable angina. *Circulation* 2002;106:24-30.

85. Wood D, Joint European Societies Task Force: Established and emerging cardiovascular risk factors. *Am Heart J* 2001;141(2 suppl):S49-S57.

CHAPTER 13

Special Populations

Although the risk factors and interventions for coronary heart disease (CHD) are similar for all people, risk factor prevalence, onset of risk, and benefits from treatment are different in different groups. Populations that require special consideration when developing prevention strategies include children and adolescents, women, the elderly, and various ethnic groups.

Children and Adolescents

Because the behaviors associated with cardiovascular risk factors—dietary habits, attitudes toward physical activity, use of tobacco—begin in childhood,[1-5] identifying children and adolescents who are at high risk for cardiovascular disease (CVD) is an important first step in prevention. There have been no controlled clinical trials comparing the effect of risk reductions beginning in childhood on the subsequent development of CVD because such trials would take many years to demonstrate event reduction. However, trials and programs aimed at reducing risk factors in childhood have produced substantial evidence of successful intervention. They include the Dietary Intervention Study in Children trial (DISC),[6] which demonstrated the safety and efficacy of a low-fat diet in children with hypercholesterolemia; the Child and Adolescent Trial for Cardiovascular Health Study (CATCH),[7] which used elementary school-based programs to increase physical activity levels in children; skill-training programs in smoking prevention in adolescents; and long-term, family-based treatment programs aimed at childhood obesity.

Based on this evidence, the American Heart Association (AHA) has developed guidelines for promoting, identifying, and managing known risk factors for CVD. Table 13-1 presents guidelines for cardiovascular health promotion in children.[8] These guidelines and the intervention guidelines presented in Table 13-2 are meant to complement a cardiovascular health schedule developed by the AHA's Council on Cardiovascular Disease in the Young that allows risk factor identification and modification within the framework of routine pediatric care.[9]

Obesity in children is an important issue, not only because it is rapidly increasing in incidence and prevalence, but also because obese children are likely to become obese adults.[10] The prevalence of excess weight in children has tripled since the 1960s, and more than 30% of children are above what is considered the appropriate 85th percentile for weight.[11] Population-based approaches that encourage children to be more physically active, consume fewer calories (especially fast food, soda, and snack food), and spend less time watching television and playing video games are essential to address this epidemic. Physicians play a critical role by identifying overweight children early and initiating effective treatments such as family-based behavior therapies, reduced sedentary behavior, improved nutrition, and additional physical activity.[10] Ensuring that all family members receive professional nutritional evaluation and counseling, work together to reduce children's video time, and increase activity has been proven to help children lose weight.[12,13]

Women

Despite many advancements in treatment, CVD is still the leading killer of women in the United States and in most developed areas of the world.[14,15] In the United States, more than half a million women die of CVD every year. This exceeds the number of CVD deaths in men and the next seven causes of death in women combined and translates into approximately one death every minute.[14] Most CVD deaths in women are caused by CHD, which also disproportionately afflicts racial and ethnic minorities and is a prime target for prevention.[14,16] Prevention of CHD is essential because CHD is often fatal and because two thirds of women who die suddenly from CHD have no previously recognized symptoms.[14] Yet women are far less likely to receive life-saving prevention therapies than men.[17]

Recent reports of results from the Women's Health Initiative and the Heart and Estrogen/Progestin Replacement Study (HERS) showing that combination hormone replacement therapy was associated with adverse CVD effects heightened the need to develop new strategies to prevent CVD in women.[18,19] To this end, the AHA created a panel of recognized experts in CVD prevention who had particular knowledge about women. The panel's objective was to develop the first set of evidence-based guidelines for preventing CVD in adult women with a broad range of cardiovascular risk. The resulting recommendations are grouped into five categories (Tables 13-3 through 13-7) and are ordered by class, level of supporting evidence, and generalizability index.

Prevention Strategies for Clinical Practice

Overwhelming evidence suggests that CVD can be prevented in women as well as in men. Evidence gathered by the AHA expert panel shows that while several prevention strategies are likely to have considerably greater benefit than risk, other strategies are associated with greater risk than benefit. Physicians should keep patients informed about the risks and benefits of potentially lifesaving preventive therapies and encourage them to take appropriate action to lower their risk. However, the risk of taking no action seems to be far greater than any risk that might be associated with applying knowledge to prevent CVD.[20] In conjunction with the CVD prevention guidelines for

Table 13-1: Guidelines for Cardiovascular Health Promotion for All Children and Adolescents

Health Promotion Goals	Recommendations
Diet	
• An overall healthy eating pattern • Appropriate body weight • Desirable lipid profile • Desirable blood pressure	• Assess diet at every health maintenance visit. • Match energy intake with energy needs for normal growth and development. • Make appropriate changes to maintain a healthy weight and achieve weight loss when indicated. • Advocate consumption of a variety of fruits, vegetables, whole grains, dairy products, fish, legumes, poultry, and lean meat. • Do not restrict fat intake in children younger than 2 years. After age 2, limit foods high in saturated fat (<10% of calories per day) and trans-fatty acids. • Limit salt intake to <6 g/d. • Limit intake of sugar.

(continued on next page)

Table 13-1: Guidelines for Cardiovascular Health Promotion for All Children and Adolescents

(continued)

Health Promotion Goals	Recommendations
Smoking	
• No new initiation of cigarette smoking	• Question tobacco use by parents at every visit.
• No exposure to environmental tobacco smoke	• Question tobacco use by children at every visit starting at age 10.
• Complete cessation for those who do smoke	• Advise avoidance of secondhand smoke at home, with friends, at school, or at work.

Health Promotion Goals	Recommendations
Physical Activity	
• Be physically active every day • Reduce sedentary time (eg, watching TV, playing computer video games, talking on the phone)	• Assess physical activity at every health maintenance visit. • Advise young people to participate in at least 60 minutes of moderate to vigorous physical activity (including exercise and play) daily. • Suggest physical activity that can be fun for children. • For adolescents, recommend an overall activity program that combines resistance training (10 to 15 repetitions of moderate intensity) with aerobic activity. • Recommend limiting sedentary time. Suggest limiting total video time to, at most, 2 hours daily.

Kavey et al, *Circulation* 2003;107:1562-1566.

Table 13-2: Guidelines for CVD Risk Reduction: Interventions for Children and Adolescents With Identified Risks

Risk Intervention Goals

Blood Cholesterol Management

- LDL-C <110 mg/dL
- For patients with diabetes, LDL-C <100 mg/dL
  Note: LDL >190 mg/dL is likely familial hypercholesterolemia (genetic cause)—requires medical treatment

Recommendations

- If LDL-C is above goals, initiate additional therapeutic lifestyle changes, including diet (<7% of calories from saturated fat; <200 mg/d cholesterol), in conjunction with a trained dietitian.
- Consider LDL-lowering dietary options (increases in soluble fiber by using age [in years] plus 5 to 10 g up to age 15, when the total remains at 25 g/d) in conjunction with a trained dietitian.
- Emphasize weight management and increased physical activity.
- If LDL-C is persistently above goals, evaluate for secondary causes (thyroid-stimulating hormone, liver function tests, renal function tests, urinalysis).
- Consider pharmacologic therapy for individuals with LDL-C >190 mg/dL (familial hypercholesterolemia) and no other risk factors for CVD or >160 mg/dL with other risk factors present (blood pressure elevation, diabetes, obesity, strong family history of premature CVD).
- Bile acid-binding resins or statins are usual first-line agents.
- Pharmacologic intervention for dyslipidemia should be accomplished in collaboration with a physician experienced in treatment of cholesterol disorders in pediatric patients.

(continued on next page)

Table 13-2: Guidelines for CVD Risk Reduction: Interventions for Children and Adolescents With Identified Risks *(continued)*

Risk Intervention Goals

Other Lipids and Lipoprotein

- Fasting TG <150 mg/dL
- HDL-C >40 mg/dL

Management of Blood Pressure Elevation

- Systolic and diastolic blood pressure <95th percentile for age, sex, and height

Recommendations

- Elevated fasting TG and reduced HDL-C are often seen in overweight, insulin-resistant patients. Therapeutic lifestyle changes should include weight management with appropriate energy intake and expenditure. Decrease intake of simple sugars.
- If fasting TG are persistently elevated, evaluate for secondary causes such as diabetes, thyroid disease, renal disease, and alcohol abuse.
- Pharmacologic interventions may be recommended for children with elevation of fasting TG if it is marked (>400 mg/dL to protect against postprandial TG of 1,000 mg/dL or greater, which may be associated with an increased risk of pancreatitis), or treatment may be initiated at TG >200 mg/dL in children with low HDL-C.

- Promote achievement of appropriate weight.
- Reduce sodium in the diet. Emphasize increased consumption of fruits and vegetables.
- If blood pressure is persistently above the 95th percentile, consider possible secondary causes (eg, renal disease, coarctation of the aorta).

(continued on next page)

Table 13-2: Guidelines for CVD Risk Reduction: Interventions for Children and Adolescents With Identified Risks *(continued)*

Risk Intervention Goals

Management of Blood Pressure Elevation (continued)

Weight Management

- Achieve and maintain BMI <95th percentile for age and sex

Recommendations

- Consider pharmacologic therapy for individuals above the 95th percentile if lifestyle modification brings no improvement and there is evidence of target organ changes (left ventricular hypertrophy, microalbuminuria, retinal vascular abnormalities). Start blood pressure medication individualized to other patient requirements and characteristics (eg, age, race, need for drugs with specific benefits).
- Pharmacologic management of hypertension should be accomplished in collaboration with a physician experienced in pediatric hypertension.

- For children who are at risk of overweight (>85th percentile) or obesity (>95th percentile). A weight management program should be initiated with appropriate energy balance achieved through changes in diet and physical activity.
- For children of normal height, a secondary cause of obesity is unlikely.
- Weight management should be directed at all family members who are overweight, using a family-centered behavioral management approach.
- Weight management should be done in collaboration with a trained dietitian.

(continued on next page)

Table 13-2: Guidelines for CVD Risk Reduction: Interventions for Children and Adolescents With Identified Risks *(continued)*

Risk Intervention Goals

Diabetes Management

- Near-normal fasting plasma glucose (<120 mg/dL)
- Near-normal Hb A_{1c} (<7%); goals for fasting glucose and Hb A_{1c} should take into consideration age and risk of hypoglycemia.

Cigarette Smoking

- Complete cessation of smoking for children and parents who smoke

Recommendations

- Management of type 1 and type 2 diabetes in children and adolescents should be accomplished in collaboration with a pediatric endocrinologist.
- For type 2 diabetes, the first step is weight management with improved diet and exercise.
- Because of risk for accelerated vascular disease, other risk factors (eg, blood pressure, lipid abnormalities) should be treated more aggressively in patients with diabetes.

- Advise every tobacco user (parents and children) to quit, and be prepared to provide assistance (eg, counseling, referral to develop a plan for quitting using available community resources).

BMI = body mass index, CVD = cardiovascular disease, HDL-C = high-density lipoprotein cholesterol, LDL-C = low-density lipoprotein cholesterol, TG = triglycerides

Kavey et al, *Circulation* 2003;107:1562-1566.

women, the AHA expert panel offered the following CVD prevention strategies for clinicians.[20]

1. Assess and stratify women into high, intermediate, lower, or optimal risk categories.
2. Use lifestyle approaches (smoking cessation, regular exercise, weight management, heart-healthy diet) to prevent CVD in all women. Lifestyle approaches are class I recommendations and a top priority in clinical practice.
3. Prioritize other CVD risk-reducing interventions on the basis of the strength of the recommendation (class I > class IIa > class IIb) and, within each class of recommendation, on the basis of the level of evidence (A > B > C).
4. Use risk stratification to prioritize risk intervention (high risk > intermediate risk > lower risk > optimal risk).
5. Avoid interventions designated as class III.

Table 13-8 prioritizes prevention practices based on risk group.

Elderly

Advancing age is one of the strongest risk factors for CHD. In 1995, the prevalence of chronic ischemic heart disease in people aged 65 years and older in the United States was 83 per 1,000 men and 90 per 1,000 women. Among those aged 75 years or older, the prevalence was 217 per 1,000 men and 129 per 1,000 women.[21] Thirty-nine percent of all Americans living with CVD are older than 65 years; of the population aged 65 years and older, more than 65% are dealing with some form of CVD.[22] Clinically, CHD in older patients represents the effects of heart disease superimposed on the physiologic effects of age.[23] Obstructive coronary artery disease is present at autopsy in almost 50% of elderly women and 70% to 80% of elderly men. In addition, although only 5% of the US population is older than 80 years, this group accounts for 20% of all hospitalizations for myocardial infarction (MI) and 30% of all MI-related deaths.[24] Until recently, clini-

Table 13-3: Clinical Recommendations for Lifestyle Interventions

Intervention	Recommendation	Class and GI
Cigarette smoking	Consistently encourage women not to smoke and to avoid environmental tobacco.	Class 1, Level B, GI = 1
Physical activity	Consistently encourage women to accumulate a minimum of 30 minutes of moderate-intensity physical activity (eg, brisk walking) on most, and preferably all, days of the week.	Class 1, Level B, GI = 1
Cardiac rehabilitation	Women with a recent acute coronary syndrome or coronary intervention or with new onset or chronic angina should participate in a comprehensive risk-reduction regimen, such as cardiac rehabilitation or a physician-guided home- or community-based program.	Class 1, Level B, GI = 2

(continued on next page)

Table 13-3: Clinical Recommendations for Lifestyle Interventions

(continued)

Intervention	Recommendation	Class and GI
Heart-healthy diet	• Consistently encourage an overall healthy eating pattern that includes intake of a variety of fruits, vegetables, grains, low-fat or nonfat dairy products, fish, legumes, and sources of protein low in saturated fat. • Limit saturated fat intake to <10% of calories • Limit cholesterol intake to <300 mg/d. • Limit trans-fatty acids.	Class I, Level B, GI = 1
Weight maintenance/ reduction	Consistently encourage weight maintenance/ reduction through an appropriate balance of physical activity, caloric intake, and normal behavioral programs when indicated to maintain/achieve a BMI between 18.5 and 24.9 kg/m^2 and a waist circumference <35 in.	Class I, Level B, GI = 1

BMI = body mass index, CVD = cardiovascular disease, GI = generalizability index

Intervention	Recommendation	Class and GI
Psychosocial factors	Women with CVD should be evaluated for depression and referred or treated when indicated.	Class IIa, Level B, GI = 2
ω-3 fatty acids	As an adjunct to diet, ω-3 fatty-acid supplementation may be considered in high-risk* women.	Class IIb, Level B, GI = 2
Folic acid	As an adjunct to diet, folic acid supplementation may be considered in high-risk* women (except after revascularization procedure) if a higher-than-normal level of homocysteine has been detected.	Class IIb, Level B, GI = 2

* High risk is defined as coronary heart disease (CHD) or risk equivalent, or 10-year absolute CHD risk >20%.

Mosca et al, *Circulation* 2004;109:672-693.

Table 13-4: Clinical Recommendations for Major Risk Factor Interventions

Intervention	Recommendation	Class and GI
Blood pressure—lifestyle	Encourage an optimal blood pressure of <120/80 mm Hg through lifestyle approaches.	Class I, Level B, GI = 1
Blood pressure—drugs	• Pharmacotherapy is indicated when blood pressure is ≥140/90 mm Hg or at a lower blood pressure in patients with blood pressure-related target-organ damage or diabetes. • Thiazide diuretics should be part of the drug regimen for most patients unless contraindicated.	Class I, Level A, GI = 1
Lipid, lipoproteins	The following optimal levels of lipids and lipoproteins for women should be encouraged through lifestyle approaches: • LDL-C <100 mg/dL • HDL-C >50 mg/dL • Triglycerides <150 mg/dL • Non-HDL-C <130 mg/dL	Class 1, Level B, GI = 1

Intervention	Recommendation	Class and GI
Lipids—diet therapy	• In high-risk women or when LDL-C is elevated, saturated fat intake should be reduced to <7% of calories. • Cholesterol should be reduced to <200 mg/d. • Trans-fatty acid intake should be reduced.	Class I, Level B, GI = 1
Lipids—pharmacotherapy—high risk*	• Initiate LDL-C-lowering therapy (preferably a statin) simultaneously with lifestyle therapy in high-risk women with LDL-C ≥100 mg/dL.	Class 1, Level A, GI = 1
	• Initiate statin therapy in high-risk women with LDL-C <100 mg/dL unless contraindicated.	Class 1, Level B, GI = 1
	• Initiate niacin** or fibrate therapy when HDL-C is low or non-HDL-C is elevated in high-risk women.	Class I, Level B, GI = 1

(continued on next page)

Table 13-4: Clinical Recommendations for Major Risk Factor Interventions *(continued)*

Intervention	Recommendation	Class and GI
Lipids—pharma-cotherapy—intermediate risk[†]	• Initiate LDL-C-lowering therapy (preferably a statin) if LDL-C level is ≥130 on lifestyle therapy.	Class 1, Level A, GI = 1
	• Or initiate niacin** or fibrate therapy when HDL-C is low or non-HDL-C is elevated after LDL-C goal is reached.	Class 1, Level B, GI = 1

CHD = coronary heart disease, GI = generalizability index, HDL-C = high-density lipoprotein cholesterol, LDL-C = low-density lipoprotein cholesterol

* High risk is defined as CHD or risk equivalent, or 10-year absolute CHD risk >20%.

** Dietary supplement niacin must not be used as a substitute for prescription niacin; an over-the-counter niacin should only be used if approved and monitored by a physician.

Intervention	Recommendation	Class and GI
Lipids—pharma-cotherapy—lower risk[‡]	• Consider LDL-C-lowering therapy in low-risk women with 0 or 1 risk factor when LDL-C level is ≥190 mg/dL or if multiple risk factors are present when LDL-C is ≥160 mg/dL.	Class IIa, Level B
	• Or consider niacin** or fibrate therapy when HDL-C is low or non-HDL-C is elevated after LDL-C goal is reached.	Class IIa, Level B, GI = 1
Diabetes	Lifestyle and pharma-cotherapy should be used to achieve near normal Hb A_{1c} (<7%) in women with diabetes.	Class I, Level B, GI = 1

[†] Intermediate risk is defined as 10-year absolute CHD risk 10% to 20%.

[‡] Lower risk is defined as 10-year absolute CHD risk <10%.

Mosca et al, *Circulation* 2004;109:672-693.

Table 13-5: Clinical Recommendations for Preventive Drug Interventions

Intervention	Recommendation	Class and GI
Aspirin—high risk	Aspirin therapy (75 to 162 mg), or clopidogrel if patient is intolerant to aspirin, should be used in high-risk women unless contraindicated.	Class I, Level A, GI = 1
Aspirin—intermediate risk	Consider aspirin therapy (75 to 162 mg) in intermediate-risk women as long as blood pressure is controlled and benefit is likely to outweigh risk of gastrointestinal side effects.	Class IIa, Level B, GI = 2
β-Blockers	β-Blockers should be used indefinitely in all women who have had a myocardial infarction or who have chronic ischemic syndromes, unless contraindicated.	Class I, Level A, GI = 1

cal trials have not addressed risk factor control in the elderly with or without established vascular disease, but there is increasing evidence that vascular risk reduction can benefit the older population.[23,25]

Secondary CVD Prevention

The goal of CVD prevention in the elderly is to improve quality of life by preventing morbidity and mortality, preserving function and preventing frailty, keeping the well

Intervention	Recommendation	Class and GI
ACE inhibitors	ACE inhibitors should be used (unless contra-indicated) in high-risk women.	Class I, Level A, GI = 1
ARBs	ARBs should be used in high-risk women who have clinical evidence of heart failure or an ejection fraction <40% and are intolerant to ACE inhibitors.	Class I, Level B, GI = 1

ACE = angiotensin-converting enzyme, ARB = angiotensin receptor blocker, GI = generalizability index

Mosca et al, *Circulation* 2004;109:672-693.

elderly well, and preventing the frail elderly from deteriorating. Cardiac rehabilitation programs are especially well suited to providing secondary prevention services, but many older patients who would benefit from these interventions do not participate in them because of lack of referral or because of societal and other barriers.[26] Relatively few data have been reported about the effectiveness of interventions to reduce risk factors associated with secondary events in

Table 13-6: Clinical Recommendations for Atrial Fibrillation and Stroke Prevention

Intervention	Recommendation	Class and GI
Warfarin—atrial fibrillation	Warfarin should be used to maintain the INR at 2.0 to 3.0 in women with chronic or paroxysmal atrial fibrillation unless they are considered to be at low risk for stroke (<1%/y) or high risk of bleeding.	Class I, Level A, GI = 1
Aspirin—atrial fibrillation	Aspirin (325 mg) should be used in women with chronic or paroxysmal atrial fibrillation who have a contraindication to warfarin or are at low risk for stroke (<1%/y).	Class I, Level A, GI = 1

GI = generalizability index, INR = international normalized ratio

Mosca et al, *Circulation* 2004;109:672-693.

older patients with CHD. However, it seems that strategies similar or identical to those used in younger patients have benefit when used in the elderly.

Smoking

Continued smoking after MI or other cardiac events is associated with serious harmful effects on the cardiovascular system that can result in angina pectoris, MI, stroke, and death. Strong physician advice, behavioral counseling, buddy support programs, self-help materials, telephone counseling, and pharmacologic therapies (eg, nicotine replacement therapy[27]) can all be used to aid smoking cessation in elderly cardiovascular patients. Interventions found to be effective in younger individuals have also proved effective.[28,29] Cardiac rehabilitation programs offer a unique opportunity to provide smoking cessation counseling for older patients.

Hypertension

More than two thirds of people older than 65 years have hypertension,[30] which is a major risk factor for CHD, CVD, and peripheral arterial disease and is the most common antecedent of heart failure and chronic renal failure. Despite the high prevalence of hypertension in this population and the substantial associated morbidity, treatment and control of hypertension are suboptimal in the elderly. Two thirds of people aged 75 years or older have uncontrolled hypertension (systolic blood pressure ≥140 mm Hg and diastolic blood pressure ≥90 mm Hg).[31] However, because isolated systolic hypertension (≥149 mm Hg with diastolic ≥90 mm Hg) is the most common type of hypertension in the elderly, a wide pulse pressure (≥50 mm Hg) may be a better marker for CVD and heart failure in this group than mean diastolic blood pressure.[32]

Treatment of hypertension in the elderly should follow the guidelines of the seventh Joint National Committee on Prevention, Detection, Evaluation, and Treatment of High Blood Pressure report (see Chapter 12). Nonpharmacologic therapy, including weight reduction, decreased sodium and alcohol intake, and exercise, is more effective in older populations when compared with younger age groups.[33] Selection of pharmacologic therapy should be based on severity of hypertension, presence of risk factors, and target organ damage. Controlling hypertension, specifically isolated systolic hypertension, has been clearly associated with reduction in morbidity and mortality from stroke, CHD, heart failure, and chronic renal failure.[34] Meta-analysis has dem-

Table 13-7: Clinical Recommendations for Class III Interventions

Intervention	Recommendation	Class and GI
Hormone therapy*	• Combined estrogen plus progestin hormone therapy should not be initiated to prevent CVD in postmenopausal women.	Class III, Level C
	• Combined estrogen plus progestin hormone therapy should not be continued to prevent CVD in postmenopausal women.	Class III, Level C
	• Other forms of menopausal hormone (eg, unopposed estrogen) should not be initiated or continued to prevent CVD in postmenopausal women, pending the results of ongoing trials.	Class III, Level C

CVD = cardiovascular disease

* Hot flashes are a considerable problem related to the quality of a postmenopausal woman's life. The trials that now demonstrate increased risk of thrombotic events and cancer prove that hormone replacement therapy (HRT) is not a therapy for coronary heart disease prevention, but HRT does reduce menopausal symptoms, and the overall absolute risk of adverse events is small but important.[18] There are other treatment options for hot flashes, such as regular physical activity, isoflavones, vitamin E, black cohosh, venlafaxine, paroxetine, fluoxetine, or gabapentin, but they are not as effective as HRT.[19]

Intervention	Recommendation	Class and GI
Antioxidant supplements	Antioxidant vitamin supplements should not be used to prevent CVD, pending the results of ongoing trials.	Class III, Level A, GI = 1
Aspirin—lower risk	Routine use of aspirin in lower-risk women is not recommended, pending the results of ongoing trials.	Class III, Level B, GI = 2

Mosca et al, *Circulation* 2004;109:672-693.

Table 13-8: Priorities for Prevention in Practice According to Risk Group

High-risk Women (>20% risk)

Class I Recommendations

- Smoking cessation
- Physical activity/cardiac rehabilitation
- Diet therapy
- Weight maintenance or reduction
- Blood pressure control
- Lipid control/statin therapy
- Aspirin therapy
- β-Blocker therapy
- ACE inhibitor therapy (ARBs, if contraindicated)
- Glycemic control in diabetic patients

Class IIa Recommendations

- Evaluate/treat for depression

Class IIb Recommendations

- ω-3 fatty-acid supplementation
- Folic acid supplementation

CVD = cardiovascular disease

Mosca et al, *Circulation* 2004;109:672-693.

Intermediate-risk Women (10% to 20% risk)

Class I Recommendations

- Smoking cessation
- Physical activity
- Heart-healthy diet
- Weight maintenance/reduction
- Blood pressure control
- Lipid control

Class IIa Recommendations

- Aspirin therapy

Lower-risk Women (<10% risk)

Class I Recommendations

- Smoking cessation
- Physical activity
- Heart-healthy diet
- Weight maintenance/reduction
- Treat individual CVD risk factors as indicated

Stroke Prevention Among Women With Atrial Fibrillation

Class I Recommendations

- High-intermediate risk of stroke: Warfarin therapy
- Low risk of stroke (<1%/y) or contraindication to warfarin: Aspirin therapy

onstrated that the benefits of antihypertensive therapy are especially high in patients 60 to 80 years old.[35]

Large, randomized hypertension treatment studies have not included enough older patients to draw conclusions for patients older than 80 years.[23] However, results from a recent study[36] and a subgroup meta-analysis of randomized controlled antihypertensive drug trials[37] demonstrated the benefits of active treatment in patients older than 80 years, including reduction of risk for stroke, major cardiovascular events, and heart failure. There was no reduction in cardiovascular death or total mortality. An international trial (Hypertension in the Very Elderly Trial [HYVET]) evaluating the effect of antihypertensive therapy on incidence of stroke and cognitive function in patients older than 80 years may provide answers regarding risks and benefits.[23]

Abnormal lipid levels

There is reason to believe that lipid-lowering therapy should be extended to very old coronary patients. The National Cholesterol Education Program Adult Treatment Panel III (NCEP ATP III) guidelines should be followed to lower low-density lipoprotein cholesterol (LDL-C) levels to <100 mg/dL and raise high-density lipoprotein cholesterol (HDL-C) levels to >40 mg/dL, if possible.[38] Recommendations for appropriate levels of triglycerides in the elderly are not specifically addressed by NCEP ATP III because few data relative to this age group are available.[23] The AHA/American College of Cardiology guidelines for secondary prevention suggest that, in general, when the triglyceride level is ≥200 mg/dL, the non-HDL-C level should be <130 mg/dL.[39]

Data suggest that older patients with CHD will benefit from treatment of abnormal lipid levels and that the benefit is likely to be even greater than that seen in younger patients because of older patients' greater absolute risk. A post ad-hoc analysis of the Scandinavian Simvastatin Survival Study (4S) demonstrated that cholesterol lowering with simvastatin (Zocor®) produced reductions in relative risk for major coronary events in patients aged 65 years or older similar to those in younger patients.[40] A similar analysis from the Cholesterol and Recurrent Events (CARE) trial demonstrated that statin therapy in the elderly was equally effective when applied to older patients with known CHD whose total cholesterol was not above 240 mg/dL.[41] The Pravastatin Pooling Project, which compared younger patients to patients aged 65 years or older, demonstrated identical benefits in the elderly.[42] Two ongoing studies are specifically focusing on the value of statin therapy in the elderly: the Prospective Study of Pravastatin in the Elderly at Risk (PROSPER) and the Fluvastatin Assessment of Morbi-Mortality in the Elderly (FAME).[43]

Obesity

According to data from the Framingham Study,[43] obesity is a risk factor for secondary coronary events in older men and women with CHD because of the clustering of dyslipidemia, hypertension, and insulin resistance in older overweight individuals, particularly those with abdominal obesity. Weight loss therefore may act as a multifactor risk reduction intervention in the elderly. However, few data describing the effect of either increased physical activity or low-calorie diets in older patients with CHD are available. The effect of exercise training without calorie reduction on measures of obesity and abdominal adiposity in older CHD patients has been minimal.[44,45] Altering the exercise prescription to include more frequent and more prolonged walks as a means to increase exercise-related energy expenditure is promising as an adjunct to dietary therapy in older obese patients with CHD.[46]

Diabetes

The prevalence of insulin resistance and diabetes mellitus increases with age, especially in the presence of abdominal obesity.[47] The presence of diabetes mellitus is a strong predictor for the occurrence of secondary coronary events in older CHD patients.[48] Management of diabetes mellitus in older CHD patients should extend beyond exercise programming and weight management programs and should include blood glucose screening for undiagnosed diabetes and surveillance of patients in treatment. Risk factor assessment should include fasting glucose and glycosylated hemoglobin. Appropriate hypoglycemic therapy should achieve near-normal fasting plasma glucose (a glycosylated hemoglobin level <7% is recommended).[39]

Patients with diabetes need to be informed about the short-term hypoglycemic effects of exercise. Exercise training is known to improve insulin resistance and diabetic control in healthy older people.[49,50] In older coronary patients, glucose and insulin levels are more closely related to total body fat mass than to measures of fitness or exercise training response.[44] This suggests that the effect of exercise programming on glycemic control in older diabetic patients may relate more to its favorable effects on fat mass or body fat distribution than to its effect on fitness.[44,45]

Physical activity

Clinicians must strongly and repeatedly encourage patients to exercise, taking into consideration appropriate, individualized recommendations for the exercise prescription. Exercise improves functional capacity and reduces activity-related abnormal signs or symptoms. Prescribing exercise to increase physical activity and fitness for elderly patients with heart disease has been an essential component of secondary prevention for 20 years.[51] Published methods of prescribing exercise for cardiac patients generally do not require significant modification for elderly patients.[52]

The recommendations for increasing participation in physical activity programs should not be limited to structured exercise but should include a broader interpretation of exercise programming, consider the differences in needs between women and men, and include occupational, leisure, and daily living activities.[53] Clinicians should consider modifying components of the exercise prescription for elderly patients, especially those aged 75 years or older and those with significant comorbidities that limit mobility. Strength training to improve neuromuscular function, muscular strength, and endurance is essential to improving responses to the physical demands of daily living as well as occupational and recreational activities and should be a component of the overall exercise prescription.[54]

Increases of 10% to 60% in functional capacity and decreases of 10% to 25% in myocardial work at standardized exercise workloads have been observed after 12 weeks of early exercise training following hospitalization.[45,55-59] Extended periods of training have resulted in modest further gains.[58,60] Expected outcomes are similar to those for younger patients, but absolute levels of functional capacity in the elderly are lower, and results may take longer to achieve, particularly for patients aged 75 years or older.[51-53] As with younger people, including exercise in a multidisciplinary approach to secondary prevention may have a positive impact on other heart disease risk factors.[25,45,59] Although it has not yet been established whether exercise training as part of secondary prevention is associated with a reduction of morbidity and mortality in older patients, one study of older patients with heart disease and several others of older persons without known heart disease have suggested that physical activity has a positive effect on mortality.[61-64]

Psychosocial Interventions

Although few studies have examined the specific psychosocial needs of elderly patients with CHD who are participating in secondary prevention or cardiac rehabilitation, research from younger populations and elderly populations with noncardiac illnesses has helped to define the issues important to cardiac patients.[25,65] General areas that need assessment or intervention include socioeconomic status, depression, social support/isolation, cognitive functioning, and issues related to work, sexual activity, and well-being.

Income and education may have a serious effect on morbidity and mortality. Low socioeconomic status is a risk factor for CHD mortality in men and women, and it influences participation in secondary prevention or rehabilitation programs.[65] When designing secondary prevention programs for elderly patients, clinicians should assess each patient's educational and economic resources and make adjustments and recommendations as needed.

Studies indicate that depression also has a major effect on morbidity, mortality, and functional recovery of patients with CVD.[66] Because safe and effective treatments for depression are available, all elderly patients should be evaluated for depression and offered treatment as appropriate.[23] Elderly people, especially those aged 75 years and older, are likely to suffer significant personal, financial, and other types of losses. For example, among patients aged 65 years and older, 51% of women and 13% of men are widowed.[67] Loss of spouse may lead to depression, isolation, and other problems. Lack of social support and social isolation have been associated with increased morbidity and mortality in elderly men and women who have had an MI.[68] The National Heart, Lung, and Blood Institute (NHLBI) Enhancing Recovery in Coronary Heart Disease (ENRICHD) trial is evaluating the effects of interventions to reduce depression and social isolation in a large sample of post-MI patients, half of whom are aged 65 years or older.[66]

An important issue when dealing with elderly CHD patients is a potential change in sensory function that may make it difficult for them to read health information or hear instructions. Many elderly people are also likely to have significant cognitive impairment. For example, dementia is present in 15% to 20% of those older than 85 years.[69] Although alcohol and substance abuse seem to diminish with age, they are still common in older patients and should be assessed.[70]

Assessing desire for physical functioning, including helping individuals continue to remain sexually active, is an important part of the psychosocial assessment and intervention. Simple screening tools can help identify most major problems and can be followed up with additional assessments and referral for treatment as needed.[71] It is also important for clinicians to address end-of-life issues with patients who have terminal CVD, including determining advance directives.[72]

Ethnic Populations

Although race does appear to be a factor in heart disease, the overall risk of any racial group can be reduced through lifestyle changes and the other interventions examined in this book.

African Americans

CVD is the leading cause of death in African-American men and women, taking the lives of more than 100,000 every year.[73] According to the Centers for Disease Control and Prevention of the National Center for Health Statistics, CVD accounted for 33.5% of deaths among African-American men and 40.6% of deaths among African-American women in 2000. The AHA has reported that African Americans are at greater risk for CVD and stroke death than whites and that, compared with whites, young African Americans have a two- to three-fold greater risk of ischemic stroke and African-American men and women are more likely to die of stroke. The prevalence of high blood pressure in African Americans in the United States is among the highest in the world. Among African Americans aged 20 years and older, 36.7% of men and 36.6% of women have high blood pressure.

Among all African Americans, 45% of men and 46% of women have total blood cholesterol levels over 200 mg/dL; 77.3% of women are overweight and 49.7% are obese; and 60.7% of men are overweight and 28.1% are obese. Among African Americans, 44.1% of men and 55.2% of women are sedentary, with no leisure-time physical activity. In terms of overall physical activity, African Americans are one of the least active ethnic groups.

Hispanic Americans

CVD is the number-one killer of Hispanic Americans, accounting for more than 30% of all deaths in Hispanic Americans each year. Approximately 138 per 10,000 Hispanic Americans had a CVD event last year, compared with 178 per 10,000 in the white population.[74] Nearly 30% of Hispanic-American adults (older than 30 years) have some form of CVD.[74] Hispanic Americans tend to have higher cholesterol and to exercise less often than do African Americans and whites.

Obesity, type 2 diabetes, hypertension, hyperlipidemia, and elevated lipoprotein (a) are all more common in African Americans, Hispanic Americans, and other races in America. Risk factor screening, counseling, and early intervention are essential in these higher-risk patients. Special statements on the facts related to ethnicity and CVD are available through the AHA's Web site (http://www.americanheart.org).

Prevention Programs

Clinicians should make sure that high-risk patients are aware of their increased risk of heart disease and stroke and encourage them to do everything they can to reduce their personal risk. The AHA has a number of national programs and activities in which African Americans and others can participate, including the Cholesterol Low Down, a program that provides year-round support to help participants reach their health goals; the Heart of Diabetes℠ Understanding Insulin Resistance program, which can help patients with type 2 diabetes reduce their risk for heart disease through physical activity, weight control, nutrition, and cholesterol management; and cardiopulmonary resuscitation (CPR) training courses, which teach participants how to use an automated external defibrillator and how to perform CPR.

The AHA also offers a faith-based program designed specifically to educate African Americans and Hispanic Americans through hands-on prevention, including health screenings, workshops and activities. This program, Search Your Heart, contains six modules highlighting physical activity and weight management; nutrition, including recipes and tips on eating out and eating on the run; high blood pressure, high cholesterol, and diabetes management; stroke prevention; stress reduction; and advocacy, which teaches participants how to become advocates of good health and take issues to lawmakers to make changes.

References

1. Relationship of atherosclerosis in young men to serum lipoprotein cholesterol concentrations and smoking. A preliminary report from the Pathobiological Determinants of Atherosclerosis in Youth (PDAY) Research Group. *JAMA* 1990;264:3018-3024.

2. McGill HC Jr, McMahan CA, Zieske AW, et al: Effects of nonlipid risk factors on atherosclerosis in youth with a favorable lipoprotein profile. *Circulation* 2001;103:1546-1550.

3. Newman WP 3rd, Freedman DS, Voors AW, et al: Relation of serum lipoprotein levels and systolic blood pressure to early atherosclerosis. The Bogalusa Heart Study. *N Engl J Med* 1986;314:138-144.

4. Berenson GS, Srinivasan SR, Bao W, et al: Association between multiple cardiovascular risk factors and atherosclerosis in children and young adults. The Bogalusa Heart Study. *N Engl J Med* 1998;338:1650-1656.

5. Mahoney LT, Burns TL, Stanford W, et al: Coronary risk factors measured in childhood and young adult life are associated with coronary artery calcification in young adults: the Muscatine Study. *J Am Coll Cardiol* 1996;27:277-284.

6. Efficacy and safety of lowering dietary intake of fat and cholesterol in children with elevated low-density lipoprotein cholesterol. The Dietary Intervention Study in Children (DISC). The Writing Group for the DISC Collaborative Research Group. *JAMA* 1995;273:1429-1435.

7. Lytle LA, Stone EJ, Nichaman MZ, et al: Changes in nutrient intakes of elementary school children following a school-based intervention: results from the CATCH Study. *Prev Med* 1996; 25:465-477.

8. Kavey RE, Daniels SR, Lauer RM, et al: American Heart Association guidelines for primary prevention of atherosclerotic cardiovascular disease beginning in childhood. *Circulation* 2003;107:1562-1566.

9. Williams CL, Hayman LL, Daniels SR, et al: Cardiovascular health in childhood: a statement for health professionals from the Committee on Atherosclerosis, Hypertension, and Obesity in the Young (AHOY) of the Council on Cardiovascular Disease in the Young, American Heart Association. *Circulation* 2002;106: 143-160.

10. Fowler-Brown A, Kahwati LC: Prevention and treatment of overweight in children and adolescents. *Am Fam Physician* 2004;69:2591-2598.

11. Center for Disease Control and Prevention, National Center for Health Statistics: Prevalence of overweight among children and adolescents: United States, 1999-2000. 2004. Available at: http://www.cdc.gov/nchs/products/pubs/pubd/hestats/overwght99.htm. Accessed August 30, 2004.

12. Summerbell CD, Ashton V, Campbell KJ, et al: Interventions for treating obesity in children. *Cochrane Database Syst Rev* 2003;(3):CD001872.

13. The President's Council on Physical Fitness and Sports: Motivating kids in physical activity. *The President's Council on Physical Fitness and Sports Research Digest* 2000;3(11). Available at: http://www.fitness.gov/activity/activity2/digest_sept2000/digest_sept2000.html. Accessed August 30, 2004.

14. American Heart Association: Heart disease and stroke statistics—2003 update. Dallas, TX, American Heart Association, 2002.

15. Yusuf S, Reddy S, Ounpuu S, et al: Global burden of cardiovascular diseases: part I: general considerations, the epidemiologic transition, risk factors, and impact of urbanization. *Circulation* 2001;104:2746-2753.

16. Mosca L, Grundy SM, Judelson D, et al: Guide to preventive cardiology for women. AHA/ACC scientific statement. Consensus panel statement. *Circulation* 1999;99:2480-2484.

17. Miller AP, Oparil S: Secondary prevention of coronary heart disease in women: a call to action. *Ann Intern Med* 2003;138:150-151.

18. Solomon CG, Dluhy RG: Rethinking postmenopausal hormone therapy. *N Engl J Med* 2003;348:579-580.

19. Neff MJ: NAMS releases position statement on the treatment of vasomotor symptoms associated with menopause. *Am Fam Physician* 2004;70:393-394, 396, 399.

20. Mosca L, Appel LJ, Benjamin EJ, et al: Evidence-based guidelines for cardiovascular disease prevention in women. *Circulation* 2004;109:672-693.

21. National Center for Health Statistics. Current Estimates from the National Health Interview Survey, 1995. Hyattsville, MD, US Department of Health and Human Services, 1998. DHS publication no. (PHS) 98-1527.

22. American Heart Association: *Heart Disease and Stroke Statistics—2004 Update.* Dallas, TX, American Heart Association, 2003.

23. Williams MA, Fleg JL, Ades PA, et al: Secondary prevention of coronary heart disease in the elderly (with emphasis on patients ≥75 years of age): an American Heart Association scientific statement from the Council on Clinical Cardiology Subcommittee on Exercise, Cardiac Rehabilitation, and Prevention. *Circulation* 2002;105:1735-1743.

24. Wenger NK, ed. *Cardiovascular Disease in the Octogenarian and Beyond.* London, Martin Dunitz, Ltd, 1999.

25. Wenger NK, Froelicher ES, Ades PA, et al: Cardiac rehabilitation. Clinical Practice Guideline No. 17. Rockville, MD, Agency for Health Care Policy and Research, 1995. AHCPR publication no. 96-0672.

26. Ades PA, Waldmann ML, McCann WJ, et al: Predictors of cardiac rehabilitation participation in older coronary patients. *Arch Intern Med* 1992;152:1033-1035.

27. Fiore MC, Bailey WC, Cohen SJ, et al: Treating tobacco use and dependence. Clinical Practice Guideline. Rockville, MD, US Department of Health and Human Services Public Health Service, 2000.

28. Morgan GD, Noll EL, Orleans CT, et al: Reaching midlife and older smokers: tailored interventions for routine medical care. *Prev Med* 1996;25:346-354.

29. Vetter NJ, Ford D: Smoking prevention among people aged 60 and over: a randomized controlled trial. *Age Ageing* 1990;19:164-168.

30. Chobanian AV, Bakris GL, Black HR, et al: The seventh report of the Joint National Committee on Prevention, Detection,

Evaluation, and Treatment of High Blood Pressure: the JNC 7 Report. *JAMA* 2003;289:2560-2572.

31. Black HR: Isolated systolic hypertension in the elderly: lessons from clinical trials and future directions. *J Hypertens* 1999;17(suppl 5):S49-S54.

32. Glynn RJ, Chae CU, Guralnik JM, et al: Pulse pressure and mortality in older people. *Arch Intern Med* 2000;160:2765-2772.

33. Whelton PK, Appel LJ, Espeland MA, et al: Sodium reduction and weight loss in the treatment of hypertension in older persons: a randomized controlled trial of nonpharmacologic interventions in the elderly (TONE). TONE Collaborative Research Group. *JAMA* 1998;279:839-846.

34. 1999 World Health Organization-International Society of Hypertension guidelines for the management of hypertension. Guidelines Subcommittee. *J Hypertens* 1999;17:151-183.

35. MacMahon S, Rodger A: The effects of blood pressure reduction in older patients: an overview of five randomized controlled trials in elderly hypertensives. *Clin Exp Hypertens* 1993;15:967-978.

36. Staessen JA, Fagard R, Thijs L, et al: Randomised double-blind comparison of placebo and active treatment for older patients with isolated systolic hypertension. The Systolic Hypertension in Europe (Syst-Eur) Trial. *Lancet* 1997;350:757-764.

37. Gueyffier F, Bulpitt C, Boissel JP, et al: Antihypertensive drugs in very old people: a subgroup meta-analysis of randomised controlled trials. INDANA Group. *Lancet* 1999;353:793-796.

38. Third Report of the National Cholesterol Education Program (NCEP) Expert Panel on Detection, Evaluation, and Treatment of High Blood Cholesterol in Adults (Adult Treatment Panel III). Executive Summary. Rockville, MD, National Heart, Lung, and Blood Institute, 2001. NIH publication no. 01-3670.

39. Smith SC Jr, Blair SN, Bonow RO, et al: AHA/ACC scientific statement: AHA/ACC guidelines for preventing heart attack and death in patients with atherosclerotic cardiovascular disease: 2001 update. A statement for healthcare professionals from the American Heart Association and the American College of Cardiology. *Circulation* 2001;104:1577-1579.

40. Miettinen TA, Pyorala K, Olsson AG, et al: Cholesterol-lowering therapy in women and elderly patients with myocardial in-

farction or angina pectoris: findings from the Scandinavian Simvastatin Survival Study (4S). *Circulation* 1997;96:4211-4218.

41. Lewis SJ, Moye LA, Sacks FM, et al: Effect of pravastatin on cardiovascular events in older patients with myocardial infarction and cholesterol levels in the average range. Results of the Cholesterol and Recurrent Events (CARE) trial. *Ann Intern Med* 1998;129:681-689.

42. Sacks FM, Tonkin AM, Shepherd J, et al: Effect of pravastatin on coronary disease events in subgroups defined by coronary risk factors: the Prospective Pravastatin Pooling Project. *Circulation* 2000;102:1893-1900.

43. Vokonas PS, Kannel WB: Epidemiology of coronary heart disease in the elderly. In: Tresch DD, Aronow WS, eds. *Cardiovascular Disease in the Elderly Patient.* New York, NY, Marcel Dekker, 1994, pp 91-123.

44. Brochu M, Poehlman ET, Savage P, et al: Coronary risk profiles in men with coronary artery disease: effects of body composition, fat distribution, age and fitness. *Coron Artery Dis* 2000;11:137-144.

45. Lavie CJ, Milani RV: Effects of cardiac rehabilitation programs on exercise capacity, coronary risk factors, behavioral characteristics, and quality of life in a large elderly cohort. *Am J Cardiol* 1995;76:177-179.

46. Mertens DJ, Kavanagh T, Campbell RB, et al: Exercise without dietary restriction as a means to long-term fat loss in the obese cardiac patient. *J Sports Med Phys Fitness* 1998;38:310-316.

47. Kohrt WM, Kirwan JP, Staten MA, et al: Insulin resistance in aging is related to abdominal obesity. *Diabetes* 1993;42:273-281.

48. Vokonas PS, Kannel WB: Diabetes mellitus and coronary heart disease in the elderly. *Clin Geriatr Med* 1996;12:69-78.

49. Kirwan JP, Kohrt WM, Wojta DM, et al: Endurance exercise training reduces glucose-stimulated insulin levels in 60-to 70-year-old men and women. *J Gerontol* 1993;48:M84-M90.

50. Ruderman N, Devlin JT, eds. *The Health Professional's Guide to Diabetes and Exercise.* Alexandria, VA, American Diabetes Association, 1995.

51. Williams MA, Fardy PS: *Exercise Testing and Training In the Elderly Cardiac Patient.* Champaign, IL, Human Kinetics, 1994.

52. Williams MA: Exercise testing in cardiac rehabilitation. Exercise prescription and beyond. *Cardiol Clin* 2001;19:415-431.

53. Ades PA, Hanson JS, Gunther PG, et al: Exercise conditioning in the elderly coronary patient. *J Am Geriatr Soc* 1987;35:121-124.

54. National Center for Chronic Disease Prevention and Health Promotion: *Physical Activity and Health: a Report of the Surgeon General.* Atlanta, GA: US Department of Health and Human Services, 1995.

55. Pollock ML, Franklin BA, Balady GJ, et al: AHA science advisory. Resistance exercise in individuals with and without cardiovascular disease: benefits, rationale, safety, and prescription. An advisory from the Committee on Exercise, Rehabilitation, and Prevention, Council on Clinical Cardiology, American Heart Association; Position paper endorsed by the American College of Sports Medicine. *Circulation* 2000;101:828-833.

56. Williams MA, Maresh CM, Esterbrooks DJ, et al: Early exercise training in patients older than age 65 years compared with that in younger patients after acute myocardial infarction or coronary artery bypass grafting. *Am J Cardiol* 1985;55:263-266.

57. Ades PA, Grunvald MH: Cardiopulmonary exercise testing before and after conditioning in older coronary patients. *Am Heart J* 1990;120:585-589.

58. Ades PA, Waldmann ML, Poehlman ET, et al: Exercise conditioning in older coronary patients. Submaximal lactate response and endurance capacity. *Circulation* 1993;88:572-577.

59. Lavie CJ, Milani RV, Littman AB: Benefits of cardiac rehabilitation and exercise training in secondary coronary prevention in the elderly. *J Am Coll Cardiol* 1993;22:678-683.

60. Williams MA, Maresh CM, Esterbrooks DJ, et al: Characteristics of exercise responses following short and long term aerobic training in elderly cardiac patients. *J Am Geriatr Soc* 1987;35:904.

61. Wannamethee SG, Shaper AG, Walker M: Physical activity and mortality in older men with diagnosed coronary heart disease. *Circulation* 2000;102:1358-1363.

62. Hakim AA, Petrovitch H, Burchfiel CM, et al: Effects of walking on mortality among nonsmoking retired men. *N Engl J Med* 1998;338:94-99.

63. Kushi LH, Fee RM, Folsom AR, et al: Physical activity and mortality in postmenopausal women. *JAMA* 1997;277:1287-1292.

64. Fried LP, Kronmal RA, Newman AB, et al: Risk factors for 5-year mortality in older adults: the Cardiovascular Health Study. *JAMA* 1998;279:585-592.

65. Brezinka V, Kittel F: Psychosocial factors of coronary heart disease in women: a review. *Soc Sci Med* 1996;42:1351-1365.

66. Enhancing recovery in coronary heart disease patients (ENRICHD): study design and methods. The ENRICHD investigators. *Am Heart J* 2000;139(1 pt 1):1-9.

67. Gallagher-Thompson D, Thompson LW: Bereavement and adjustment disorders. In: Busse EW, Blazer DG, eds. *Textbook of Geriatric Psychiatry*. 2nd ed. Washington, DC, American Psychiatry Press, 1996, pp 313-328.

68. Krumholz HM, Butler J, Miller J, et al: Prognostic importance of emotional support for elderly patients hospitalized with heart failure. *Circulation* 1998;97:958-964.

69. Regier DA, Boyd JH, Burke JD Jr, et al: One-month prevalence of mental disorders in the United States. Based on five Epidemiologic Catchment Area sites. *Arch Gen Psychiatry* 1988;45:977-986.

70. Blazer DG: Alcohol and drug problems. In: Busse EW, Blazer DG, eds. *Textbook of Geriatric Psychiatry.* 2nd ed. Washington, DC, American Psychiatry Press, 1996, pp 341-356.

71. Knox D, Mischke L, Williams RE: Heart failure patient and family education. In: Moser DK, Riegel BJ, eds. *Improving Outcomes In Heart Failure: An Interdisciplinary Approach.* Gaithersburg, MD, Aspen Publishers, Inc, 2001, pp 178-196.

72. Quaglietti SE, Atwood JE, Ackerman L, et al: Management of the patient with congestive heart failure using outpatient, home, and palliative care. *Prog Cardiovasc Dis* 2000;43:259-274.

73. American Heart Association. Facts about African Americans, Heart Disease, and Stroke. 1999. Available at: http://www.americanheart.org. Accessed on March 1, 2004.

74. American Heart Association: Heart facts 2004: Latino/Hispanic Americans. Cardiovascular diseases still no. 1. Available at: http://www.americanheart.org/downloadable/heart/1073973326774Heart%20Facts%202004%20Latino-Hisp.pdf. Accessed August 26, 2004.

CHAPTER 14

Putting Prevention Into Practice

Abundant clinical evidence demonstrates the efficacy of a variety of interventions for both primary and secondary prevention of coronary disease. The importance of these interventions is summarized in consensus statements from the American Heart Association (AHA) and the American College of Cardiology (ACC) on the primary and secondary prevention of coronary artery disease (CAD).[1,2] The AHA guidelines for the primary prevention of cardiovascular disease and stroke are summarized in Appendix C. Although substantial evidence supports the potential to reduce recurrent cardiovascular events in individuals with coronary heart disease (CHD) and to prevent coronary disease in high-risk individuals, there is also substantial evidence that these interventions are underused, particularly for female patients.[3]

Preventive services, including counseling, are provided less often than recommended and less frequently than patients and their physicians prefer. In a study of 1,495 US hospitals, of more than 138,000 patients discharged post-myocardial infarction (MI), only 32% were discharged on cholesterol therapy, despite the significant impact of this intervention on short-term and long-term outcomes.[4] This rate was only slightly higher than those found in the evaluation of primary care practices.[5] The National Committee for Quality Assurance (NCQA) study found that lipid profiles were available for only 69% of patients with diabetes and that lipids were controlled in only 37% of this group. In addition, only 62% of patients who smoked were advised to quit.[5] Regarding hypertension, despite the fact that 79% of patients report taking action to control their blood pressure, less than 20% of them are considered to be under adequate control.[6]

Barriers to Implementation

Numerous barriers to successfully implementing preventive services have been identified:[7]

- A shortage and inadequate distribution of primary care physicians
- Busy practices with overwhelming acute care demands
- Lack of reimbursement for many preventive services
- Limited access to community resources necessary for providing routine and comprehensive prevention services
- Gaps in physician and staff training
- Inadequate organizational support and incentives
- Patient resistance to change
- Lack of adequate follow-up.

These barriers can be divided into four general categories: the patient, the physician, the health-care setting, and community or society (Table 14-1). Any one barrier in the chain can result in a lack of provision of preventive services. Considering each factor when attempting to improve the delivery of services can improve health-care quality.[7]

Although patients consistently report that preventive services are a high priority for their health care, and they want physicians to provide lifestyle and prevention recommendations, physicians frequently believe that patients are unmotivated or noncompliant. On the other hand, patients often mention the physician's failure to order tests, provide information, or communicate results as the reasons they do not request preventive services. Patient demand for service is still the most powerful determinant of whether a physician addresses the patient's problem.[8] In the final analysis, the effectiveness of risk factor manage-

Table 14-1: Barriers to Implementation of Preventive Services[1]

Patient	*Physician*
• Lack of knowledge and motivation • Lack of access to care • Cultural factors • Social factors	• Problem-based focus • Feedback on prevention is negative or neutral • Time constraints • Lack of incentives, including reimbursement • Lack of training – Poor knowledge of benefits – Perceived ineffectiveness – Lack of skills • Lack of specialist-generalist communication • Lack of perceived legitimacy

ment is reduced when the physician fails to optimize patient compliance. It is also important that family members take an active role in the patient's compliance. Family members can help improve compliance by supporting the patient's treatment program.[9]

From the physician's perspective, both primary care physicians and cardiologists have limited time to carry out additional assessments and interventions because their primary focus is on acute problems. Acute and chronic problems rather than health screening or prevention primarily drive practice schedules. In addition, there is immediate gratification from a patient's improvement after an acute intervention, and reimbursement is better than

Health-Care Setting	*Community/Society*
• Acute-care priority • Lack of resources and facilities • Lack of systems for preventive services • Time and economic concerns • Poor communication between specialty and primary care providers • Lack of policies and standards	• Lack of policies and standards • Lack of reimbursements

for risk factor management, which has traditionally been poorly reimbursed.

Physicians often cite lack of training and confidence—limitations in training, skills, and experience—as major barriers to using prevention strategies. A survey of primary care physicians found that 69% of them felt qualified to provide smoking cessation counseling, but only 32% felt confident about providing dietary counseling and 36% felt confident about using medications to lower cholesterol.[10] Also, because the treatment recommendations for a patient hospitalized for an MI often do not include recommendations for managing risk factors, the patient is left with the perception that preventive interventions are not important. It is often not clear which physician will take the lead in prescribing treatment for risk reduction for CHD patients, so clear communication is vital. The specialist and primary care physician need to support each other's efforts to provide a consistent and strong recommendation for the management of risk factors.

Hospitals, managed care organizations, and primary care and specialty practices may raise obstacles to even well-trained, skillful physicians and their patients. Providing risk factor management in a hospital or practice setting can be particularly difficult because acute illness care poses logistic problems, there is often no infrastructure to enable health-care professionals to focus on prevention, and there may be a lack of reimbursement for some prevention services. Management of chronic disease, using case management and disease state management, is an example of a successful chronic disease care strategy for long-term prevention.

The external factors affecting the provision of risk factor management primarily involve the lack of clear standards for preventive services and the lack of financial reimbursement for these services. Health-care professionals have not traditionally been paid to provide preventive services, so the financial focus on acute care rather than prevention diminishes the likelihood that health-care organizations will commit resources and personnel for preventive services until prevention becomes a priority.

Practice-based Intervention Systems

Appropriate risk factor management is critical for the optimal care of both patients with established cardiovascular disease and patients at high risk of developing CHD. Patients identify physicians as their primary source of health information and indicate that they would try to improve their health habits if their doctors told them it was important. This puts primary care physicians and other primary care clinicians, in particular, on the front line for screening for and treating cardiovascular risk factors in millions of Americans.

The Health Education and Research Trial (HEART) project, which was funded by the National Institutes of Health (NIH), demonstrated that it is possible to deliver effective heart disease prevention services in the primary care setting. Experience with the HEART project showed that when office-based prevention programs are established, they are effective.[11] Other studies found that using computerized reminders increased prevention tests and counseling between 9% and 31%,[12] and a plan that emphasized office organization increased cancer screening and prevention counseling by 10% to 20%.[13] Organized programs of physician education and practice organization can assist physicians in helping patients to improve nutrition and lose weight.[14]

A clearly defined, well-established office system of routine screening, management, and monitoring is the key to successful prevention programs. Most practices already have these systems in place for routine blood pressure checks, screening virtually all patients for high blood pressure at each visit.[15] The same approach can be expanded to include other cardiovascular risk factors. However, if they are to be successful, heart disease prevention systems cannot require large amounts of physician or staff time.

Developing a prevention system can provide an opportunity to review the general efficiency of your office and eliminate some of the typical 'time wasters,' allowing you to regain time needed to provide important preventive services. Examples of time wasters include duplication of information entered in the medical record, vital signs that are not vital (eg, respiration or temperature for all patients), and poorly organized patient education. Designing a prevention system that is more efficient than your current routines enables you to establish it with a modest initial time investment and to maintain it with a minimum amount of staff time. To increase cost-effectiveness and better use resources, consider using office staff rather than physicians whenever possible.

The Fundamentals

The goal of a prevention system is to make sure all patients seen in your practice are appropriately screened, managed, and monitored at every visit, not just when it is convenient or when a member of the practice remembers to do it.

Screening for Risk Factors

The first step in the process is to develop an office routine for risk factor screening. This could include giving a self-administered questionnaire to patients when they check in. The questionnaire should ask about heart disease risk factors as well as medical, social, and family history, and the information should be updated every 2 years. A staff nurse can review the questionnaire with the patient, enter any pertinent data on a 'problem' list, and file the questionnaire in the designated spot in the medical record. When the physician sees the patient, he or she can review the nurse's entries on the problem list and look at the questionnaire in more detail if desired. It is a good idea to change the color of the questionnaire at 2-year intervals. This makes it easy to recognize when the information needs to be updated.

Another way to facilitate routine screening is to include important risk factors—such as smoking habits, physical activity status, and waist circumference at the iliac crest—as vital signs. This information is potentially more valuable than respiration, which takes time to collect, is usually not accurate when taken by staff, and often has limited clinical benefit. Respiration information should only be collected when it is important. Only patients with an infectious complaint need have their temperatures recorded. On the other hand, more than 40% of adults are overweight and have the metabolic syndrome, which is why measur-

Table 14-2: Suggested Roles of the Preventive Services Team

Physician

- Direct office system changes to provide appropriate preventive services
- Train office staff
- Support efforts of office staff
- Determine what counseling a patient needs and endorse the patient education process
- Deliver a clear message to patients about the importance of prevention and the capabilities of the staff members who are providing the counseling

Office Nurse

- Organize patient education services
- Provide direct counseling and patient education
- Provide routine preventive services
- Assist or direct case-management programs
- Assist or direct prevention programs (eg, smoking cessation, lipid treatment, dietary, weight loss)

Medical Assistant

- Carefully select, conveniently organize (eg, in each examination room for common problems), maintain, and order educational materials
- Collect risk factor information
- Review education information with patients at the end of visits
- Assist with referral process and follow-up

Receptionist

- Organize and collect patient questionnaires
- Be responsible for mailing appropriate information related to the patient's scheduled visits
- Assist in scheduling preventive services or facilitating referrals

ing waist circumference is helpful (see Chapter 8). More than 25% of teens and adults use tobacco. Identified risks can be flagged with a colored sticker to alert the staff.

Managing Risk Factors

Managing CHD risk factors involves recommending behavior change, providing counseling and, in some cases, prescribing medications. Patient education, an important part of behavior change, is most effectively conducted using a team approach. Each team member can fulfill specific roles (Table 14-2).

When a physician prescribes medication, a staff member can save the physician time by explaining how to use the medication and its potential side effects. To make this process more efficient, the staff member can give the patient a one-page outline of the purpose of the medication and its potential side effects. This sheet can even be personalized with dosage information for the patient. Drug information sheets are available at most pharmacies or can be obtained from Internet sources such as MedlinePlus (www.medlineplus.com).

Monitoring Risk Factors

After a plan to manage CHD risk factors has been established, a patient's progress needs to be monitored. To help encourage compliance with the plan, a schedule of follow-up appointments should be established. This schedule can be transferred from the physician's charge slip to a computer or card file and monitored by a staff person who is responsible for sending out reminder cards. Patients are more likely to recognize the importance of managing risk factors when they are addressed in a routine and consistent way.

To monitor a patient's progress, it may be helpful to use a flow sheet in an easy-to-read format to record pertinent information from several visits. Table 14-3 is a sample health monitoring flow sheet that features the important factors to include when tracking a patient's health over several visits. Some practices use flow sheets to summa-

Table 14-3: Health Monitoring Flow Sheet[16]

Name ________________ Birth date ________________

Height ________________

Date

Weight

Body mass index

Blood pressure

Total cholesterol

Triglycerides

High-density-lipoprotein cholesterol

Low-density-lipoprotein cholesterol

Tobacco use (type, amount)

Exercise

Nutrition

Alcohol

Medications, dose

Patient history update

Assessment

Plan

Provider initials

rize screening tests or immunizations, or to track chronic conditions such as diabetes, high cholesterol, and hypertension. When using a tool like this, it is important to define when and how the information will be included and who will be responsible for data collection and updating. This will save time and eliminate mistakes.

Recommendations for Monitoring Risk Factors in Practice

In addition to using a flow sheet (see above) to track changes in therapy and results for chronic conditions (eg, blood pressure, cholesterol, hemoglobin A_{1c}, creatinine), carefully plan follow-up, including having follow-up visits within 4 to 6 weeks after a change in therapy to reinforce the effectiveness of the treatment. Waiting longer will reduce adherence to therapy. At the same time, planning long-term, routine follow-up will help the patient understand that you consider his or her treatment an important issue. Follow-up visits for initial lab testing can be conducted by office staff such as nurses or physician assistants, or be visits for labs only with a follow-up phone call by the office staff.

Risk Reduction Strategies

The following CHD risk reduction strategies should be implemented for patients with established cardiovascular disease. Some of these strategies, which have been endorsed by the AHA and ACC, can be used to create key measures for risk factor management and to monitor quality of care.

1. Smoking status should be documented in all patients with coronary or other vascular disease.
2. A smoking cessation program should be encouraged for the smoking patient and his or her family.
3. The offer of physician advice and self-help materials to stop smoking should be documented for all eligible patients hospitalized with coronary or other vascular disease.
4. A fasting lipoprotein profile should be ordered and documented for all patients with coronary or other vascular disease within the first 3 months after onset of disease, if diet or pharmacologic intervention is deemed appropriate for the patient.
5. Nutritional evaluation and counseling should be offered to all patients with coronary or other vascular

disease and documented in the medical record at the time of diagnosis.

6. Lipid-lowering pharmacologic therapy should be prescribed and documented in the medical record for all patients with coronary or other vascular disease who have an LDL cholesterol level higher than 130 mg/dL after nutritional therapy, if intervention is deemed appropriate for the patient.
7. All patients with coronary or other vascular disease should be assessed and provided with an exercise counseling prescription at the time of diagnosis or as a component of routine health maintenance.
8. Aspirin therapy should be offered to all eligible patients who are diagnosed with coronary or other atherosclerotic disease. If aspirin therapy is not indicated, the contraindications should be documented in the medical record.
9. All patients with coronary or other vascular disease should have a blood pressure measurement documented at every visit.
10. If an average of two or more blood pressure measurements is equal to or greater than 140 mm Hg systolic or 90 mm Hg diastolic, or is greater than 135/85 in a patient with diabetes mellitus or chronic kidney disease, lifestyle and pharmacologic therapy plans should be offered and documented at the time of diagnosis.

Patient Education Strategies for Primary Prevention

The two main objectives of patient education and counseling are to change health behavior and improve health status. When considering an approach to patient education, knowledge about the health consequences of a particular behavior is necessary, but it is not enough to change the behavior. Following are some recommendations from the US Preventive Services Task Force (USPSTF) that may be useful in changing your patients' health behaviors.[17]

Table 14-4: Stages of Change and Suggested Physician Intervention[23,24]

Stage	Patient
Precontemplation	
Goal: Patient will begin thinking about change	Not thinking about change May be resigned Feeling of no control Denial: does not believe it applies to self Believes consequences are not serious
Contemplation	
Goal: Patient will examine benefits and barriers to change	Weighing benefits and costs of behavior, proposed change
Preparation	
Goal: Patient will discover the elements necessary for decisive action	Experimenting with small changes

Physician

Use relationship-building skills
Personalize risk factors
Give data about patient's vital signs, laboratory results, etc, compared with norm
Rather than use scare tactics, express your caring concern
Use teachable moments (the symptoms as a message)
Educate in small bits, repeatedly, over time
Ask, "How would you know if your ____ was a problem for you?"
Ask, "If you were to decide to change, what do you imagine might be some advantages?"

Elicit from patient the reasons to change and the consequences of changing
Explore ambivalence; praise the patient for considering the difficulties of change
Restate both sides of ambivalence
Question possible solutions for one barrier at a time
Pose advice gently as "a solution that has been effective for some patients might be adaptable to you" to avoid patient's natural resistance

Encourage the patient's efforts
Ask what strategies the patient has selected for risk situations
Ask for a change date

(continued on next page)

Table 14-4: Stages of Change and Suggested Physician Intervention[23,24] *(continued)*

Stage	Patient
Action	
Goal: Patient will take decisive action	Taking a definitive action to change
Maintenance	
Goal: Patient will incorporate change into daily lifestyle	Maintaining new behavior over time
Relapse	
Goal: Learn from the temporary success and reengage patient in the change process	Experiencing normal part of the process of change Usually feels demoralized

- Frame the teaching to match the patient's perceptions. Where possible, consider and incorporate the beliefs and concerns of the patient.
- Fully inform patients of the purposes and expected effects of interventions and when to expect these effects. This may prevent discouragement when benefits are not immediately evident.
- Suggest small changes rather than large ones. For example, to a patient who is extremely overweight, losing 50 or 100 pounds might seem impossible, but losing 3 to 5 pounds in a month seems reachable.
- Give specific and informational instructions. Explaining a regimen and the rationale behind it–in writing so the patient can take it home–improves adherence.

Physician

Reinforce the decision
Delight in even small successes
View problems as helpful information
Ask what else is needed for success

Continue reinforcement
Ask what strategies have been helpful and what situations cause problems. This provides more information to use with other patients as well

Reframe from 'failure' to 'successful for a while,' plus new lessons for continued success

- Try suggesting a new behavior. It is sometimes easier to add a new behavior than to get rid of an established one. For example, if weight is an issue, you might suggest that a patient begin moderate physical exercise rather than try to change his or her eating pattern.
- Connect new behaviors to old behaviors. For example, you might suggest that the patient take prescribed medication twice a day before or after brushing his or her teeth.
- Use the power inherent in your profession. Patients view clinicians as health experts and consider what they say as important. Do not hesitate to tell a patient, "I want you to reduce the amount of fat in your diet because..." and describe how excess fat contributes to the patient's specific health issues or medical problems.

Table 14-5: Internet Resources With Supporting Materials for Specific Recommendations

Clinical Recommendation	Recommended Web Site
Cigarette smoking	http://www.surgeongeneral.gov/tobacco/treating_tobacco_use.pdf
Diet	http://www.cfsan.fda.gov/~frt/sea-mehg.html
Weight management	http://www.nhlbi.nih.gov/guidelines/obesity/ob_home.htm
Lipids	http://www.medicine.wisc.edu/naa
Blood pressure	http://www.medicine.wisc.edu/naa
	http://www.nhlbi.nih.gov/health/public/heart/hbp/dash/index/htm
Diabetes	http://www.diabetes.org/home.jsp http://www.medicine.wisc.edu/naa
Atrial fibrillation/stroke prevention	http://www.nhlbi.nih.gov/about/framingham/stroke.htm http://www.americanheart.org/downloadable/heart/222_ja22017993p_1.pdf
Absolute CHD risk calculation	http://www.nhlbi.nih.gov/guidelines/cholesterol/index.htm http://www.heartdecision.com
Cardiovascular health	http://www.dhfs.wisconsin.gov/health/cardiovascular

Comments

Treating tobacco use and dependence

Mercury levels in seafood

Clinical guidelines and the identification, evaluation, and treatment of overweight and obesity in adults

Third Report of the National Cholesterol Education Program Adult Treatment Panel III (NCEP ATP III) and many other resources

Seventh Report of the Joint National Committee on Prevention, Detection, Evaluation, and Treatment of High Blood Pressure (JNC 7) and many other resources

Dietary Approaches to Stop Hypertension (DASH) eating plan

American Diabetes Association
AHA Conference Proceedings: Prevention Conference VI: Diabetes and Cardiovascular Disease and many other resources

Framingham Stroke Risk Scoring System

ACC/AHA/ESC Guidelines for Management of Patients with Atrial Fibrillation

Framingham CHD Risk Scoring System

Physician tool of preventive cardiology information, office flow sheet, and patient card for tracking blood pressure, cholesterol levels, etc.

- Get specific commitments from patients by asking them to describe how they intend to follow the recommended regimen.
- Use a combination of strategies such as individual counseling, group classes, written materials, audiovisual aids, and community resources. Patient education efforts that integrate several different approaches are more likely to be effective.
- Take a team approach to patient education by involving office staff. Patient education is facilitated by involving physicians, nurses, clinical nurse specialists, health educators, dietitians, and other related health professionals, as appropriate.
- Refer when necessary. It is not always possible for a busy practice to handle complete patient education and counseling and, in some situations, the patients may be better served by an appropriate referral, such as referral to a dietitian for case management of secondary prevention from cardiac rehabilitation. Sources of referral include hospital resources, community agencies, national voluntary health organizations, such as the AHA, instructional materials such as books and videotapes, and even other patients. An excellent way to change health behavior is to connect the patient with someone with the same problem who has successfully made changes and can serve as a role model.
- Monitor progress by scheduling follow-up contact by an appointment or a telephone call within a few weeks. Provider-initiated contact may be more effective than patient-initiated phone calls.[18] Calls made by the provider to the patient have been shown to reinforce behavior change effectively.[19-22]

Stages of Change

Obviously, it is unreasonable to expect that patients—even highly motivated patients—will change behaviors overnight. Table 14-4 summarizes the stages of change and suggests interventions you can use at each stage.

The ACC and the AHA also publish excellent resources, including their joint Continuous Quality Improvement Project guidelines[25,26] and the AHA's Get With The Guidelines program, which is helpful in setting up a hospital discharge and monitoring program that hospitals and practices can use to improve adherence to secondary prevention guidelines. There are also several Web resources and books[27] for guidelines.

Practice Tools

The Internet is an excellent source of information and tools to help you put prevention into practice. Table 14-5 lists risk factors and recommended sites where you and your patients can find valuable information.

References

1. Pearson TA, McBride PE, Miller NH, et al: 27th Bethesda Conference: matching the intensity of risk factor management with the hazard for coronary disease events. Task force 8. Organization of preventive cardiology service. *J Am Coll Cardiol* 1996;27:1039-1047.

2. Pearson TA, Blair SN, Daniels SR, et al: AHA guidelines for primary prevention of cardiovascular disease and stroke: 2002 update: consensus panel guide to comprehensive risk reduction for adult patients without coronary or other atherosclerotic vascular diseases. American Heart Association Science Advisory and Coordinating Committee. *Circulation* 2002;106:388-391.

3. Stein JH, McBride PE: Implementing strategies for the secondary prevention of coronary heart disease. In: Douglas PS, ed. *Clinical Coronary Heart Disease.* 2nd ed. Orlando, FL, WB Saunders, 2002, pp 383-401.

4. Fonarow GC, French WJ, Parsons LS, et al: Use of lipid-lowering medications at discharge in patients with acute myocardial infarction: data from the National Registry of Myocardial Infarction 3. *Circulation* 2001;103:38-44.

5. Hibbard H, Nutting PA, Grady MI, eds: Primary care research: theory and methods: conference proceedings. Rockville, Md: Agency for Health Care Policy and Research. 1991; ACHPR publication no. 91-0011.

6. Healthy People 2000: National health promotion and disease prevention objectives. Washington, DC: US Department of Health

and Human Services, Public Health Service, 1991; DHHS publication no. (PHS)91-50213.

7. McBride PE: Overcoming the barriers to preventive care: the 5 Ps. *Med Econ* 2001;78(suppl):18-24.

8. Kottke TE, Brekke ML, Soilberg LI: Making "time" for preventive services. *Mayo Clin Proc* 1993;68:785-791.

9. Pearson T, Rapaport E, Criqui M, et al: Optimal risk factor management in the patient after coronary revascularization. A statement for healthcare professionals from an American Heart Association Writing Group. *Circulation* 1994;90:3125-3133.

10. Shea S, Gemson DH, Mossel P: Management of high blood cholesterol by primary care physicians: diffusion of the National Cholesterol Education Program Adult Treatment Panel guidelines. *J Gen Intern Med* 1990;5:327-334.

11. McBride P, Underbakke G, Plane MB, et al: Improving prevention systems in primary care practices: the Health Education and Research Trial (HEART). *J Fam Pract* 2000;49:115-125.

12. McPhee SJ, Detmer WM: Office-based interventions to improve delivery of cancer prevention services by primary care physicians. *Cancer* 1993;72(suppl 3):1100-1112.

13. Carney PA, Dietrich AJ, Keller A, et al: Tools, teamwork, and tenacity: an office system for cancer prevention. *J Fam Pract* 1992;35:388-394.

14. Ockene IS, Hebert JR, Ockene JK, et al: Effect of training and a structured office practice on physician-delivered nutrition counseling: the Worcester-Area Trial for Counseling in Hyperlipidemia (WATCH). *Am J Prev Med* 1996;12:252-258.

15. McBride PE, Underbakke G, Plane MB: Heart disease prevention practices of primary care physicians. *Circulation* 1992;86:1-402.

16. Underbakke MS, McBride PE: Preventing heart disease: a practice-based program that works. *Your Patient and Fitness* 1996;10:6-12.

17. US Preventive Services Task Force. *Guide to Clinical Preventive Services*, 2nd ed. Washington, DC: US Department of Health and Human Services, Office of Disease Prevention and Health Promotion, 1996.

18. Schofield MJ, Sanson-Fisher R, Halpin S, et al: Notification and follow-up of Pap test results: current practice and women's preferences. *Prev Med* 1994;23:276-283.

19. Weinberger M, Kirkman MS, Samsa GP, et al: A nurse-coordinated intervention for primary care patients with non-insulin-dependent diabetes mellitus: impact on glycemic control and health-related quality of life. *J Gen Intern Med* 1995;10:59-66.

20. van Elderen-van Kemenade T, Maes S, van den Broek Y: Effects of a health education programme with telephone follow-up during cardiac rehabilitation. *Br J Clin Psychol* 1994;33(Pt. 3): 367-378.

21. Ahring KK, Ahring JP, Joyce C, et al: Telephone modem access improves diabetes control in those with insulin-requiring diabetes. *Diabetes Care* 1992;15:971-975.

22. Department of Health and Human Services, Public Health Service, Office of Disease Prevention and Health Promotion. "Put Prevention into Practice" education and action kit. Washington, DC, Government Printing Office, 1994.

23. Zimmerman GL, Olsen CG, Bosworth MF: A 'staging change' approach to helping patients change behavior. *Am Fam Phys* 2000;61:1409-1416.

24. Prochaska JO, DiClemente CC, Norcross JC: In search of how people change. Applications to addictive behaviors. *Am Psychol* 1992;47:1102-1104.

25. Gibbons RJ, Smith S, Antman E, et al: The American College of Cardiology/American Heart Association clinical practice guidelines: Part I: where do they come from? *Circulation* 2003;107: 2979-2986.

26. Gibbons RJ, Smith SC Jr, Antman E, et al: The American College of Cardiology/American Heart Association clinical practice guidelines: Part II: evolutionary changes in a continuous quality improvement project. *Circulation* 2003;107:3101-3107.

27. Miller WR, Rollnick S: *Motivational Interviewing: Preparing People to Change Addiction Behavior*. New York, Guilford, 1991, pp 191-202.

CHAPTER 15

Secondary Prevention of Cardiovascular Events: Summary of Recommendations for Primary Care Physicians

Secondary prevention in cardiovascular disease (CVD) refers to preventing recurrent CVD events in patients with established atherosclerotic vascular disease, including those with coronary artery disease (CAD), cerebrovascular disease, or peripheral arterial disease (including abdominal aortic aneurysm). There is no doubt that patients with established atherosclerotic vascular disease are at the highest risk for cardiovascular events such as myocardial infarction (MI), stroke, or cardiovascular death. Accordingly, targeting these high-risk patients with proven secondary prevention measures is the most therapeutic and cost-effective approach to preventing the consequences of atherosclerosis. Nevertheless, proven therapies for secondary prevention remain underprescribed by physicians. This chapter will review the most important secondary prevention strategies for preventing heart disease in patients with established atherosclerosis (Table 15-1).

According to the National Cholesterol Education Program Adult Treatment Panel III (NCEP ATP III) guidelines, patients without established vascular disease, but with an estimated 10-year risk of MI or dying of CAD, also should be treated from a prevention standpoint with the same level of aggressiveness as patients with established vascular disease. This includes patients with diabetes mellitus, and some guidelines also suggest that patients with chronic kidney disease should be treated in this manner.

Antiplatelet Agents and Anticoagulation

Aspirin is recommended for all patients with acute MI, unstable angina pectoris, or chronic CAD. Use of aspirin is a Class 1 recommendation in most guidelines based on the results of several randomized clinical trials.[1-3] Its use is associated with 20% to 25% reductions in the risk of recurrent cardiovascular events. In the setting of an acute MI, aspirin saves a life at the cost of $13 per year and is one of the most effective and inexpensive interventions for the treatment of CAD.[4]

Current recommendations for use of aspirin in the setting of an acute MI are to administer 325 mg immediately and to continue this dose daily for the duration of the initial hospitalization, then to use 75 to 325 mg daily indefinitely. Adding dipyridamole (Persantine®) to aspirin is not more effective than using aspirin alone.[5] Clopidogrel (Plavix® [75 mg daily]) is as effective as aspirin for secondary prevention and may have some advantages over aspirin in very high-risk patients, such as those with peripheral vascular disease, those who have had recurrent cardiovascular events while on aspirin therapy, those who have undergone coronary artery bypass graft surgery, and possibly those with diabetes mellitus.[6] Clopidogrel should be started in conjunction with aspirin in patients with an acute coronary syndrome at the time of presentation, unless there is a high suspicion that the patient will need cardiac graft surgery. It should be continued at least for 30 days after an acute coronary syndrome and in patients

Table 15-1: Summary of Prevention Strategies for Patients With Cardiovascular Disease

Antiplatelet agents/ anticoagulants	• Start aspirin 325 mg daily, then continue indefinitely a dose of 75 to 162 mg daily, unless aspirin allergy. • Consider clopidogrel 75 mg daily or warfarin if aspirin is contraindicated. • Use clopidogrel for 30 days in patients with stents (6 months if a drug-eluting stent). • Consider long-term clopidogrel therapy in patients with acute coronary syndrome, peripheral vascular disease, or coronary artery bypass graft surgery. • Manage warfarin to INR 2.5 to 3.5 after MI, when clinically indicated or in patients unable to take antiplatelet agents.
Blood pressure control	• Recommend lifestyle changes for all patients with blood pressure 120/80 mm Hg. • Target blood pressure <140/90 mm Hg; <130/80 mm Hg for patients with chronic kidney disease or diabetes mellitus.

Blood pressure control *(continued)*	• β-Blockers and inhibitors of the renin-angiotensin-aldosterone system have compelling indications. • Thiazide-type diuretics should be used in most patients.
β ***Blockade***	• Use for all patients with ST-elevation MI without contraindications. • Target heart rate 50 to 65 bpm.
Renin-angiotensin-aldosterone system blockers	• ACE inhibitors in all patients indefinitely, early in stable high-risk patients. • Angiotensin receptor blockers if intolerant of ACE inhibitors and heart failure or low ejection fraction. • Aldosterone blockade in patients with low ejection fraction and diabetes or heart failure, but without significant renal disease or hyperkalemia.
Cardiac rehabilitation	• For all patients with ST-elevation MI. • For patients at moderate to high risk needing supervised exercise training as warranted.

(continued on next page)

Table 15-1: Summary of Prevention Strategies for Patients With Cardiovascular Disease *(continued)*

Diabetes mellitus management	• Target hemoglobin A_{1c} <7%. • Preferred oral hypoglycemic agents include metformin and acarbose. • More aggressive treatment of other risk factors as indicated.
Dietary changes	• Mediterranean diet is the template for dietary composition. • Two to three servings of fatty fish per week. • Caloric intake adjusted by weight. • Reduction in saturated and trans fat, increased soluble fiber, sterol/stanol margarines for cholesterol lowering. • Salt restriction for blood pressure lowering.
Fish oil capsules	• 1 g daily in MI survivors.
Lipid management	• Therapeutic lifestyle changes (<7% of total calories are saturated fat, <200 mg cholesterol daily). • Physical activity and weight management in all patients.

Lipid management *(continued)*

- Target LDL-C <100 mg/dL.
- For very high-risk patients, target LDL-C <70 mg/dL.
- High-dose statins are first-line agents for patients with triglycerides <400 to 500 mg/dL; combination therapy with niacin and, in some cases, fibrates should be considered to optimize lipid profile.
- For patients with triglycerides >200 mg/dL, non-HDL-C <130 mg/dL is a secondary goal of therapy.

Physical activity

- Encourage a minimum of 30 to 60 minutes of activity, preferably daily, but at least 150 minutes weekly.
- Supplement physical activity by increasing daily lifestyle activities.
- See 'Cardiac rehabilitation' recommendations.

Smoking

- Strongly encourage patient to quit smoking.
- Strongly encourage family to stop smoking to avoid secondhand smoke exposure.

(continued on next page)

Table 15-1: Summary of Prevention Strategies for Patients With Cardiovascular Disease

(continued)

***Smoking** (continued)*	• Provide counseling and pharmacologic therapy using nicotine replacement and bupropion if there are no contraindications. • Use formal smoking cessation programs.
Weight management	• Determine body mass index at each visit. • Measure waist circumference at each visit. • Restrict calories by 500 to 1,000 kilocalories per day with a goal of losing 1 to 2 pounds per week. • See 'Dietary changes' and 'Physical activity' recommendations. • More exercise leads to more weight loss.

ACE = angiotensin-converting enzyme, HDL-C = high-density lipoprotein cholesterol, INR = international normalized ratio, LDL-C = low-density lipoprotein cholesterol, MI = myocardial infarction who have undergone coronary stenting. Some experts recommend continuing clopidogrel for 6 to 12 months in all patients who have had an acute coronary syndrome.[1,7] At least 6 months of combined aspirin and clopidogrel therapy is recommended for patients who have had placement of drug-eluting stents or coronary brachytherapy. Clopidogrel or ticlopidine (Ticlid®) 250 mg twice daily also are alternatives for patients with aspirin allergy.

Another alternative to antiplatelet therapy for patients with true aspirin allergy is use of warfarin (Coumadin®) with target INR of 2.5 to 3.5. This is a good option in patients younger than 75 years who are at low risk for bleeding. For patients who have received a stent but who have aspirin allergy, warfarin should be administered concomitantly with clopidogrel, 75 mg daily with a target INR of 2.0 to 3.0. Otherwise, warfarin is indicated for patients who have persistent or paroxysmal atrial fibrillation or documented left ventricular thrombus.[1]

Blood Pressure Control

The Seventh Report of the Joint National Committee on the Prevention, Detection, and Evaluation of Treatment of High Blood Pressure (JNC 7) recommends that after MI, lifestyle changes and medications should be used to target a blood pressure of less than 140/90 mm Hg.[8] A target of 130/80 mm Hg is recommended for patients with chronic kidney disease or diabetes mellitus.

JNC 7 emphasized the importance of lifestyle changes for all patients with a blood pressure of 120/80 mm Hg. The dietary changes described in the Cholesterol-Modifying Therapy section below also have beneficial effects on blood pressure. Specifically, weight loss (for patients who are overweight or obese) and following a diet that is high in fruits and vegetables and low in fat and saturated fat have been demonstrated to improve systolic blood pressure with efficacy similar to that associated with many antihypertensive medications. Additional benefits are achieved by reducing dietary sodium intake to less than 2.4 g per day.[8]

A detailed examination of the treatment of hypertension can be found in Chapter 11. For secondary prevention, ACE inhibitors and β-blockers are indicated, as are aldosterone antagonists for patients without contraindication who have left ventricular systolic dysfunction and either congestive heart failure or diabetes mellitus. These agents are examined in more detail below. Most patients will require at least two medications to reach the blood pressure goals outlined above. Indeed, combination therapy should be started if the blood pressure is >20/10 mm Hg above goal.[1,8] Although ACE inhibitors and β-blockers are indicated for most patients with atherosclerotic vascular disease, this combination is not particularly effective for lowering blood pressure in certain subgroups of patients, such as African Americans and patients with isolated systolic hypertension.[8,9] In general, most patients with hypertension should be treated with a thiazide-type diuretic (such as hydrochlorothiazide [Esidrix®] 12.5 to 25 mg daily or chlorthalidone 12.5 to 25 mg daily), either as a first- or second-line agent. For patients with renal insufficiency or congestive heart failure, a loop diuretic should be substituted for a thiazide diuretic.

Although short-acting calcium channel blockers should not be used for the treatment of hypertension in patients with atherosclerosis, long-acting calcium channel blockers may be used when other agents are not tolerated or not sufficient to reach blood pressure goals. They are especially useful in patients with angina pectoris, coronary vasospasm, and isolated systolic hypertension. Amlodipine (Norvasc®) has specifically been demonstrated to be safe in patients with reduced left ventricular systolic function, a category of patients in whom even long-acting non-dihydropyridine calcium channel blockers such as verapamil (Calan®) or diltiazem (Cardizem®) should be avoided.[8,10]

β-Blockers

β-Adrenergic blockers reduce the incidence of recurrent MI, sudden cardiac death, and overall mortality.[1] They also improve left ventricular function and survival in patients with left ventricular systolic dysfunction, contrary to old paradigms, which avoided β-blockers in patients with heart failure. β-Blockers remain significantly underused because of misunderstandings regarding the contraindications, such as fear of adverse lipid effects and concerns about central nervous system (CNS) depression. The clinical and survival benefits of β-blockers dramatically outweigh the potential adverse lipid effects, which are less common in β-1 selective agents. Similarly, CNS complaints such as fatigue, cognitive impairment, and depression are less likely to occur when moderate doses of β-1 selective agents or β-blockers with long half-lives are used. β-1 Selective agents also are less likely to cause bronchospasm. Recommended β-blockers include metoprolol (Lopressor®), 50 to 100 mg twice daily, and long-acting metoprolol (100 to 200 mg a day); atenolol (Tenormin®), 50 to 200 mg nightly; and carvedilol (Coreg®), 6.25 to 25 mg twice daily. Atenolol is dosed in the evening because its half-life does not lead to full 24-hour β-blockade. Nocturnal use may relieve nocturnal angina and prevent early morning MI. β-Blocker doses should be adjusted to achieve a resting heart rate of approximately 50 to 65 bpm, as long as hypotension, decompensated congestive heart failure, heart block greater than first degree, or obstructive pulmonary symptoms do not occur. β-Blockers have a specific benefit in patients with diabetes mellitus and are useful for the management of patients with angina pectoris, hypertension, and atrial tachydysrhythmia.

Renin-Angiotensin-Aldosterone System Blockade

Angiotensin-converting enzyme (ACE) inhibitors reduce morbidity and mortality in MI survivors, patients with asymptomatic left ventricular dysfunction, and patients with congestive heart failure (CHF).[1,8] An ACE inhibitor should be prescribed after MI in all patients without contraindications (such as pregnancy, hyperkalemia, or history of angioedema).[1-3] An angiotensin receptor blocker may be prescribed after MI for patients who are intolerant of an ACE inhibitor, if they have clinical or radiologic evidence of heart failure, and an ejection fraction <40%. Recently, the indications for ACE inhibitors have been extended to almost all patients with CAD, including those who have not had a MI but who have diabetes mellitus, even with preserved left ventricular systolic function.[8,11] In stable high-risk patients, such as those with anterior wall MI, previous MI, or CHF, ACE inhibition should be started early during hospitalization and continued chronically. ACE inhibitors should be used as chronic therapy for all other patients with coronary or other vascular diseases.

Long-term aldosterone blockade with medications such as spironolactone (Aldactone®), 12.5 to 25 mg daily, or eplerenone (Inspra®), target dose 50 mg daily, should be used in MI patients with an ejection fraction <40% and heart failure or diabetes mellitus.[1] Aldosterone antagonists should not be used in patients with significant renal dysfunction (creatinine >2.5 mg/dL in men or 2.0 mg/dL in women) or hyperkalemia (>5.0 mEq/L).

Cardiac Rehabilitation

Cardiac rehabilitation is a comprehensive, long-term cardiovascular health maintenance program that involves medical evaluation of patients with atherosclerotic vascular disease and prescribes exercise, risk factor modification, patient education, and counseling. Its goals are to limit the physiologic and psychological effects of cardiovascular disease, decrease the risk of sudden cardiac death, decrease cardiac symptoms, and improve psychosocial and vocational function.

Regular exercise is a critical component of heart disease prevention; however, cardiac rehabilitation involves more than physical activity. It includes comprehensive education, counseling, and management of risk factors. In meta-analysis, enrollment in cardiac rehabilitation is associated with a 24% reduction in all-cause mortality, primarily as a result of reduction in sudden cardiac death, recurrent MI, and other cardiac causes of death.[12-14] Cardiac rehabilitation improves quality of life, shortens post-MI convalescence, and increases rates of return to work. It is also safe and cost-effective, yet highly underused.[12-14]

Cardiac rehabilitation and secondary prevention programs are recommended for patients with MI and moderate- to high-risk patients in whom supervised exercise training is warranted. However, it cannot be emphasized enough that cardiac rehabilitation is more than just exercising. Cardiac rehabilitation programs involve setting goals related to physical activity; managing dyslipidemia, hypertension, and diabetes mellitus; smoking cessation; nutrition and weight loss education; and psychosocial counseling, using a case management approach.[12] The case management approach allows for patient and provider continuity, is more effective for targeting risk factor and treatment goals, improves communication between patients and their team of health care providers, and helps individualize the patient's rehabilitation goals. Communication with the patient's health care providers and family members is an essential part of the program.

Diabetes Mellitus Management

In patients with diabetes mellitus, strict glycemic control with insulin has been shown to lower both acute and 1-year mortality rates during acute ST segment elevation MI and in the year following. Strict glycemic control is defined as a hemoglobin A_{1c} of <7% and has also been shown to reduce long-term microvascular disease.[1] The relationship between glycemic control and macrovascular disease remains controversial; however, in overweight patients without contraindications to its use, metformin (Glucophage®) reduces cardiovascular events. Similarly, in patients with impaired glucose tolerance, metformin reduces the development of type 2 diabetes mellitus, and acarbose reduces the risk of cardiovascular events, including MI and new cases of hypertension.[15,16]

Although commonly used, sulfonylureas may interfere with ischemic preconditioning and generally should be avoided in patients with atherosclerotic vascular disease, in whom metformin, α-glucosidase inhibitors, intensive insulin therapy, and even thiazolidinediones (TZDs) are preferred, when contraindications are not present.[17] Because of their ease of use and relatively low cost, however, sulfonylureas are used widely. One sulfonylurea, glimepiride (Amaryl®), appears to have less effect on cardiac and vascular potassium-gated ATP channels and should be the preferred sulfonylurea, when possible. TZDs are helpful for treating insulin resistance but remain second-line therapy for improving glycemic control in patients with vascular disease because they may be associated with fluid retention and edema, which in some cases can cause CHF, especially in patients with pre-existing Class 3 or Class 4 heart failure. Nevertheless, their beneficial vascular and neurohormonal effects may eventually prove to reduce atherosclerotic progression. This is an area of intensive current evaluation, so use of TZDs cannot be recommended routinely at this time.

Fish Oil

Low-dose fish oil therapy (1 g of docosahexaenoic acid and eicosapentaenoic acid daily) is recommended for patients who have experienced an acute MI. It reduces the risk of sudden cardiac death and prevents atherosclerosis progression, independent of effects on serum lipid levels.[18] At the low doses used for sudden cardiac death prevention, side effects are uncommon but can include bruising because they are platelet inhibitors. At higher doses, fish oils lower triglycerides, but can also cause weight gain, eructation, and a 'fishy' smell. A diet that contains 2 to 3 servings of fatty fish per week also is encouraged.

Lipid Management

In patients with CAD, lipid-lowering therapy is one of the most thoroughly investigated and efficacious interventions for preventing recurrent cardiovascular events.[19,20] Although most studies have used hydroxymethylglutaryl-coenzyme A (HMG-CoA) reductase inhibitors (statins), evidence for improving lipids with other classes of agents, including nicotinic acid and fibrates, is strong. Therapeutic lifestyle changes, as examined below, also are an essential component of the management of lipids (Table 15-2). Recent trials have confirmed the benefit of cholesterol-modifying therapy in patients with established CAD and support a target low-density lipoprotein cholesterol (LDL-C) goal of <100 mg/dL.[20] These recommendations also extend to patients with cerebrovascular disease, peripheral vascular disease, and diabetes mellitus, and should be considered in patients with increased levels of high-sensitivity C-reactive protein, chronic kidney disease, or extensive subclinical atherosclerosis. Non-high-density lipoprotein cholesterol (non-HDL-C) is a secondary target of therapy for patients whose triglycerides are 200 mg/dL. It is calculated as the difference between total cholesterol and HDL-C (total cholesterol-HDL-C). The appropriate non-HDL-C target is 130 mg/dL in high-risk patients.[19,20]

A more aggressive LDL-C goal of <70 mg/dL is a therapeutic option, especially for patients with baseline LDL-C <100 mg/dL or individuals who are considered

Table 15-2: Summary of Lipid-lowering Medication Choices

Medication Sequence	TG <200 mg/dL
1st	High-dose statin
2nd	Add ezetimibe
3rd	Add niacin or resin

to be at very high risk.[20] Those include individuals with atherosclerotic vascular disease and multiple major risk factors (especially diabetes mellitus), severe poorly controlled risk factors (especially smoking), or multiple risk factors of the metabolic syndrome (especially triglycerides 200 or HDL-C <40 mg/dL). This alternate target also is appropriate for patients with an acute coronary syndrome and should be considered in patients with chronic kidney disease. To achieve these levels, most patients will require high doses of higher-potency statins, such as atorvastatin (Lipitor®) or simvastatin (Zocor®), frequently in combination with other agents such as ezetimibe (Zetia®) or niacin. A detailed examination of lipid-lowering therapy is in Chapter 10.

Use of treatment algorithms is encouraged, because treatment algorithms that provide definitions of lipid goals, as well as specific recommendations for lifestyle changes and medication use, improve prescribing habits and increase the number of patients at target levels. Standard discharge orders that include preventive therapies also improve use and reduce adverse cardiovascular events. Patients with acute coronary syndromes should start intensive lipid-lowering therapy during the hospital admission. Although obtaining a fasting lipid

Lipid Pattern	
TG 200-499 mg/dL	**TG 500 mg/dL**
High-dose statin	Fibrate or niacin
Add niacin	Fibrate + niacin
Add ezetimibe	Add statin or fish oils

panel in patients with acute coronary syndromes has been recommended, it is important to keep in mind that total cholesterol, LDL-C, and HDL-C levels may be artificially low because of acute phase response, and that triglyceride levels may be inaccurate, even within 24 hours of admission. Interpretation of in-hospital lipid panels should be performed with caution. For patients with acute coronary syndromes, early initiation of aggressive lipid-lowering therapy, usually with a high-dose statin, is indicated. Hepatic transaminases and a repeat fasting lipid panel should be measured 6 weeks later to assure achievement of targets and the absence of hepatotoxicity.

For patients with LDL-C values above goal, drug therapy, usually with a statin, should be initiated in conjunction with lifestyle changes.[19,20] For individuals with high triglycerides and low HDL-C, consider combining nicotinic acid or a fibrate with LDL-C lowering. In general, combining prescription niacin with a statin is safer than combining a fibrate with a statin and has a richer evidence base for preventing cardiovascular events. When combining a fibrate with a statin, fenofibrate (Tricor®, Lofibra®) appears to be safer; however, gemfibrozil (Lopid®) can be used in conjunction with low doses of statins (<20 mg daily) in individuals who are at lower risk for rhabdomyolysis.[21] Risk factors for rhabdomyolysis include combination drug therapy, advanced age, concomitant use of medications that impair catabolism or clearance of lipid-lowering drugs, renal insufficiency, and hypothyroidism.

Optimal diets for prevention of coronary heart disease have three major components: substituting nonhydrogenated unsaturated fats for saturated and trans fats, eating more ω-3 fats from fish, fish oil supplements, or plants, and following a diet that is high in fruits, vegetables, nuts, and whole grains, but low in refined grain products. The Mediterranean diet has been proven to reduce cardiac death in survivors of MI.[22,23] Foods that represent the most caloric intake include breads and cereals (especially whole grains), roots and green vegetables, nuts and legumes, daily fruit, and fish. Eating less red meat and replacing butter with olive oil is suggested. Although the Mediterranean diet is not necessarily associated with improvement in the lipid panel, it provides a context for dietary changes that have been proven to prevent cardiac events. The Therapeutic Lifestyle Change diet suggested by the National Cholesterol Education Program (NCEP), which will help improve the lipid profile, includes reducing saturated and trans fats to less than 7% of total calories, reducing dietary cholesterol to less than 200 mg per day, eating 10 to 25 g of viscous (soluble) fiber each day, and eating approximately 2 g of plant stanol and sterol margarines.[19] These changes can lead to improvements in LDL-C and triglycerides that are close to the improvements caused by lower doses of statins, and results are magnified by weight reduction and increased physical activity.

Smoking Cessation

Tobacco abuse is a powerful risk factor for recurrent cardiovascular events. Individuals who continue to smoke after a MI have nearly a threefold increased risk of a recurrent event.[24,25] Smoking as few as one to four cigarettes daily doubles the risk of a cardiac event.[25,26] Tobacco smoking can trigger coronary spasm, reduce the efficacy of anti-ischemic medications, and double the mortality after MI.[1] Smoking cessation reduces rates of reinfarction and death within 1 year of cessation, but relapse rates after MI are high.[1-3] Environmental (secondhand) smoke also increases cardiovascular risk.[1] Individuals who stop smoking after a cardiac event rapidly reduce their risk of future events.[1-3] Smoking cessation is a highly cost-effective intervention for patients with a history of MI and should be included in cardiac rehabilitation programs and health care coverage by insurance companies. Despite these benefits, only 50% of patients report being asked about tobacco use by their primary physicians, and less than 50% report being advised to stop smoking.

Many physicians believe that smoking cessation therapy is ineffective and that efforts are futile. The effectiveness of smoking cessation has been demonstrated in several clinical trials in patients with coronary disease. Early trials, before effective pharmacologic therapy was introduced, demonstrated only 12% to 15% abstinence rates; however, use of nicotine replacement therapies improves abstinence rates by 17% to 26% and cessation rates of approximately 70% have been reported after acute coronary syndromes.[27] This emphasizes the importance of routinely monitoring smoking status in all patients with atherosclerotic vascular disease and offering pharmacologic smoking cessation therapy. Hospitalization for acute MI is a critical stage during which significant behavior change can take place. Nicotine replacement therapy is safe and does not increase cardiovascular events, even in high-risk patients. If nicotine replacement therapy is not successful or is contraindicated, bupropion (Wellbutrin®) can be used.

Bupropion should be avoided in patients with a history of seizures or eating disorders, or those concomitantly taking another antidepressant medication. The combination of bupropion and nicotine replacement therapy is especially effective. Enrolling in a formal smoking cessation program is recommended and family members also should be encouraged to stop smoking to avoid secondhand smoke.

Weight Management

Achieving an optimal body weight (body mass index [BMI] 18.5 to 24.9 kg/m^2) is recommended for all patients.[1] Also recommended is achieving an ideal waist circumference of less than 35 inches in women and less than 40 inches in men.[1] Reaching targets for weight management improves lipid parameters and blood pressure, reduces insulin resistance, and prevents the development of type 2 diabetes mellitus. Body mass index and waist circumference should be part of all evaluations, and the response of these parameters to dietary and exercise interventions should be monitored. Dietary changes, as discussed above, should be initiated for patients with an increased waist circumference or heavier than the ideal body weight.

Weight loss should be initiated by caloric restriction by 500 to 1,000 kilocalories per day, with a goal of losing 1 to 2 pounds per week.[28] For most men, this results in a target of 1,200 to 1,600 kilocalories per day; for most women, a target of 1,000 to 1,200 kilocalories per day. As examined above, optimal strategies for dietary change include reducing intake of saturated and trans fats, increasing intake of ω-3 and monounsaturated fats, and eating a diet that is high in fruits, vegetables, nuts, and whole grains, but low in refined grain products. Although very low-fat (<10% of calories) diets reduce progression of coronary atherosclerosis and cardiac events, they are difficult to adhere to long term. Very low-carbohydrate diets also are not recommended. Between these two extremes, there is great room for moderation, common sense, and dietary variety, using the Mediterranean diet and components of the LDL-lowering Therapeutic Lifestyle Change diet as templates for weight loss in the context of caloric restriction.

Weight management is most successful when combined with physical activity. For sedentary patients, a starting point of 20 minutes of physical activity 3 to 5 days per week is recommended. To avoid injury, patients should start with simple exercises at a slow pace, such as walking, and reducing sedentary time. For weight loss, a minimum of 30 minutes of exercise, 5 times per week (150 minutes per week) will improve fitness, but weight loss will result only if it is performed in the presence of caloric restriction.[29] A goal of 60 minutes daily 5 to 7 days per week will lead to more weight loss. Exercise should be of moderate intensity (10 to 14 on a scale of 20) and should be supplemented by increased activities of daily living.[29]

Cardiac rehabilitation programs (examined above) are recommended for patients with ST elevation MI or for patients who are at moderate to high risk, in whom supervised exercise training is warranted, as examined below.

Therapies That Are No Longer Recommended

Several interventions that previously were recommended for patients with atherosclerotic vascular disease have been proven to be ineffective and, in some cases, harmful.

Hormone replacement therapy with estrogen plus a progestin should not be initiated in postmenopausal women after MI for secondary prevention of coronary events.[1,3] Postmenopausal women who are already taking estrogen plus progestin at the time of MI should not continue hormone therapy; however, women who are beyond 1 to 2 years after initiation of hormone therapy and wish to continue therapy for noncardiovascular reasons should weigh the risks and benefits, recognizing that there is an increased risk of cardiovascular events.[1,3] Hormone replacement therapy should not be continued while patients are on bed rest in the hospital.[1] There are fewer data regarding the use of unopposed estrogen, but in general it also is not recommended for the prevention of cardiovascular disease and is associated with other health risks. As examined above, dipyridamole is not a useful adjunct to aspirin for the prevention of cardiovascular events.[5]

Finally, antioxidant vitamins such as vitamin E and/or vitamin C should not be prescribed to prevent cardiovascular events in patients with atherosclerotic vascular disease.

References

1. Antman EM, Anbe DT, Armstrong PW, et al: ACC/AHA guidelines for the management of patients with ST-elevation myocardial infarction: a report of the American College of Cardiology/American Heart Association Task Force on Practice Guidelines (Committee to Review the 1999 Guidelines for the Management of Patients With Acute Myocardial Infarction). Available at: www.acc.org/clinical/guidelines.stemi/index.pdf. Accessed August 3, 2004.

2. Smith SC Jr, Blair SN, Bonow RO, et al: AHA/ACC Scientific Statement: AHA/ACC guidelines for preventing heart attack and death in patients with atherosclerotic cardiovascular disease: 2001 update: A statement for healthcare professionals from the American Heart Association and the American College of Cardiology. *Circulation* 2001;104:1577-1579.

3. Mosca L, Appel LJ, Benjamin EJ, et al: Evidence-based guidelines for cardiovascular disease prevention in women. *Circulation* 2004;109:672-693.

4. Hennekens CH, Jonas MA, Buring JE: The benefits of aspirin in acute myocardial infarction. Still a well-kept secret in the United States. *Arch Intern Med* 1994;154:37-39.

5. Fuster V, Dyken ML, Vokonas PS, et al: Aspirin as a therapeutic agent in cardiovascular disease. Special Writing Group. *Circulation* 1993;87:659-675.

6. A randomised, blinded, trial of clopidogrel versus aspirin in patients at risk of ischaemic events (CAPRIE). CAPRIE Steering Committee. *Lancet* 1996;348:1329-1339.

7. Yusuf S, Zhao F, Mehta SR, et al: Effects of clopidogrel in addition to aspirin in patients with acute coronary syndromes without ST-segment elevation. *N Engl J Med* 2001;345:494-502.

8. Chobanian AV, Bakris GL, Black HR, et al: The Seventh Report of the Joint National Committee on Prevention, Detection, Evaluation, and Treatment of High Blood Pressure: the JNC 7 report. *JAMA* 2003;289:2560-2572.

9. Major outcomes in high-risk hypertensive patients randomized to angiotensin-converting enzyme inhibitor or calcium channel blocker vs diuretic: The Antihypertensive and Lipid-Lowering Treatment to Prevent Heart Attack Trial (ALLHAT). *JAMA* 2002;288:2981-2997.

10. Packer M, O'Connor CM, Ghali JK, et al: Effect of amlodipine on morbidity and mortality in severe chronic heart failure. Prospective Randomized Amlodipine Survival Evaluation Study Group. *N Engl J Med* 1996;335:1107-1114.

11. Yusuf S, Sleight P, Pogue J, et al: Effects of an angiotensin-converting-enzyme inhibitor, ramipril, on cardiovascular events in high-risk patients. The Heart Outcomes Prevention Evaluation Study Investigators. *N Engl J Med* 2000;342:145-153.

12. Wenger NK, Froelicher ES, Smith LK, et al: Cardiac rehabilitation. 1995. Rockville, MD, US Department of Health and Social Services, Public Health Service, Agency for Health Care Policy and Research and The National Heart, Lung, and Blood Institute, pamphlet.

13. Oldridge N, Furlong W, Feeny D, et al: Economic evaluation of cardiac rehabilitation soon after acute myocardial infarction. *Am J Cardiol* 1993;72:154-161.

14. O'Connor GT, Buring JE, Yusuf S, et al: An overview of randomized trials of rehabilitation with exercise after myocardial infarction. *Circulation* 1989;80:234-244.

15. Effect of intensive blood-glucose control with metformin on complications in overweight patients with type 2 diabetes (UKPDS 34). UK Prospective Diabetes Study (UKPDS) Group. *Lancet* 1998;352:854-865.

16. Chiasson JL, Josse RG, Gomis R, et al: Acarbose treatment and the risk of cardiovascular disease and hypertension in patients with impaired glucose tolerance: the STOP-NIDDM trial. *JAMA* 2003;290:486-494.

17. Brady PA, Terzic A: The sulfonylurea controversy: more questions from the heart. *J Am Coll Cardiol* 1998;31:950-956.

18. Hopper L, Ness A, Higgins JP, et al: GISSI-Prevenzione trial. *Lancet* 1999;354:1557.

19. Executive Summary of The Third Report of The National Cholesterol Education Program (NCEP) Expert Panel on Detection, Evaluation, and Treatment of High Blood Cholesterol in Adults (Adult Treatment Panel III). *JAMA* 2001;285:2486-2497.

20. Grundy SM, Cleeman JI, Merz CN, et al: Implications of recent clinical trials for the National Cholesterol Education Program Adult Treatment Panel III guidelines. *Circulation* 2004;110:227-239.

21. Ballantyne CM, Davidson MH: Possible differences between fibrates in pharmacokinetic interactions with statins. *Arch Intern Med* 2003;163:2394-2395.

22. de Lorgeril M, Salen P, Martin JL, et al: Mediterranean diet, traditional risk factors, and the rate of cardiovascular complications after myocardial infarction: final report of the Lyon Diet Heart Study. *Circulation* 1999;99:779-785.

23. Hu FB: The Mediterranean diet and mortality—olive oil and beyond. *N Engl J Med* 2003;348:2595-2596.

24. McBride PE: The health consequences of smoking. Cardiovascular diseases. *Med Clin North Am* 1992;76:333-353.

25. Willett WC, Green A, Stampfer MJ, et al: Relative and absolute excess risks of coronary heart disease among women who smoke cigarettes. *N Engl J Med* 1987;317:1303-1309.

26. Glantz SA, Parmley WW: Passive smoking and heart disease. Epidemiology, physiology, and biochemistry. *Circulation* 1991;83:1-12.

27. Fiore MC, Bailey WC, Cohen SJ, et al: Smoking cessation. 1996. Rockville, MD, US Department of Health and Human Services, Public Health Service, Agency for Health Care Policy and Research, pamphlet.

28. The Practical Guide: Identification, Evaluation, and Treatment of Overweight and Obesity in Adults. 2000. US Department of Health and Human Services, Public Health Service, National Institutes of Health, National Heart, Lung, and Blood Institute. NIH Publication No. 00-4084, pamphlet.

29. Lee IM: Physical activity in women: how much is good enough? *JAMA* 2003;290:1377-1379.

APPENDIX A

Identifying and Reducing Cardiovascular Disease Risk in Children and Adolescents

Guidelines for Identifying Children and Adolescents at High Risk for Cardiovascular Disease

Goals for Pediatric Care Providers

- Timed, targeted risk factor assessment
- Appropriate interpretation of results and communication to families
- Recognition of obesity and cardiovascular risk factors, especially family history

Risk Factors to Evaluate

- Family history: Update regularly (parents, grandparents, aunts, and uncles) regarding obesity, hypertension, dyslipidemia, diabetes, cigarette smoking, and cardiovascular disease (CVD) before age 55 in men and age 65 in women.
- Height, weight, body mass index (BMI): Assess at every examination.
- Blood pressure: Measure at every examination after age 3 years; chart for age/sex/height.
- Diet and physical activity: Assess at every visit.
- Tobacco use: Evaluate starting at 9 to 10 years of age and update regularly.

- Lipids and lipoproteins: Perform targeted screening of fasting lipids in children >2 years of age with a family history of dyslipidemia or premature CVD. For children in whom family history is unknown and other risk factors are present, assess lipids and lipoproteins. If averaged results of two fasting lipid profiles are above cut points, refer to Table 7-2.

Abnormal Cholesterol Levels for Children and Adolescents (in mg/dL)

- Total cholesterol >170
- Low-density lipoprotein cholesterol (LDL-C) >110 is borderline; >130 is elevated
- Triglycerides >150
- High-density lipoprotein cholesterol (HDL-C) <40

Blood Pressure

- Know appropriate blood pressure measurement techniques, including appropriate cuff size.
- Interpret blood pressure measurements on the basis of age, sex, and height. Blood pressure percentiles based on these parameters have been published in the 1996 National High Blood Pressure Education Program report, Update on the Task Force Report (1987) on High Blood Pressure in Children and Adolescents, which is available for download at http://www.nhlbi.nih.gov/health/prof/heart/hbp/hbp_ped.htm.
- Systolic and diastolic blood pressure >90th percentile for age, sex, and height may indicate hypertension.

Body Size (Height/Weight/BMI)

- Body size should be charted by BMI. Norms for BMI percentiles are available at http://www.cdc.gov/growthcharts/.
- BMI >85th percentile is at risk of overweight; >95th percentile is overweight. After age 9 years, the 95th percentile can be approximated by the age (in years) + 13 for boys and the age (in years) + 14 for girls.

Guidelines for Cardiovascular Risk Reduction: Intervention for At-Risk Children and Adolescents

Blood Cholesterol Management

Before initiating therapy, consider secondary causes of LDL-C elevation if LDL-C is persistently above goals. Possible secondary causes include hypothyroidism (test thyroid-stimulating hormone), liver disease (perform liver function tests), and nephrosis (perform renal function tests and urinalysis for protein). Check for use of steroids.

Goals

- LDL-C <110 mg/dL, TG <150 mg/dL, and HDL-C >40 mg/dL.
- For patients with diabetes, LDL-C <100 mg/dL

Recommendations

- If LDL-C is above goals, initiate additional therapeutic lifestyle changes, including diet (<7% of calories from saturated fat; <200 mg cholesterol per day) in conjunction with a trained dietitian.
- Consider LDL-lowering dietary options (increase soluble fiber by using age [in years] plus 5 to 10 g up to age 15, when the total remains at 25 g per day) in conjunction with a trained dietitian.
- Emphasize weight management and increased physical activity.
- Consider pharmacologic therapy for patients with LDL >190 mg/dL but no other risk factors for CVD and for patients with LDL >160 mg/dL plus other risk factors (blood pressure elevation, diabetes, obesity, strong family history of premature CVD).
- Use of statins, bile acid binding resins, or niacin is approved in children and adolescents with significant hypercholesterolemia.
- Pharmacologic intervention for dyslipidemia should be accomplished in collaboration with a physician experienced in treating cholesterol disorders in pediatric patients.

Elevated Triglyceride and Low HDL-C

Recommendations

- Elevated triglyceride and reduced HDL-C are often seen in the context of overweight with insulin resistance. Therapeutic lifestyle changes should include weight management with appropriate energy intake and expenditure and decreased intake of simple sugars.
- If fasting triglyceride is persistently elevated, evaluate for secondary causes such as diabetes, thyroid disease, renal disease, and alcohol abuse.
- No pharmacologic interventions are recommended in children for isolated elevation of fasting triglyceride unless it is very marked; treatment may be initiated at triglyceride >400 mg/dL to protect against postprandial triglyceride levels of 1,000 mg/dL or greater, which may be associated with an increased risk of pancreatitis.

Management of Blood Pressure Elevation

Goal

- Systolic and diastolic blood pressure <95th percentile for age, sex, and height (usually <120/80 mm Hg in children and adolescents).

Recommendations

- Promote achievement of appropriate weight.
- Reduce sodium in the diet. Emphasize increased consumption of fruits and vegetables (highly effective).
- If blood pressure is persistently above the 95th percentile, consider possible secondary causes (eg, renal disease, coarctation of the aorta).
- Consider pharmacologic therapy for patients above the 95th percentile if lifestyle modification brings no improvement and there is evidence of target organ changes (left ventricular hypertrophy, microalbuminuria, retinal vascular abnormalities). Start blood pressure medication individualized to other patient requirements and characteristics (eg, age, race, need for drugs with specific benefits).
- Pharmacologic management of hypertension should be accomplished in collaboration with a physician experi-

enced in pediatric hypertension and after secondary causes have been ruled out.

Weight Management

Goal

- Achieve and maintain BMI <95th percentile for age and sex.

Recommendations

- For children who are at risk of overweight (>85th percentile) or obesity (≥95th percentile), a weight management program should be initiated with appropriate energy balance achieved through changes in diet and physical activity. For children of normal height, a secondary cause of obesity is unlikely.
- Weight management should be directed at all family members who are overweight, using a family-centered, behavioral management approach.
- A trained dietitian should work with the family, especially members responsible for food shopping and preparation.
- Reduce total dietary caloric intake, reduce dietary fat calories, and improve nutritional quality.
- Reduce television, video, and computer time.
- Increase physical activity; consider family activity.

Diabetes Management

Goals

- Near normal fasting plasma glucose (<120 mg/dL).
- Near normal HbA_{1c} (<7%) goals for fasting glucose. Target HbA_{1c} should take into consideration patient age and risk of hypoglycemia.

Recommendations

- Management of type 1 and type 2 diabetes in children and adolescents may require consultation with a pediatric endocrinologist.
- For type 2 diabetes, the first step is weight management with improved diet and exercise.
- Because of risk for accelerated vascular disease, other risk factors (eg, blood pressure, lipid abnormalities) should be treated more aggressively in patients with diabetes.

Tobacco/Smoking Cessation

Goal

- Complete cessation of smoking for children and parents who smoke. Secondhand smoke has significant effects on children and adolescents living in the household with a person who smokes.

Recommendation

- Advise every tobacco user (parents and children) to quit, and be prepared to provide assistance, such as counseling/referral to develop a plan for quitting, using available community resources to help with smoking cessation.

APPENDIX B

Online Resources

Obesity and Nutrition

Web Sites for Patients

- www.americanheart.org/grfw.htm
- www.eatright.org/Public/
- www.nhlbi.nih.gov/health/public/heart
- www.obesity.org
- www.shapeup.org

Diet Evaluation Assistance

- www.atkinsdietalert.org
- www.consumer.gov/weightloss
- win.niddk.nih.gov/publications/myths.htm
- www.pcrm.org/news/health010109.html

Web Sites for Physicians/Health-care Providers

- www.americanheart.org/grfw.htm

American Heart Association Web site; good for patients and professionals. Go to the Science and Professionals Library section for outstanding guidelines and scientific statements on every topic in cardiovascular disease.

- www.eatright.org/Public/

The Partnership for Healthy Weight Management Web site. The partnership has developed guidelines for providers of weight loss products or services and also provides useful resources to evaluate weight loss programs. The guidelines can be downloaded from www.ftc.gov/bcp/conline/pubs/buspubs/wgtguide.pdf.

• www.naaso.org

Great interactive Web site with self-learning modules, links to other Web sites with very useful educational materials, great office patient education materials, and more.

• www.obesity.org

American Obesity Association Web site; excellent set of obesity guidelines.

Physical Activity

Web Sites for Patients

• www.cdc.gov/nccdphp/dnpa/physical/

Centers for Disease Control and Prevention Physical Activity Web site.

• www.infoaging.org/l-exer-4-healthy.html

Exercise Information Center: "How do you choose a healthy exercise program?" The American Federation for Aging Research.

• www.walkinginfo.org/walkingchecklist.htm

Walkability checklist and neighborhood assessment. Partnership for a Walkable America, US Department of Transportation.

Web Sites for Physicians/Health-care Providers

• www.aahperd.org/naspe

National Association for Sport and Physical Education Web site.

• www.brightfutures.org/physicalactivity/about.htm

Bright Futures in Practice: Physical Activity (2001) provides developmental guidelines on physical activity for the period of infancy through adolescence as well as current information on screening, assessment, and counseling to promote physical activity and to meet the needs of health professionals, families, and communities.

- www.cdc.gov/nccdphp/dnpa/kidswalk/resources.htm.

Centers for Disease Control and Prevention Kids Walk-to-School Guide.

- www.cdc.gov/nccdphp/dnpa/pahand.htm

US Department of Health and Human Services. *Promoting Physical Activity: A Guide for Community Action. A Step-by-Step Guide to Community-wide Behavior Change.* Atlanta, GA, US Department of Health and Human Services, Centers for Disease Control and Prevention, 1999. Available from: Human Kinetics, PO Box 5076, Champaign, IL 61825-5076; phone: (800) 747-4457 or (217) 351-5076.

- www.cdc.gov/nccdphp/dnpa/physical/handbook/index.htm

US Department of Health and Human Services. *Physical Activity Evaluation Handbook.*
US Department of Health and Human Services, Centers for Disease Control and Prevention, 2002.

- www.fitness.gov

The President's Council on Physical Fitness and Sports Web site.

- www.thecommunityguide.org/pa/default/htm

The Guide to Community Preventive Services. Systematic reviews and evidence-based recommendations. Physical activity.

APPENDIX C

Guide to Primary Prevention of CVD and Stroke: Risk Intervention

Risk Prevention	Goals
Smoking	Complete cessation. No exposure to environmental tobacco smoke.
Blood pressure control	• <140/90 mm Hg • <130/80 mm Hg if diabetes, congestive heart failure, or renal failure is present[1]

Recommendations

- Ask about tobacco use status at every visit.
- In a clear, strong, and personalized manner, advise every tobacco user to quit.
- Assess the tobacco user's willingness to quit.
- Assist by counseling and developing a plan for quitting.
- Arrange follow-up referral to special programs or pharmacotherapy.
- Urge avoidance of exposure to secondhand smoke at work or home.

- Promote healthy lifestyle modification.
- Advocate weight reduction; reduction of sodium intake; consumption of fruits, vegetables, and low-fat dairy products; moderation of alcohol intake; and physical activity in patients with BP of ≥120 mm Hg systolic or 80 mm Hg diastolic.
- For patients with renal insufficiency, heart failure, or diabetes, initiate medication if BP is ≥130 mm Hg systolic or 80 mm Hg diastolic.

(continued on next page)

Risk Prevention	Goals
Blood pressure control *(continued)*	
Dietary intake	Overall healthy eating pattern
Aspirin	Low-dose aspirin in persons at higher CHD risk (especially those with 10-year risk of CHD ≥10%)

Recommendations

- Initiate medication for those with BP ≥140/90 mm Hg if 6 to 12 months of lifestyle modification is not effective, depending on the number of factors present.
- Add BP medications, individualized to other patient requirements and characteristics (eg, age, race, need for medication with specific benefits).

- Advocate consumption of a variety of fruits, vegetables, grains, low-fat or nonfat dairy products, fish, legumes, poultry, and lean meats.
- Match energy intake with energy needs and make appropriate changes to achieve weight loss when indicated.
- Modify food choices to reduce saturated fats (<10% of calories), cholesterol (<300 mg/d), and *trans*-fatty acids by substituting grains and unsaturated fatty acids from fish, vegetables, legumes, and nuts.
- Limit salt intake to <6 g/d.
- Limit alcohol intake (≤2 drinks/d in men, ≤1 drink/d in women) among those who drink.

- Do not recommend for patients with aspirin intolerance.
- Low-dose aspirin increases risk for gastrointestinal bleeding and hemorrhagic stroke. Do not use in patients at increased risk for these diseases.
- Benefits of cardiovascular risk reduction outweigh these risks in most patients at higher coronary risk.[2,3]
- Doses of 75-160 mg/d are as effective as higher doses. Therefore, consider 75-160 mg aspirin per day for patients at higher risk (especially those with 10-year risk of CHD of ≥10%).

(continued on next page)

Risk Prevention	Goals
Lipid management	*Primary goal:* • LDL-C <160 mg/dL if ≤1 risk factor is present • LDL-C <130 mg/dL if ≥2 risk factors are present and 10-year CHD risk is <20% • LDL-C <100 mg/dL if ≥2 risk factors are present and 10-year CHD risk is ≥20% or if patient has atherosclerosis or diabetes (optional goal: LDL-C >70 mg/dL for very high risk patients) *Secondary goals* (if LDL-C is at goal range): • If triglycerides are >200 mg/dL, then use non-HDL-C as a secondary goal: – Non-HDL-C <190 mg/dL for ≤1 risk factor – Non-HDL-C <160 mg/dL for ≥2 risk factors and 10-year CHD risk ≤20% – Non-HDL-C <130 mg/dL for atherosclerotic or diabetic patients or for ≥2 risk factors and 10-year CHD risk >20% (optional non-HDL-C <100 mg/dL for very high risk patients) • Other targets for therapy: – Triglycerides >150 mg/dL – HDL-C <40 mg/dL in men and <50 mg/dL in women

Recommendations

- If LDL-C is above goal range, initiate additional therapeutic lifestyle changes consisting of dietary modifications to lower LDL-C (<7% of calories from saturated fat, cholesterol <200 mg/d) and, if further LDL-C lowering is required, dietary options such as plant stanols/sterols (not to exceed 2 g/d) and/or increased viscous (soluble) fiber (10-25 g/d) and additional emphasis on weight reduction and physical activity.
- If LDL-C is above goal range, rule out secondary causes (liver function test, thyroid stimulating hormone level, urinalysis).
- After 12 weeks of therapeutic lifestyle change, consider LDL-lowering drug therapy if:
  - ≥2 risk factors are present, 10-year risk is >10%, and LDL-C is ≥130 mg/dL;
  - ≥2 risk factors are present, 10-year risk is <10%, and LDL-C is ≥160 mg/dL; or
  - ≤1 risk factor is present and LDL-C is ≥190 mg/dL.
- Start medications and advance dose to bring LDL-C to goal range, usually a statin, but also consider CAI or niacin.
- If LDL-C goal is not achieved, consider combination therapy (statin+CAI, statin+niacin).
- After LDL-C goal has been reached, consider triglyceride level.
  - If 150-199 mg/dL, treat with therapeutic lifestyle changes.
  - If 200-499 mg/dL, treat elevated non-HDL-C with therapeutic lifestyle changes and, if necessary, consider higher doses of statin or adding niacin or fibrate.
  - If >500 mg/dL, treat with fibrate or niacin to reduce risk of pancreatitis.
  - If HDL-C is <40 mg/dL in men and <50 mg/dL in women, initiate or intensify therapeutic lifestyle changes.
- For higher-risk patients, consider medications that raise HDL-C (eg, niacin, fibrates, statins).

(continued on next page)

Risk Prevention	Goals
Physical activity	At least 30 minutes of moderate-intensity physical activity on most (and preferably all) days of the week
Weight management	Achieve and maintain desirable weight (body mass index 18.5 to 24.9 kg/m^2). When body mass index is ≥25 kg/m^2, waist circumference at iliac crest level ≤40 inches in men and ≤35 inches in women.
Diabetes management	Normal fasting plasma glucose (<110 mg/dL) and near-normal HbA_{1c} (<7%)

Recommendations

- If cardiovascular, respiratory, metabolic, orthopedic, or neurologic disorders are suspected, or if patient is middle-aged or older and is sedentary, consult physician before initiating vigorous exercise program.
- Moderate-intensity activities (40% to 60% of maximum capacity) are equivalent to a brisk walk (15-30 min per mile).
- Additional benefits are gained from vigorous-intensity activity (>60% of maximum capacity) for 20-40 min on 3-5 days a week.
- Recommend resistance training with 8-10 different exercises, 1-2 sets per exercise, and 10-15 repetitions of moderate intensity ≥2 days a week.
- Flexibility training and an increase in daily lifestyle activities should complement this regimen.

- Initiate weight-management program through caloric restriction and increased caloric expenditure as appropriate.
- For overweight/obese persons, reduce body weight by 10% in first year of therapy.

- Initiate appropriate hypoglycemic therapy to achieve near-normal testing plasma glucose or as indicated by near-normal HbA_{1c}.
- First step is diet and exercise.
- Second-step therapy is usually metformin with ancillary use of acarbose and thiazolidinediones.
- Third-step therapy is sulfonylureas or insulin.
- Treat other risk factors more aggressively (eg, change BP goal to <130/80 mm Hg and LDL-C goal to <100 mg/dL).

(continued on next page)

Risk Prevention	Goals
Chronic atrial fibrillation	Normal sinus rhythm, rate control, or, if paroxysmal or chronic atrial fibrillation is present, anticoagulation with INR 2.0 to 3.0 (target 2.5).

BP = blood pressure, CAI = cholesterol absorption inhibitor, CHD = coronary heart disease, CVD = cardiovascular disease, HDL-C = high-density lipoprotein cholesterol, INR = international normalized ratio, LDL-C = low-density lipoprotein cholesterol

References

1. Chobanian AV, Bakris GL, Black HR, et al: The Seventh Report of the Joint National Committee on Prevention, Detection, Evaluation, and Treatment of High Blood Pressure: the JNC report. *JAMA* 2003;289:2560-2572.

2. Grundy SM, Balady GJ, Criqui MH, et al: Guide to primary prevention of cardiovascular diseases. A statement for healthcare professionals from the Task Force on Risk Reduction. American

Recommendations

- Irregular pulse should be verified by an electrocardiogram.
- Conversion of appropriate individuals to normal sinus rhythm.
- For patients in chronic or intermittent atrial fibrillation, use warfarin anticoagulants to INR 2.0 to 3.0 (target 2.5).
- Aspirin (325 mg/d) can be used as an alternative in those with specific contraindications to oral anticoagulation.
- Patients <65 years of age without high risk may be treated with aspirin.

Adapted from Pearson TA, Blair SN, Daniels SR, et al: AHA guidelines for primary prevention of cardiovascular disease and stroke: 2002 update: consensus panel guide to comprehensive risk reduction for adult patients without coronary or other atherosclerotic vascular diseases. *Circulation* 2002;106:388-391.

Heart Association Science Advisory and Coordinating Committee. *Circulation* 1997;95:2329-2331.

3. Smith SC Jr, Blair SN, Bonow RO, et al: AHA/ACC Scientific Statement: AHA/ACC guidelines for preventing heart attack and death in patients with atherosclerotic cardiovascular disease: 2001 update: a statement for healthcare professionals from the American Heart Association and the American College of Cardiology. *Circulation* 2001;104:1577-1579.

Index

B

C

D

F

G

H

L

M

O

P

Q

R

S

T

U

V

W

X

Z

NOTES